# HEALTH PROMOTION
# IN NURSING PRACTICE

With a chapter by:

Albert R. Pender, Ph.D.
Associate Professor
College of Business
Northern Illinois University
DeKalb, Illinois

# HEALTH PROMOTION IN NURSING PRACTICE

NOLA J. PENDER, R.N., PH.D., F.A.A.N.
Professor
School of Nursing
Northern Illinois University
DeKalb, Illinois

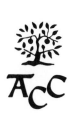

APPLETON-CENTURY-CROFTS/Norwalk, Connecticut

To Andrea and Brent
healthy children today,
healthier adults tomorrow

Copyright © 1982 by APPLETON-CENTURY-CROFTS
A Publishing Division of Prentice-Hall, Inc.

All rights reserved. This book, or any parts thereof,
may not be used or reproduced in any manner without
written permission. For information, address
Appleton-Century-Crofts, 25 Van Zant Street, East Norwalk,
CT. 06855.

82  83  84  85  86    /    10  9  8  7  6  5  4  3  2  1

Prentice-Hall International, Inc., London
Prentice-Hall of Australia, Pty. Ltd., Sydney
Prentice-Hall of India Private Limited, New Delhi
Prentice-Hall of Japan, Inc., Tokyo
Prentice-Hall of Southeast Asia (Pte.) Ltd., Singapore
Whitehall Books Ltd., Wellington, New Zealand

**Library of Congress Cataloging in Publication Data**

Pender, Nola J., 1941–
    Health promotion in nursing practice.

    Bibliography: p.
    Includes index.
    1. Health. 2. Preventive health services.
3. Nursing. I. Title. [DNLM: 1. Health promotion.
2. Nursing care. WY 100 P397h]
RT67.P56         613         81-10867
ISBN 0-8385-3668-9          AACR2

Cover and text design: Gloria J. Moyer

PRINTED IN THE UNITED STATES OF AMERICA

# Contents

# Preface

Emphasis on prevention and health promotion as integral aspects of client care in all types of service settings represents the most exciting development in health care in many years. Changing patterns of disease within the American population, disillusionment with medical technology, inflation in health-care costs, and renewed interest in self-care and self-responsibility have motivated the public to demand changes in the present health-care system. The "medical model" that serves as the current prototype for health-care delivery is being challenged. In response, more innovative approaches to the provision of health services are evolving. Examples of new approaches include primary care in occupational and school settings, increased emphasis on ambulatory and home care, physical fitness and nutritional awareness programs for the elderly, and self-care education for children and adults. With increased awareness of the impact of ecological, psychological, sociological and physiological factors on human health, a more comprehensive approach to health care is imperative.

Restructuring of the present health-care system toward a balance between prevention/health promotion services and care in illness will require new points of access to health care, changes in working relationships among health professionals, greater client involvement in self-care, and modification of current policies for third-party pay. In addition, the nature of prevention and health-promotion services will need to be identified clearly so that health-care consumers are aware of the various types of care available to them. If high-quality health care is to be economically feasible, the "pay structure" for health services must provide incentives for people to stay well and to detect illness in its early stages. While almost everyone would accept the philosophical premise that it is more desirable to keep people well than to provide care only after illness, the present health-care system is not economically or operationally structured to function in that way. Fortunately, the American people are coming to realize that the wealth and productivity of any people depends not only on *decreasing morbidity and mortality* but also on *increasing the level of physical, psychological, social, and environmental well-being of all groups within society.*

The role of professional nurses in the evolving health-care system is yet to be determined. Despite an expressed commitment to the prevention of illness and promotion of health, the major emphasis of professional nursing education has been, and continues to be, on the knowledge and skills needed to provide care in illness or health crises. While coronary care following myocardial infarction or surgical care after a radical mastectomy challenge professional nurses and demand scientific intervention, promotion of healthful lifestyles and the prevention or early detection of illness present equally exciting nursing care demands. The opportunity is ripe for nurses to provide leadership in generating the knowledge and skills essential to the provision of competent prevention and health-promotion services to individuals and families. Nurse researchers must undertake the formidable task of developing and testing empirically theories that describe and explain health behavior and that prescribe appropriate nursing interventions to assist clients in achieving health goals. Evidence of such leadership within the nursing community is emerging. Examples of nurses actively involved in the provision of innovative prevention and health-promotion services will be shared with the reader throughout the following chapters.

The purpose for writing this book is twofold: (1) to provide nurses with a conceptual framework for understanding the many factors that affect the health behavior of individuals and families, and (2) equally important, to present specific nursing strategies for providing prevention and health-promotion services to clients. My interest in this area is long-standing and has been fueled by discussions with nursing colleagues, contact with undergraduate and graduate students in hospital and community settings, and by my private practice with clients in a comprehensive hypertension management program. I am convinced that the public is not only interested in, but is actively and aggressively seeking sources of, prevention and health-promotion care within their own communities. Interdisciplinary efforts among health professionals and lay involvement will be critical for the ultimate success of such services.

The content of this book is organized into four areas. In Part I, the human quest for health is explored. Critical dimensions of human behavior that affect health-seeking are examined, various definitions of health are analyzed, and models for understanding health-protecting (preventive) behavior and health-promoting behavior are presented. This provides the conceptual framework for the rest of the content.

Health-protecting and health-promoting behaviors are divided into the decision-making phase and the action phase. Strategies useful during the decision-making phase are presented in Part II and include bio-psychosocial assessment, values clarification, health education for self-care, and the development of a health protection/promotion plan. These specific interventions have been selected for presentation because they place prevention and health-promotion care in a holistic context that takes into consideration not only individual clients but the social support groups and environments in which they live. Part II stresses the critical need to consider the personal values, knowledge, and skills of clients and families in developing a meaningful health protection/ promotion plan.

In Part III, strategies for the action phase are discussed in detail and include: modification of lifestyle, exercise and physical fitness, nutrition and weight control, stress management, and building social support systems. These specific strategies were selected by the author because of formidable evidence from research literature that consideration of such areas is critical to improving human health.

Part IV provides the reader with an overview of sociopolitical dilemmas and economic issues related to health promotion and prevention. Changes in public policy and economic structures are essential if major impact is to be realized from prevention and health-promotion activities within the American population. In essence, then this section is the "other side of the coin" and complements consideration of individual and family responsibility for health discussed in previous sections.

Throughout the book, assessment tools and intervention strategies have been presented and outlined in detail. This provides practical assistance for nurses in clinical settings, nursing students, and instructors responsible for teaching prevention and health-promotion concepts. Readers must select from the many strategies described those that they will incorporate into their own nursing practice or include in nursing curricula. While care of the sick will always be an important role of the nurse, the vast majority of the population spend most of their lives as the "essentially" well or worried well. Assisting individuals, regardless of their illness state, in moving toward their maximum health potential is a critical dimension of the nursing role. This book has been written to enhance the competence of nurses to fulfill that role and responsibility to society.

The word *client* rather than *patient* will be used throughout the book because of its more appropriate application to individuals who are well and to groups that are also the recipients of preventive/promotive care. Health and wellness will be used as interchangeable terms, as both are considered by the author to be comprehensive and holistic in orientation.

I am deeply indebted to the many individuals for whom I have provided care throughout my nursing career and from whom I have learned so much, particularly to my current clients who keep me in contact with the realities of professional practice. A special word of thanks is extended to graduate students at Northern Illinois University and Rush University for providing intellectual stimulation supportive of thought and conceptualization.

Appreciation is extended to Debbie Lovell for superb typing of the manuscript and assistance with the many illustrations, and to Leslie Boyer, former nursing editor at Appleton-Century-Crofts, and John Allison, present nursing editor, for direction and support throughout the writing of this book. I particularly want to thank my husband, Al, for contributing the chapter on economic issues in prevention and health promotion and for his unwavering support of my writing efforts; and Andrea and Brent, our children, who make the quest for knowledge about prevention and health promotion personally worthwhile.

NOLA J. PENDER

# Introduction

The changing patterns of disease within the American population are a major factor behind the shift in emphasis from treatment of illness to prevention and health promotion. Chronic illnesses are responsible for an increasing share of the ill health experienced by adults. Eighty percent of individuals over 65 years of age have one or more chronic health problems. More than 45 percent of this group experience limitations in mobility and social pursuits because of chronic disease. Chronic illnesses do not respond to efforts for a medical cure, and almost all such health problems are caused or aggravated by inappropriate health habits. Experts have estimated that at least half the deaths in the United States each year result from health-damaging lifestyles. Habits, often established in early childhood or adolescence, such as overeating, sedentary existence, use of alcohol and tobacco, and high levels of occupational and domestic stress, represent the many threats to health from everyday patterns of living.

Considering current evidence on the etiologic and epidemiologic characteristics of illness and disease, it is apparent that significant improvements in the health status of individuals and families will not come about through greater emphasis on the treatment of existing illness but through aggressive prevention and health-promotion efforts. At present, the major means of prevention for chronic diseases and improvement of health status include risk appraisal, health education, health counseling, anticipatory guidance, stress management, and lifestyle modification.

While congressional priorities for health planning (P.L. 93-641) have shifted to include the development of programs for community health education, health-maintenance organizations (dedicated to a wellness as opposed to an illness model for health care), and expansion of preventive services, progress has been slow. The future roles of government, health professionals, and the public in promoting good health are still unclear. Obviously, there are ethical limits to the extent that government can legislate good health practices. Individuals and families must be prepared to assume considerable responsibility for health maintenance and disease control. Health professionals bear the primary responsibility for assisting clients to achieve competence in self-care and for promoting the establishment of national health policy supportive of healthful lifestyles.

1

Nurses, because of their recognized expertise and frequent, continuing contact with clients, have the unique opportunity of promoting better personal health among those they care for and of serving as role models for health-promoting lifestyles. Nurses must be aware of the danger of becoming so pressed by demands for diagnostic, treatment, and illness care services that they fail to give adequate time to health education, health counseling, and other health-promoting interventions.

While there is much to be learned through continuing research and clinical work regarding effective health-promoting interventions, health providers cannot afford to wait for optimum solutions before beginning to act. A great deal of knowledge already exists about the benefits of health actions, motivation of health behavior, and barriers to selection of health-promoting options and lifestyles. This knowledge can provide the basis for beginning intervention efforts. Many factors that increase the risk of illness and premature death can be ameliorated without expensive medical treatment. Individuals and groups have a great deal of unrecognized potential for changing their health status for the better. In fact, many adult health problems can only be effectively controlled through intelligent self-care. It can be said unequivocally that a significant reduction in inactivity, overnutrition, alcoholism, and hypertension could save more lives in the 40-to-64 age range than the best current medical practices.

Health-promotion efforts have the potential long-term benefits of enhancing the quality of life from childhood through the adult years, increasing longevity, reducing health care costs, and increasing national productivity through reduced illness and absenteeism.[1] In a series of studies in California, Belloc and Breslow[2] found empirical evidence that lifestyle contributes significantly to longevity. Individuals who exercised regularly, maintained normal weight, ate breakfast, did not snack between meals, avoided smoking, limited alcohol consumption, and slept at least seven hours a night had a longer life span than individuals who did not engage in these practices. The higher the number of health habits reported by individuals, the longer their potential life span. A nine-year follow-up study of the same population group[3] indicated that the significant relationship of five of the health habits to longevity persisted over time. Eating breakfast daily and avoiding snacks between meals were the only health behaviors originally explored that were unrelated to *long-term* health outcomes.

At this point, it is important to differentiate between the terms *health promotion* and *prevention*:

- *Health promotion* refers to activities directed toward developing the resources of clients that maintain or enhance well-being.
- *Prevention* refers to activities that seek to protect clients from potential or actual health threats and their harmful consequences.

While the two terms are conceptually distinct, they are frequently used as synonyms in health literature. This confusion is easy to understand when an attempt is made to categorize a given behavior as either a health-promotion or a prevention activity. For instance, in a study by Heinzelmann and Bagley[4] regarding sources of motivation for participating in a program of physical activity, participants cited the desire to feel better and more invigorated (health promotion) and the desire to decrease chances of having a heart attack (prevention) as reasons for involvement in the program. Both health promotion and prevention were anticipated outcomes.

To date, scientists have expended much more energy in exploring various aspects of prevention than in explicating the dimensions of health promotion. This reflects the logical link between the prevailing medical orientation to health care and preventive activities that focus on a particular disease entity. At present, it is easier to talk concretely about preventing a specific health problem than about the promotion of health or well-being among individuals, groups, and communities. The target variables are more clearly identified in prevention than in health promotion, and the potential influences are less diverse.

Historically, it is interesting to note that therapeutic methods for dealing with disease and rituals directed toward preventing illness have for decades been institutionalized as part of all societies, even the most primitive cultures. This is not true of health-promotion methods or strategies. History indicates that a society must be well advanced before attention is given to positive approaches for improving the level of health and quality of life for its citizens. Prerequisites for any national focus on health promotion appear to be the following:

• Recognition of the dignity of a person *as* an individual
• A belief that illness is not an inevitable part of the lot of human beings
• A future orientation or vision beyond that of immediate survival
• Awareness of the close relationship between individual health assets and the well-being and productivity of society as a whole
• Widespread acceptance of health care as a basic human right

Health-promotion and prevention services have a different focus from that of the treatment of illness. Preventive/promotive care is directed toward (1) increasing the free and open expression of human potential unhampered by discrete or prolonged experiences of illness or (2) facilitating the ongoing actualizaton of human potential in the presence of illness. In order to achieve these goals, health-promotion and prevention activities must be integrated with existing health services, humanistic in orientation, positive in approach, and comprehensive in scope.

## INTEGRATION OF HEALTH PROMOTION AND PREVENTION CARE WITH EXISTING SERVICES

Medical services within the United States have become fragmented and narrow in scope, resulting in segregation of the services provided to a single individual and even greater lack of continuity in services provided to families. An individual may be seen by as many as five to seven different health specialists, all in varying locations, with little if any means of contact with each other. Families may see as many as 15 different health professionals. A single integrated record of services to a given individual or family is in most instances impossible to locate.

If the health care system of the United States is to be significantly restructured and health-promotion and prevention services are to become an integral part of health care delivery, coordination of services is essential in order to focus on individuals and groups rather than on specific problems of pathology. Such services should be offered by collaborating professionals with differing areas of expertise that complement each other. Better systems of communication must exist between these providers in order to promote a sense of caring, security, and well-being among recipients of care. Individual clients and families must be an important part of the communication network since they will assume a great deal of responsibility for the day-to-day management of their own health.

Health professionals also face the difficult task of dispelling expectations of passivity in personal health care that have been instilled in the American public by the current medical care system.[5] Individuals must be assisted in overcoming the learned tendency to balk at active involvement in examining their current lifestyles and changing personal or family habits that are health damaging. Acceptance of personal responsibility for health status is critical to any significant movement away from the current paternalistic system of health care toward individual competence in self-direction and self-care.

## A HUMANISTIC ORIENTATION TO HEALTH CARE

Perceptions of dehumanization of individuals in illness-oriented treatment programs may well be a primary cause of the distressing lack of compliance with medical regimens and other failures of the existing health system. Compliance rates as low as 25 percent have been reported in the literature.[6-8] It is possible that a depersonalized approach with little, if any, information given concerning how to integrate the therapeutic regimen into activities of daily living as well as lack of appropriate health counseling follow-up may account for low compliance rates.

Humanism as a philosophical context for providing health care emphasizes the basic striving of individuals for fulfillment and actualization. This "striving" characteristic of all human beings is frequently referred to as the *growth principle,* since the effect of such striving is to move one continuously toward greater levels of maturity and personal health. Humanism recognizes the importance of the inner experience of human beings and their personal goals, feelings, beliefs, attitudes, and values. In discussing the determinants of health behavior within a humanistic context, perception emerges as a key concept. It is not the external event that directly affects behavior but the meaning that an individual gives to any object or event. Success in assisting individuals or groups to change personal health habits or health-service use patterns depends primarily on an accurate understanding of cultural and personal perceptions, attitudes, and values relevant to the target behaviors.

Assumptions that stem from a humanistic view of health include the following:

- The need for actualization and fulfillment is characteristic of all human beings.
- The behavior of a person is purposive and selective.
- A person engages in behavior that is perceived as instrumental in achieving fulfillment.
- Illness interferes with the movement of a person toward growth and health.

Recognition of individual rights is an important component of humanism. The content of this book is based on acceptance of the following rights for all human beings:

- The right to personal fulfillment
- The right to make decisions about health as long as the health of others is not endangered
- The right to accurate information about personal health status as a basis for informed decision making
- The right to accurate information regarding the action alternatives with the highest probability of enhancing health and/or minimizing health threats
- The right of access to comprehensive health care
- The right to nursing care for health promotion and illness prevention

A humanistic orientation to health care by nurses mandates that the profession accept their social responsibility to develop knowledge and skills useful in facilitating and supporting the health-seeking behaviors of the clients they serve.

## A POSITIVE APPROACH TO HEALTH CARE

Treatment of illness has developed a negative connotation associated with threat, discomfort, embarrassment, and loss of control. Anticipation of negative consequences results in avoidance of health care services even when use would be most appropriate and perhaps critical to continuing good health. Avoidance behavior indicates the presence of fear and feelings of frustration. Apprehension concerning curative care probably stems from the patient focusing on the immediate negative consequences of behavior, such as inconvenience, time loss, discomfort, and unpleasantness, rather than on the positive outcomes, such as the amelioration of symptoms, return to health, and control of personal health status.

Emphasis on promoting health rather than curing disease provides a positive orientation for health care. Illness need no longer be the primary focus for nurse–client relationships. Expectations of control, participation, involvement, and influence facilitate approach rather than avoidance of health services.

The sources of satisfaction and reinforcement from health-promoting behaviors need to be more clearly identified to facilitate a positive milieu for client care. Questions that remain only partially answered include the following:

- What are the perceived positive and negative consequences of health-promoting behaviors?
- What are the perceived positive and negative consequences of health-damaging behaviors?
- How can negative consequences of health-promoting behaviors be attenuated and positive consequences strengthened?
- What are the potential sources of immediate gratification from health-promoting behaviors?
- What part do individual attitudes, interpersonal relationships, societal norms, and environmental factors play in generating and sustaining healthful lifestyles?

Nursing strategies that are positively oriented, such as goal-setting techniques and change-inducing interventions, must be developed and evaluated clinically for their client appeal and effectiveness in facilitating more healthful lifestyles among individuals and families of all ages.

### THE COMPREHENSIVE SCOPE OF HEALTH PROMOTION

Distortions in the behavior of individuals and families cannot entirely explain all existing health problems, nor should health promotion be completely an individual responsibility. Approaches to health promotion and prevention are highly complex and require consideration of behavioral patterns of organizations, communities, and nations, in addition to individual behavior. Milio[9] has identified the impact of decisions or policy choices made by governmental/nongovernmental and for-profit/nonprofit organizations on the range of options available to individuals and families for personal choice making in the area of health. Decisions made at all levels of the bureaucratic pyramid characteristic of Western society affect the ease with which individuals can select health-promoting options as opposed to health-damaging ones.

Victor Fuchs, in his book, *Who Shall Live? Health, Economics, and Social Choice,*[10] concluded that in addition to individual decisions about diet, exercise, and smoking, collective decisions affecting pollution, quality of food products, stress levels, and other aspects of the environment are critical to altering the health status and increasing significantly the longevity of any group of people. Coordination of broad policy decisions, organizational behavior, community changes, and individual lifestyles will be critical if health promotion is to become a dominant theme in health care delivery in the future.

Social and commercial determinants of health-damaging behavior offer many possibilities for scientific investigation. Questions that ought to be addressed include the following:

- What roles do social groups play in perpetuating unhealthy lifestyles?
- Can health habits of entire groups be changed more effectively than health practices of individuals?
- How can health-promoting behaviors be maintained by persons with membership in nonsupportive groups?
- What impact do advertising and marketing strategies of business and industry have on individual and family health practices?

Contradictions that directly affect the nation's health exist currently in both government and private enterprise. For instance, the Department of Agriculture continues to subsidize tobacco farmers although national statistics clearly support the position that smoking is health threatening. Since the tobacco industry represents a significant source of tax revenues and employs a sizable labor force, cigarettes continue to be freely accessible to anyone with the money or inclination to buy them. Meanwhile, the federal government invests millions of dollars in support of antismoking campaigns.

Another puzzling contradiction is found in the amount of money spent in educating children and adolescents concerning good nutrition while the schools themselves provide a wide array of foods in vending machines and school cafeterias that are high in carbohydrates, cholesterol, and sodium. Little governmental pressure is applied to encourage schools to offer foods that are more nutritious, lower in calories, and contain fewer harmful chemical agents.

Yet another conflict is evident in the expressed need of the American public for more physical exercise and the portrayal by commercial advertising of the affluent lifestyle as the owning of two or more cars, so that one can drive with ease from one destination to another. Not only are Americans encouraged to make extravagant investments in motorized vehicles, but most streets and highways are unsafe for other means of transportation that would require greater expenditures of human rather than fossil-fuel energy.

One final problem should not escape attention. American business and industry provide time each day for employees to ingest caffeine during the traditional "coffee break," yet few establishments provide exercise breaks for employees in sedentary jobs or set aside facilities to allow employees to maintain physical fitness or release emotional and muscular tension during the work day.

Slowly, things are changing. More emphasis is being placed on self-care, natural support systems (nuclear and extended families) as buffers against disease, management of stress, nutrition and weight control, modification of lifestyle, organized physical activity programs, and the prevention, early detection, and treatment of chronic illness. Whether the pressures for change are primarily humanitarian or economic could be the subject of lengthy debate. At any rate, the changes being made in health care appear to be in the best interest of the American people. In this period of increasing inflation, the lesser cost of individual and group health-promotion and prevention services in comparison to illness care lends support to large-scale efforts focused on further development of health-promoting services for the public.

## NURSING CARE FOR PREVENTION AND HEALTH PROMOTION

Nursing has entered a new era in health care that offers many opportunities to expand the parameters of professional practice and the visibility and significance of the contribution of nursing to the nation's health. Traditional roles of nurses have frequently led to discontent, low self-esteem, and feelings of powerlessness within the health care system. This problem has become particularly acute with the increasing level of educational preparation among professional nurses. The desire for a collaborative relationship with physicians, interdependence with other health professionals, direct access to clients, and autonomy in making nursing decisions will continue to press nurses toward the realization of their own potential.

Many states have already revised their nursing practice acts to allow professional nurses to perform comprehensive patient assessments, provide anticipatory guidance and monitoring to chronically ill patients, and implement health education and health counseling without physician supervision. Increasing autonomy among professional nurses will allow them to more fully develop health-promotion and prevention strategies that will be effective in a variety of clinical settings.

The expected outcomes of nursing care directed toward promoting health include:

- Increased levels of health and well-being among individuals, families, and communities
- Decreased incidence of illness and disability for individuals and families
- Increased personal competence and control in minimizing the barriers that prevent personal growth and fulfillment
- Improvement in the abilities of clients or families to make rational health-relevant decisions
- Competence on the part of clients and families in self-care
- Increased ability among clients to assess accurately personal or family needs for professional health care
- Judicious use of health care services for health promotion, prevention, and treatment of illness
- Greater availability and convenience of health-promoting as opposed to health-damaging options
- Greater prevalence of health-promoting personal and family lifestyles

The complex nature of health promotion and prevention will require the best investigative efforts of individuals with expertise in many different fields. Nursing as a practice discipline must identify priorities for research in prevention and health promotion consistent with the expanding knowledge base within the discipline and the changing domain of professional practice. The challenge of developing new health care strategies offers the scientific and professional excitement of venturing into areas of human health that at present are undeveloped and unexplained.

## REFERENCES

1. Kristein, M.M., Arnold, C.B., & Wynder, E.L. Health economics and preventive care. *Science,* 1977, *195,* 457–462.
2. Belloc, N.B., & Breslow, L. Relationship of physical health status and health practices. *Preventive Medicine,* 1972, *1,* 409–421.
3. Wiley, J.A., & Comacho, T.C. Life style and future health: Evidence from the Alemeda County study. *Preventive Medicine,* 1980, *9,* 1–21.
4. Heinzelmann, F., & Bagley, R.W. Response to physical activity programs and their effects on health behavior. *Public Health Reports,* 1970, *85,* 905.
5. Fielding, J.E. Successes of prevention. *Milbank Memorial Fund Quarterly,* 1978, *56,* 274–302.
6. Sackett D.L., & Haynes, R.B. *Compliance with therapeutic regimens.* Baltimore: Johns Hopkins University Press, 1976.
7. Becker, M.H., Drachman, R.H., & Kirscht, J.P. Predicting mothers' compliance with pediatric medical regimens. *Journal of Pediatrics,* 1972, *81,* 843.
8. Becker, M.H., Drachman, R.H., & Kirscht, J.P. A new approach to explaining sick-role behavior in low-income populations. *American Journal of Public Health,* 1974, *64,* 205–216.
9. Milio, N. A framework for prevention: Changing health-damaging to health-generating life patterns. *AJPH,* May 1976, *66,* 435.
10. Fuchs, V.R. *Who shall live? Health, economics, and social choice.* New York: Basic, 1974, p. 54.

# Part I
# THE HUMAN QUEST FOR HEALTH

In this section, dimensions of human behavior that influence health will be examined. In addition, various definitions of health will be contrasted, compared, and analyzed. Conceptual models for health-protecting behavior (prevention) and health-promoting behavior will be described as a basis for structuring nursing interventions. The reader will be assisted in understanding the differences between health-protecting and health-promoting behaviors and the sources of motivation for each.

# CHAPTER 1
# Human Behavior and Health

A description of human behavior as a basis for prevention and health promotion must go beyond the traditional "medical model," which focuses primarily on the physical, to a conceptualization of behavior that integrates biologic, psychologic, sociologic, and ecologic dimensions of human life. Not only intrinsic characteristics of individuals must be considered, but also the nature of the social groups and physical environments in which they reside. Professional nurses active in health promotion, while acknowledging the impact of the environment on clients, must be fully cognizant of the capacity of individuals and groups to achieve some degree of change in their lifestyle and environment if they choose to do so. Nursing care that results in better health and more productive living for individuals and families can only be delivered by professionals who believe in the growth potential of the clients they serve. In this chapter, five dimensions of human behavior that strongly influence observed health behaviors of clients will be discussed. The five dimensions to be considered are purpose, motivation, awareness, control, and complexity.

## PURPOSE

Goal-directed behavior is an important characteristic of human beings. Past experiences, present internal state, and the immediate environment determine the hierarchy of goals evident in a specific individual at any point in time. A goal is an aim, a desired end, or a valued outcome. Behavior is determined by goals; therefore, behavior is always directional.[1] Purposive or goal-directed behavior has two aspects: (1) the ability to specify a purpose or goal and (2) the ability to initiate a pattern of behavior that is directed toward the achievement of that purpose. Purposiveness exists only if choices are available to individuals and if they are capable of making a choice.[2] Choice results from *problem-solving* or *decision-making* activities.

Human beings are capable of valuing and prioritizing options available to them. Internal cognitive processes determine what information will be received from the environment and how it will be interpreted and structured; this in turn

**13**

determines the goals that persons select. When a specific behavior is believed to lead to the attainment of a desired goal, the behavior will be evaluated as positive, and the probability of occurrence of the behavior will be increased.[3] Individuals exhibit those behaviors that lead to the greatest immediate or future satisfaction, given the current range of behavioral options available. In addition to establishing specific goals that give direction to behavior and existence, individuals are potentially capable of (1) modifying the environment or relevant support systems so that they can attain those goals that they have established for themselves and (2) evaluating and changing goals over time to coincide increasingly with their unique human capacities for healthful and productive living.

An important part of nursing care in health promotion and prevention involves assisting clients to recognize their values and priorities and to evaluate the extent to which daily behaviors promote or thwart the achievement of valued goals. Because purpose and direction are critical aspects of human behavior, Chapter 6 deals at length with interventions that can be used by the nurse to assist clients in values clarification. It is only as the client gains increased self-understanding of personal priorities and the nurse comes to appreciate and empathize with the goals of the client that meaningful communication and assistance can be offered in a productive nurse–client relationship.

## MOTIVATION

Motivation will be given special attention in this chapter because of its critical role in initiating and sustaining health-protecting (preventive) and health-promoting behaviors. The major sources of motivation for human behavior have been identified by the author as actualizing and stabilizing tendencies (Fig.1-1). A tendency is an active impulse or force to do something.[4] The actualizing tendency is directed toward increasing states of positive tension in order to promote change, growth, and maturation. This tendency is clearly apparent at birth but may be strengthened or weakened through interactions of individuals with their environment. Health-promoting behaviors are presented in this book as manifestations of the actualizing tendency. Health-promoting behaviors are directed toward enhancing well-being and the expression of human potential. The stabilizing tendency is evident in the functioning of homeostatic mechanisms and is directed toward maintaining balance and equilibrium. The stabilizing tendency regulates states of negative tension in order to maintain the integrity of human functions. Preventive or health-protecting behaviors reflect the stabilizing tendency and occur in reaction to a potential or actual health threat.

### The Actualizing Tendency
The actualizing tendency is evident in spontaneous, self-initiated activity directed toward increasing the amount of stimulation experienced or the impact of that stimulation on the individual. Motivated by the actualizing tendency, people seek

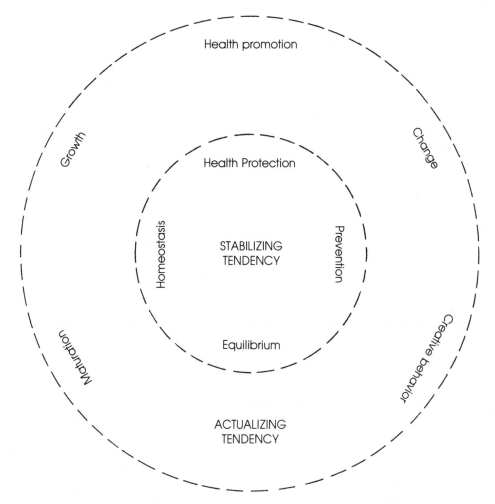

**FIGURE 1-1.** Major sources of motivation for human behavior.

to increase intensity, meaningfulness, and variation of stimuli encountered in the course of everyday living. This promotes learning, maturation, and ongoing growth through differentiation and reintegration at increasingly higher levels of complexity. Human beings find discovery both absorbing and challenging; with creative expression comes intense inner satisfaction.[5]

Empirical evidence of the spontaneous nature of human beings has resulted from the work of physiologists and psychologists. Even under relatively constant conditions and in the absence of external stimuli, people are active rather than passive. This activity is dramatically demonstrated by the human nervous system in the first movements of embryos and fetuses. The notion of activity as intrinsic to human beings is further substantiated by studies that show that brain waves are continually active, that the spontaneous firing of retinal cells increases with dark adaptation, and that there are spontaneous fluctuations in cardiac activity.[6]

Human beings are unique in exhibiting a distinct psychologic form of the actualizing tendency as the pressure to develop and behave and to experience self and the world about them. The actualizing tendency is not directed at tension reduction but at positive experiences of tension increase. Selective tension increase has been shown to be pleasurable to human beings, actively sought by them, and critical to realization of human health potential. Increased tension when serving the actualizing tendency does not result in anxiety or distress but is perceived as a positive state or experience.

In studying young children, Piaget remarked repeatedly about the enthusiastic and repeated performance of manipulation of toys and objects by children for no other apparent reason than enjoyment of the complexity of visual and tactile patterning that such an experience offers.[7] Other studies with infants, children, and adults repeatedly show a preference for stimuli that are new or novel, result in uncertainty as to their origin or nature, and are complex rather than simplistic in design.

Empirical observations of individuals of all ages indicate the persistant striving for actualization through (1) seeking experiences that increase tension level in a positive manner, (2) seeking exchanges with the environment that enhance personal control, achievement, and fulfillment, and (3) producing exchanges with the environment that provide uncertainty and challenge. Positive experiences of tension increase are perceived as growth-producing rather than as threatening and offer the potential for reward rather than the possibility of harm.

Health-promoting behaviors are self-initiated actions on the part of individuals that enhance health status in the absence of a specific health threat. The actualizing tendency is proposed as the driving force toward increased levels of well-being. Individuals are motivated to engage in health-promoting behaviors when they place a high value on personal worth, are aware of their own capacity for growth, and seek to express their own inherent and learned potentialities. A conceptual model for health-promoting behavior will be presented in Chapter 4.

### The Stabilizing Tendency
The stabilizing tendency is responsible for maintaining the value of variables in the internal and external environment within a range compatible with continuing existence. This range is known as the "steady state." Although the internal and external environments are constantly fluctuating, an input of energy or information that is less than or in excess of parameters of the steady state constitutes distress, or stress, as it is commonly called.[8] A stress is considered a *negative* form of tension increase.

Two types of stressors may occur: a *lack stress* and an *excess stress*. In a lack stress, the input or output rate falls below the standard range characteristic of the steady state. Classic studies at McGill University[9] of the reactions of individuals under conditions of minimal stimulation indicated that the subjects in the experiments developed an almost insatiable desire for variation in the environment. Few individuals could endure being shielded from stimulation more than two or three days in a laboratory setting, without exhibiting hallucinations and other forms of deviant behavior.

In an excess stress, the input or output rate goes above the range characteristic of the steady state. Examples of excess stress include high noise levels from factory machinery, loud rock music, and high glucose levels that result in diabetic coma. The impact of excess stress can be either temporary or long term. Many chronic diseases appear to be caused or aggravated by excess stress through overexposure to various chemicals, such as tars, nicotines, asbestos, or silicone dust. Intensive studies are also underway to determine the extent to which overexposure to food substances, psychologic pressure, or social chaos may predispose individuals to chronic disease.

Adaptation refers to behaviors used by individuals to maintain the steady state when faced with disruptive internal or external stimuli. Adaptive behaviors may be conscious or unconscious. Conscious modes of adaptation often involve overt behavior directed at manipulating the source of stress. Unconscious modes of adaptation include peripheral vasoconstriction, increased heart rate, hair raising, pupil dilatation, and increased blood glucose level in response to threatening stimuli. How efficiently a system adapts to its environment is determined by the strategies that are employed and the completeness with which they reduce stress without being too costly.

Man's search for psychologic stability has been described at length by the theory of cognitive dissonance.[10] According to this theory, man is motivated to maintain consistency among opinions, beliefs, and behaviors. Opinions or beliefs that are relevant to each other have either a consonant or dissonant relationship. Consonance is agreement or consistency; dissonance is disagreement or inconsistency among beliefs.

The theory makes two basic assumptions about cognitive dissonance. First, the existence of dissonance, being psychologically uncomfortable, will give rise to pressure motivating the person to reduce or eliminate it. Second, the strength of the pressure for dissonance reduction or movement toward stability depends on the magnitude of the dissonance that exists within the opinions, beliefs, and behaviors of the individual at any given point in time. The greater the degree of dissonance, the stronger the motivation to reduce it to tolerable limits. Tolerable limits represent a psychologic "steady state."

Dissonance frequently results from receiving new information that does not support present behaviors. For example, this may occur as a result of health education, health counseling, or exposure to health information in the mass media. The individual seeks to reduce dissonance either by rejecting the new information or by modifying relevant behavior or beliefs. Making decisions to take specific actions can also result in cognitive dissonance. The degree of postdecision dissonance depends on the importance of the decision being made and the attractiveness of the unchosen alternatives. The more important the decision and the greater the attractiveness of the unchosen alternatives, generally, the higher the postdecision dissonance. Given competing alternatives, consistency of behavior is particularly difficult prior to stabilization of newly acquired health habits.

All behaviors directed toward the maintenance of equilibrium are manifestations of the stabilizing tendency. Preventive or health-protecting behaviors fall within this category since they occur in response to potential or actual threats to health. Stabilizing reactions are directed toward minimizing or escaping threatening external or internal stimuli in anticipation of possible biophysical or psychosocial harm.

Many behaviors serve both health-promoting (actualizing) and health-protecting (stabilizing) functions, for example, jogging to enhance general well-being and to prevent cardiovascular disease. Thus, while some behaviors can be categorized as primarily health promotive or health protective, many health behaviors represent the integrated expression of both actualizing and stabilizing tendencies.

## AWARENESS

The capacity of human beings to interact with each other and the environment in ways that facilitate increased self-awareness is unique among species. While sensory organs serve as the major sources of information input, cognitive analysis, and interpretation of the meaning of events completes the process of perception. A given individual may interpret reality in a multiplicity of ways constrained to a degree by the parameters of language but capable of inventing new words and ideas to deal with reality in unique and creative ways. Individualized perception of the environment creates a need for introspection in order to have full understanding of the self.

Self-sensitivity and self-awareness are critical to competent self-care. Kanfer[11] states that self-awareness permits self-monitoring of psychologic and physiologic parameters. Current advances in the field of biofeedback have augmented human capacities for self-regulation by increasing awareness of subtle changes in muscle tension, body temperature, heart rate, blood pressure, and mental activity.[12] Self-monitoring increases awareness of the outcomes or consequences of differing behaviors. For example, self-awareness of feelings of tiredness and malaise during periods of prolonged inactivity may result in the evaluation of consequences of a sedentary lifestyle as unpleasant or uncomfortable. Sensitivity to feelings of satiation is important for proper nutrition and weight control. Sensitivity to increasing muscle tension promotes recognition of stress or impending fatigue.

It is highly likely that people who have taken the time to "tune in" to their own personal needs will be more receptive to learning self-care skills. Clients who exhibit a low level of self-awareness may need to be assisted in gaining greater insight into their own feelings and responses before they are ready to engage in health-protecting or health-promoting behaviors.

Self-awareness serves as the basis for many nursing interventions, including those directed toward stress management. Since stress has been associated with the development or exacerbation of many chronic diseases and with decreased productivity and a low degree of life satisfaction, Chapter 12 will be devoted to acquainting the reader with techniques that clients can use for achieving greater self-awareness and personal stress reduction. A high level of self-awareness is prerequisite to the successful handling of stressful life events and episodes of stress in everyday living.

## CONTROL

From early infancy, human beings seek to predict or control their environment and conditions of existence. The crying behavior of infants is the earliest means of communication with others in an attempt to manipulate the environment to attain human contact and proximity. The need for control of some aspects of the environment is critical to feelings of personal competence and self-esteem from childhood through old age. Lack of confidence in the efficacy or power of personal behavior to achieve desired ends can lead to feelings of frustration, powerlessness, and apathy.

Within social learning theory, the concept of "locus of control" has been used to explain the relationship between behavior and its outcomes.[13] Overt behavior is viewed as a function of expectancy that a certain outcome or reinforcement will occur as a result of behavior and the perceived personal value of that reinforcement. The generalized expectancy that reinforcement (outcome) is either under the control of the individual (internal control) or under the control of outside forces, such as chance or powerful others (external control), is referred to as internal-external locus of control. Individuals tend to hold primarily an internal or external view of power. Perceived internal control generally results in assertive behavior to shape the environment for support of growth and self-actualization. Perceptions of external control result in reliance on fate or chance for life circumstances.

Impaired "control dynamics" have been pinpointed as the source of difficulty for many low-income groups. If life events are believed to be contingent on "chance" or "powerful others" who possess more influence and control, individuals and families feel weak and helpless in shaping the present or the future. They fail to see their own behavior as instrumental to the achievement of desired goals.

Unless individuals believe that their behavior directly affects their current health state and future health outcomes, little motivation exists to engage in health-promoting and health-protecting behaviors. Wallston, Wallston, and DeVellis[14] have developed an instrument to measure the extent to which clients believe in their ability to control personal health status. The questionnaire measures the perceived impact of chance, others, and self on health and well-being. The reader is referred to Chapter 5 on health assessment for discussion of this instrument and its use in the clinical setting.

Perceptions of control of personal and family health are essential if individuals are to assume responsibility for self-care. Unfortunately, many interactions with health care personnel perpetuate feelings of helplessness on the part of clients because of condescending behavior, paternalistic attitudes, the withholding of information, and mystification of the health care experience. The client remains in awe of the "unknown" and perceives health care services as "medical temples" that must be entered with humility and deference. If clients are actively to take control of their own health, health care professionals must share knowledge openly, reinforce independent behavior, and provide an environment for health care delivery in which the uniqueness of each client is recognized, accepted, and enhanced. Further discussion of perceived control as a determinant of health behavior is presented in Chapters 3 and 4.

## COMPLEXITY

The tendency toward physiologic complexity is evident from many of the synthesis experiments in biology. Simple molecules of carbon dioxide, ammonia, methane, and water catalyzed by the energy of the sun carry out spontaneous reactions that produce many of the essential polymers found in nature. *Homo sapiens* represent the extreme of complexity among living organisms. The reason why human beings become more complex as they progress through the life cycle is not well understood.[15]

The increasing psychologic complexity of individuals as they mature is equally fascinating. The cumulative storage of information in both conscious and unconscious memory provides the basis for the elaborate thought processes of which human beings are capable. The capacities for speech, thought, and memory provide individuals with an organized set of symbols that give meaning to the external environment and prepare individuals for processing complex information. Individuals have the ability to process more information than they are aware of at any given moment. In fact, the amount of information processed outside the sphere of consciousness is much greater than the amount of information processed within consciousness.

The sociologic complexity of clients must also be considered by health professionals responsible for providing care directed toward prevention and health promotion. The support systems with which individuals interact constitute a critical aspect of their external environment. The relationship of the individual and family to their relevant support systems is illustrated in Figure 1-2. The family (nuclear and extended) or significant others (nontraditional family structure) assume primary support functions. The frequency of interaction with this level of the support system generally surpasses the frequency of interaction with all other external support levels.

The social or interactional support system consists of friends, acquaintances, and co-workers; the community incorporates all living and nonliving aspects of the environment within a restricted geographic area, while the society or culture

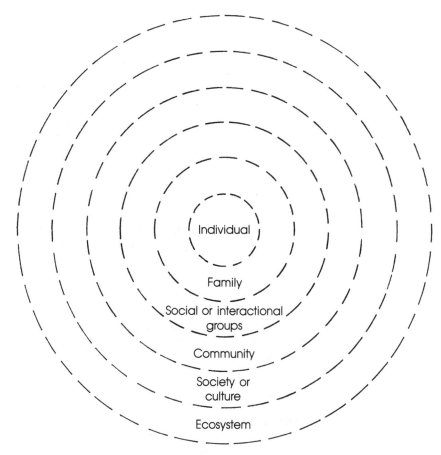

**FIGURE 1-2.** The individual in relationship to external support systems.

consists of communities within an extended geographic area and their symbolic representations of values and beliefs. The most distant suprastructure to which human beings relate, the ecosystem, consists of the world community and the nonliving environment on earth and extended into space. Events that may result in changes in the ecosystem include population explosion, industrialization, atmospheric pollution, war, and (in a more positive vein) the continuing emergence of the rich potentialities of the human species.[16]

Over time, relationships with support systems become increasingly complex. Individuals and families can choose to structure support systems that serve as protective buffers against illness and enhance their potential for fullfillment and optimum health. On the other hand, relationships with support systems can serve as barriers to continuing growth and productive survival. The reader is encouraged to give careful attention to Chapter 13 where strategies are presented for assisting clients in building and maintaining appropriate support systems.

**CONCLUSION**

Within this chapter, five dimensions of human behavior critical to understanding man's quest for health have been discussed: purpose, motivation, awareness, control, and complexity. Purpose provides direction to behavior; actualizing and stabilizing tendencies constitute the primary sources of motivation for behavior. In a fully functioning person, actualization is the dominant tendency and results in the continuing expression of inherent and learned potentialities. When stability is the dominent source of motivation, behavior is directed toward mimizing deviations from the norm or "steady state." Success in the quest for health requires a high level of self-awareness. Personal insight and perceptions of control facilitate movement toward increasing levels of health and complexity.

All health-protecting and health-promoting behaviors are carried out in the context of family, social groups, culture, and the environment. The reciprocal interactions across support systems provide a complex milieu for the delivery of preventive and health-promotive care.

**REFERENCES**

1. Rotter, J.B. *Clinical psychology.* Englewood Cliffs, N.J.: Prentice-Hall, 1971, p. 89.
2. Fraser, A.S. The evolution of purposive behavior. In Foerster, H.V. (Ed.), *Purposive systems.* New York: Spartan, 1968, p. 15.
3. Rotter, J.B. *Social learning and clinical psychology.* New York: Prentice-Hall, 1954.
4. Atkinson, J.W., & Birch, D. *The dynamics of action.* New York: Wiley, 1970, pp. 9-10.
5. Dunn, H.L. High-level wellness for man and society. From Spradley, B.W. (Ed.), *Contemporary community Nursing.* Boston: Little, Brown, 1975, p. 28.
6. Lacey, J.I., & Lacey, B.C. The relationship of resting autonomic activity to motor impulsivity. From *The brain and human behavior.* Baltimore: Williams & Wilkins, 1958, pp. 144–209.
7. Piaget, J. *The origin of intelligence in children.* New York: International Universities Press, 1962.
8. Miller, J. Living systems: Basic concepts. *Behavioral Science,* 1965, *10,* 193–237.
9. Bexton, W.H., Heron, W., & Scott, T.H. Effects of decreased variation in the sensory environment. *Canadian Journal of Psychology,* 1954, *8,* 70-76.
10. Festinger, L. *A theory of cognitive dissonance.* Stanford, Calif.: Stanford University Press, 1962.
11. Kanfer, F. Maintenance of behavior by self-generated stimuli and reinforcement. In Jacobs, A. & Sacho, L. (Eds.), *The psychology of private events: Perspective on covert response systems.* New York: Academic Press, 1971.
12. Blanchard, B., & Epstein, L.H. *A biofeedback primer.* Reading, Mass.: Addison-Wesley, 1978.
13. Rotter, 1954, op. cit.
14. Wallston, K.A., Wallston, B.S., & DeVellis, R. Development of the multi-dimensional health locus of control (MHLC) scales. *Health Education Monographs* 1978, *6,* 160–170.
15. Pattee, H.H. The evolution of self-simplifying systems. In Laszlo, E. (Ed.), *The relevance of general systems theory.* New York: George Braziller, 1972.
16. Gerard, R.W. Hierarchy, entitation and levels. In Whyte, L.I., Wilson, A., & Wilson, D. (Eds.), *Hierarchical structures.* New York: American Elsevier, 1969, p. 215.

# CHAPTER 2
# Toward a Definition of Health

Almost all nurses would agree with the statement that "the goal of nursing is health," yet few nurse scientists are actively engaged in clarification of the concept of health through investigation of its empirical dimensions. Oelbaum[1] has proposed that nurses have concerned themselves with illness rather than health because signs of maladjustment, ineptitude, and malfunction have been described in great detail by behavioral and biologic scientists, while behaviors of people with optimal health have not been similarly delineated. Mortality and morbidity have been the traditional methods used by public health and medicine for defining and measuring the level of health within a given population. Mortality-based indexes offer information on age/sex–adjusted life expectancies, while indexes of morbidity reflect the prevalence of illness in a population usually in terms of disability, dysfunction, or discomfort.[2] More recently, combined mortality/morbidity indexes have been used to provide a more comprehensive picture of the epidemiology of death and disease.

While health status indexes based on mortality and morbidity data provide information about the prevalence of illness, they do not provide direct information about the level of health within a given population. Therefore, health status indexes should be labeled *illness indexes*. Attempts to measure health in terms of mortality and morbidity are based on the assumption that only deviations from health can be measured adequately, not health itself. The following "levels of health" frequently used by the medical profession to describe client states illustrate the use of disease-oriented criteria for determining health status.

- *Level I.* No clinical evidence of disease and a low-risk profile for disease
- *Level II.* No clinical evidence of disease, but a risk profile that indicates an incubation period for disease that may emerge in the future
- *Level III.* Subclinical evidence of disease detected in the early stages and amenable to treatment, and prevention of the occurrence of illness

Recent scientific and sociocultural developments, such as stabilization of the death rate, improved methods for prevention and early detection of illness, and increased leisure time with emphasis on the esthetic dimensions of existence, mandate reexamination of the concept of health as narrowly defined by medicine. A major challenge in developing positive definitions of health is to specify measurable criteria reflective of the definitions. Many of the terms currently used to describe health lack operational specificity. Terms such as *bio-psycho-social well-being, life satisfaction, adaptation,* and *esthetic appreciation of life experiences* are highly ambiguous and need to be precisely defined in order to make health a functional concept.

The following questions illustrate some of the dilemmas that must be addressed in explicating health:

1. Does health represent a state to be reached or the characteristics of an ongoing dynamic process?
2. What is the range of individual differences in definitions of health?
3. Is the goal of health universal?
4. What conditions promote health in individuals and groups?
5. Is optimum health an ideal rather than an attainable state or process?
6. Is health a separate and distinct concept from illness?

Not only must definitions of health provide direction for policy development, they also must be clinically useful to nurses and other health professionals in evaluating the extent to which a particular client exhibits health. New health indexes and associated techniques of measurement are critically needed.

## HEALTH AS AN EVOLVING CONCEPT

A brief review of the historical development of the concept of health will provide the context for examining more recent definitions of health found in professional literature. The word *health* as it is commonly used did not appear in writing until approximately 1000 A.D. It is derived from the Old English world *hoelth,* meaning being safe or sound and whole of body.[3] Historically, physical wholeness was of major importance for acceptance in social groups. Persons suffering from disfiguring diseases like leprosy or from congenital malformations were ostracized from society and left to exist on whatever subsistence nature provided them. Not only was there fear of contagion of physically obvious disease, there was also repulsion at the grotesque appearance. Being healthy was construed as natural or in harmony with nature, while being unhealthy was thought of as unnatural or contrary to nature. The presence of disease marked the person as "unclean"; consequently, no attempt was made to affect cure or to maintain or enhance the integrity of biophysical and psychosocial functions not affected by disease.[4]

The concept of mental health as we know it did not exist until the latter part of the nineteenth century. Individuals who exhibited unpredictable, hostile, or ineffective behavior were labeled "lunatics" and ostracized in much the same way as were those with disfiguring physical ailments. Being put away with little if any human care was considered their "just due," since mental illness was often ascribed to evil spirits or satanic powers. Ostracizing the sick was a way for society to block out the painful aspects of human existence that they wished to ignore. The visibility of the ill only served to remind them of their own vulnerability. In many instances, the unhealthy individual was considered to be less than human and relegated to the status of a lower animal.

With the advent of the scientific era and the resultant increase in the rate of medical discoveries, illness came to be regarded with less disgust and society became concerned with assisting individuals to escape the catastrophic effects of illness. Health in this context was defined as "freedom from disease." Since disease was a physically or biologically defined entity, it could be diagnosed as a specific problem and treated. The notion that health was a disease-free state or condition was extremely popular into the first half of the twentieth century and was recognized by many as *the* definition of health.[5] The concept of health could not be defined except by reference to its opposite, disease. Health and illness were viewed as the extremes on a continuum. The absence of one indicated the presence of the other. This definition is still in use today. From a medical viewpoint, a person is considered healthy and the services of a physician no longer needed when the pathologic condition that served as the focus for treatment is eliminated or controlled. The assumption is frequently made that a relatively disease-free population is a healthy population.

The psychologic trauma resulting from the high-stress situations of combat during World War II increased the scope of health as a concept to include consideration of the mental status of the individual. The importance of mental health had become obscured in the rapid barrage of medical discoveries for treatment of physical disorders. Health began to be defined as a biopsychologic phenomenon; this reflected a trend toward holistic thinking. Mental health was considered to be evidenced by the ability to withstand the stresses imposed by the environment. When individuals succumbed to the rigors of life around them and could no longer carry on the functions of daily living, they were declared to be mentally or emotionally ill. Despite efforts to develop a more holistic definition of health, the dichotomy between individuals suffering from physical illness and those suffering from mental illness was very apparent in the literature of that period.

In 1974, the World Health Organization (WHO) proposed a definition of health that emphasized the positive qualities of health: "Health is a state of complete physical, mental and social well-being and not merely the absence of disease and infirmity."[6] While this definition enlarged the number of factors that needed to be taken into consideration in assessing health, it was difficult to deduce from it the criteria for recognizing health as a positive human experience. Although the WHO statement is one of the most widely accepted definitions of health today, it does not give recognition to the varying phases or levels of health that individuals may experience during their life span. However, it does have three characteristics essential to a positive conceptualization of health:

1. It reflects concern for the individual as a total person rather than as merely the sum of various parts.
2. It views health in the context of both internal and external environments.
3. It equates health with productive and creative living.

With this brief historical perspective as background, we can examine more recent definitions of health. To provide continuity with the previous chapter, the definitions of health presented will be placed in three categories: definitions focusing on actualization, definitions focusing on stability, and definitions emphasizing both actualization and stability as criteria for health. The majority of proposed definitions reflect a stability orientation. Actualization has been given less attention in definitions of health.

### Definitions of Health Focusing on Actualization

The rudiments of a definition of health emphasizing actualization appeared as early as the second century in the ideas of Galen, a Roman physician. He called health a "condition in which we neither suffer pain nor are hindered in the functions of daily life such as taking part in government, bathing, drinking, eating and doing the other things that we want." He recognized health as a state in which persons interact with the environment in ways that will produce pleasure and fulfillment.[7]

Among contemporary theorists, Halbert Dunn can be described as the leading proponent of definitions of health that emphasize actualization. Dunn coined the term *high-level wellness*, which he defined in the following way:

> *An integrated method of functioning which is oriented toward maximizing the potential of which the individual is capable. It requires that the individual maintain a continuum of balance and purposeful direction within the environment where he is functioning.*[8]

While the definition advanced by Dunn identifies balance as a dimension of health, major emphasis is on the realization of human potential through purposeful activity.

Dunn stated that high-level wellness, or optimum health, involves three components: (1) progress in a forward and upward direction toward a higher potential of functioning, (2) an open-ended and ever-expanding challenge to live at a fuller potential, and (3) progressive integration or maturation of the individual at increasingly higher levels throughout the life cycle.[9] Dunn conceptualized wellness as being a direction of progress as well as levels to be reached. In optimum health, individuals function at a high level amid a dynamic and constantly changing environment.

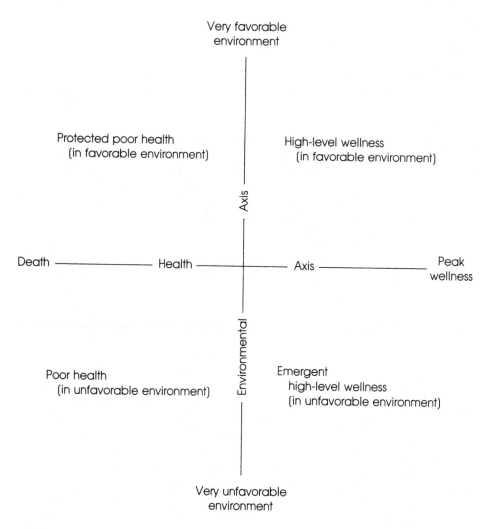

**FIGURE 2-1.** The health grid, its axes and quadrants. *(Source: U.S. Department of Health, Education and Welfare, Public Health Service, National Office of Vital Statistics.)*

According to Dunn, the essential need of an individual is freedom, if one is to realize personal uniqueness through creative expression and thereby achieve a high level of wellness. The importance of one's relationships with the environment is illustrated in Figure 2-1. In the health grid proposed by Dunn, high-level wellness can only emerge in a favorable environment. One is never isolated from the effects of surroundings.

Dunn has identified nine points of attack for promoting high-level wellness.[10]

1. Improvement of conditions of family living and community life
2. Education to assist individuals and families in application of knowledge to promote health
3. Education in principles of human relations
4. Development of high-level wellness among individuals in leadership positions
5. Maintenance of open information channels and free access to knowledge available (essential for intelligent decision making)
6. Enhancement of opportunities for creative expression
7. Promotion of caring relationships and concern for the welfare of others
8. Understanding of the concept of maturity and methods of its promotion as a realistic goal
9. Extension of the human life span with the opportunity to utilize for the benefit of society those who have become fully mature and have reached the highest attainable level of wellness

A major strength of the definition of health advanced by Dunn is the explicit rejection of the idea that health is "static," with no progression or movement. Health, according to Dunn, is not simply a "passive state of freedom from illness in which the individual is at peace with his environment or in a condition of homeostasis."[11] It is an emerging process characteristic of the entire life span. Dunn has been highly instrumental in developing and refining the concept of positive, holistic health, yet a great deal of empirical testing is needed to make operational the criteria for health that are an integral part of his definition.

Another definition that focuses on actualization as opposed to stability is the description of health by Hoyman as "optimal personal fitness for full, fruitful, creative living."[12] Hoyman states that health is a dynamic process involving the total human being, with reference to hereditary uniqueness as well as to the individual style of living. According to Hoyman, personal health is determined by three major factors: heredity, environment, and actively initiated behavior. His model focuses on the interaction of heredity, environment, and behavior and the way in which the quality and quantity of interaction determines the level of health on a continuum extending from death to optimum health. The importance of vigor, vitality, and a zest for living are emphasized as factors profoundly affecting the search of the individual for health, meaning, and fulfillment within the individual's world.

A third definition of health emphasizing actualization is that of Bauer and Schaller:

> . . . [Health is] that condition of the human organism that permits one
> to live happily and successfully. It favors efficiency but does not assure
> it. It helps towards attaining the goals and ambitions of life.[13]

This definition stresses the importance of an orientation toward growth, goal directedness, and attainment of goals as components of health.

Other definitions of health that emphasize actualization include Bermosk and Porter's definition of holistic health:

*Holistic health involves the ongoing integration of mind, body, and spirit. A person evolves from one level of wholeness to another level of wholeness.*[14]

Holistic health is defined as integrated energies of mind, body, spirit, and environment. Bermosk and Porter view ongoing integration within the human system as synonymous with healing. One is responsible for one's own state of health, and individuals evolve toward greater levels of zest and well-being as they continually heal themselves and expand their consciousness. This definition, while somewhat ambiguous, is certainly positive in orientation, with emphasis on the importance of personal fulfillment.

Hanchett, in applying general systems theory to community health assessment, described the concept of health in the following way:

*The concept of health implies energy, individuality, relationships and continuing progress toward developmental tasks.*[15]

The emergent nature of the healthy individual and the capacity for open energy exchange with other systems within the environment are characteristics of Hanchett's description of health. The nature of relationships with others is an important criterion in evaluating the level of health attained by an individual.

Many definitions of health that emphasize actualization are open-ended. Health is an asymptote, an ideal on the horizon that is often approached but seldom reached. Many of these definitions have no fixed upper limit for maximum human functioning. Given our limited ability at present to measure the character of energy exchanges, degree of self-fulfillment, and level of human wholeness, definitions emphasizing actualization provide a limited number of concrete criteria for measuring health in clients.

## DEFINITIONS OF HEALTH THAT FOCUS ON STABILITY

A great deal more attention has been given to definitions of health that focus on stability than to definitions of health that focus on actualization of human potential. The impetus for stability-based definitions derives from the physiologic concepts of homostasis and adaptation. Many of the definitions of health that emphasize stability are based on the premise that the environment is hostile to human existence. For instance, Beeson described health in the following way:

*. . . a state of interaction between self and the environment which is characterized by a ceaseless struggle between a basically hostile environment and a series of defenses we are endowed with or learn. The goal of the struggle is the homeostatic balance of forces which is accomplished by decreasing the threat of the environment or by raising the capabilities of the host to defend himself.*[16]

Life is viewed as a continuing struggle in which either the impact of the environment must be lessened or the defenses of the human being strengthened.

René Dubos, a major advocate of the stability position, defined health as a state or condition that enables the individual to adapt to his or her environment. The degree of health that one experiences is dependent on one's ability to react, accommodate, and adjust to the various internal and external tensions and stresses that one faces. The states of health and disease are the expressions of either success or failure experienced by the individual in his or her efforts to respond adaptively to environmental changes. Illness can be successful adaptation (for example, an inflammatory reaction to an invading pathogen) or unsuccessful adaptation (for example, the development of a gastric ulcer in reaction to stress). Dubos considers optimum health to be a mirage because man in the real world must face the physical, biologic, and social forces that are forever changing, frequently unpredictable, and often dangerous for the individual and for the human species as a collective. Positive health is not a state to be reached or a direction to be pursued but lies in the struggle itself and its successful waging. According to Dubos, the nearest approach to health is a physical and mental state free of discomfort and pain that permits one to function effectively as long as possible within the environment.[17]

Aubrey conceptualized health as structural wholeness, in which sensory processes are intact and function in such a way that balance and adaptability characterize the individual. Health reflects the coordinated activity of component parts, each functioning within its normal range. Aubrey defines mental health separately from physical health. Mental health is characterized by emotional stability, integration and adaptaton of the individual to surroundings so that he or she remains viable and unharmed in spite of changing conditions.

The general adaptation syndrome is of prime importance in Aubrey's definition of health in that the individual responds to the internal and external stresses of the environment with adaptive patterns of reaction that are conservative and protective. According to Aubrey, the healthy individual should experience three conditions: subjective feelings of contentment and balance, a high degree of personal efficiency, and adequate performance of those functions that societal living and human existence require of him or her. Psychologic health as a component of holistic health is characterized by cognitive efficiency, peace, and tranquility resulting from successful adaptation and open expression of affection toward others.[18]

Definitions of health based on normality can be described as stability-oriented definitions. Normality refers to the natural range of variability in structure and function of any human system and represents efficient performance and adaptation to commonly occurring stresses.[19] Statistical norms for a variety of human functions are already well defined and have been used for many years in diagnostic procedures. Many physiologic parameters are easily measured and ascertained. In contrast, the normal range for holistic dimensions of man, such as the rate of energy exchange, boundary permeability and structural complexity are not presently known, nor have many empirical data been collected on these phenomena. Thus, ambiguity persists in the scientific description of normative ranges for holistic variables.

A major problem with normative definitions of health is that they predict "what could be" on the basis of "what is," leaving little room for incorporating growth, maturation, and the evolutionary emergence of human potential into the definition of health. A norm represents the most frequently occurring phenomenon, a modicum of effectiveness rather than excellence or exceptional effectiveness in human functioning.

Defining health in terms of social norms is parallel to defining health in terms of physiologic norms. Parsons defined health in terms of social norms more than two decades ago. He described health as "the effective performance of valued roles and tasks for which an individual has been socialized."[20] Roles serve as the organizational matrix for the tasks that individuals perform. Tasks are the definitive sets of physical operations that individuals carry out in activities of daily living. According to Parsons, health status can be determined by application of normative standards of adequacy for present and future role and task performance. Specific incapacities must be evaluated relative to the tasks and roles that they affect.[21]

Health is conceptualized by Parsons as a social norm of ability to function in tasks critical to survival of the societal system at the family, society, or cultural level. In this context, health is seen as conforming behavior, illness as deviant behavior.

Similar to Parson's sociologic model of health, Patrick, Bush, and Chen[22] have identified functional norms as a major component in the definition of health that they propose. According to them, health can be defined by "those functional levels that man considers adequate or desirable." For example, physical activity is considered to be an important human function. Function levels for physical activity are as follows: (1) walks freely, (2) walks with limitations, (3) moves independently in wheel chair, and (4) remains in bed or chair. Participants in the study that they conducted were asked to evaluate each function level in terms of their preference for it.

The desirability of the immediate function level as well as the probability that the current condition or state will change to a higher or lower preference function level must be considered in assessing present health status. The probability of change in function level can be thought of as the prognosis. Prognosis is the probability that the human condition will deteriorate, remain constant, or improve with time. For example, if two individuals are confined to bed with gastrointestinal discomfort, one because of an intestinal infection, the other because of a malignancy, the functional levels for physical activity of both may be the same; however, the prognosis is very different. Therefore, the health status of the two individuals is very different. Both present function level and the probability of change to a different function level must be considered. Based on functional norms, Patrick, Bush, and Chen define health as:

> *. . . evidence of socially valued function levels in the performance of activities usual for a person's age and social roles with a minimum probability of change to less valued function levels.*[23]

The normative conception of health as proposed by Twaddle is presented in Figure 2-2. A major inadequacy of the health-illness continuum as described by Twaddle is that only one end of the continuum is attainable. He concedes that death is a possibility for everyone, yet optimum health is unattainable. He agrees with the position of Dubos that optimum health is an ideal or a mirage. One goes back and forth during one's life span, between normal health and illness. In the definition of health proffered by Twaddle, the only possible goal is mediocrity, since optimum health and higher levels of well-being are out of reach.[24]

Twaddle gives the individual very little credit for being able to assess his or her own health status. A health definer, usually the physician, is central to the definition of normal health. Twaddle labels disagreement between the opinion of the individual regarding his or her own health status and the opinion of the physician as aberrant behavior on the part of the individual.[25] Figure 2-3 vividly illustrates this point.

Within the nursing literature, the following two definitions of health, emphasizing stability, have been proposed. Hadley defined health as follows:

> *A state in which the individual of a given sex and at a given stage of growth and development is capable of meeting the minimum physical, physiological and social requirements for appropriate functioning in the sex category and at the given stage of growth and development.*[26]

Hadley emphasized that the purpose of her definition was to provide an operational description of health useful to nurses in practice. She raised the question whether health and illness are opposite poles of a single dimension or qualitatively different. Proposing that they are qualitatively different but parallel dimensions of human experience, Hadley recognized the lack of clear, operational definitions for each concept. One limitation of Hadley's definition is that criteria for measuring health

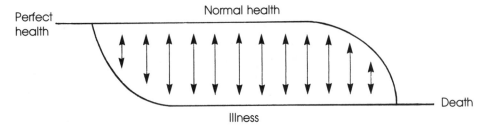

**FIGURE 2-2.** Normative conception of health. *(Reprinted with permission from Twaddle, A.C. The concept of health status.* Social Science and Medicine, 8. *Copyright © 1974, Pergamon Press, Ltd.)*

reflect the lowest end of the normative scale. Identifying varying levels of health is conceptually difficult given the nature of the definition.

In a book on nursing concepts for health promotion, Murray and Zentner presented another definition of health, also focusing on stability. They described health in the following way:

> *Health is a purposeful, adaptive response, physically, mentally, emo-tionally, and socially to internal and external stimuli in order to main-tain stability and comfort.*[27]

The external variables Murray and Zentner identified as affecting health were (1) physical variables, e.g., climate, (2) biologic variables, e.g., drugs, (3) social variables, e.g., socioeconomic status and family-life patterns, and (4) cultural variables, e.g., language, religion, and family organization. Internal variables af-fecting health included (1) personal characteristics, e.g., age, sex, and intelligence, (2) physical growth and development, (3) regulatory mechanism, e.g., homeosta-sis, biologic rhythms, and adaptation, (4) body repair mechanisms, and (5) human

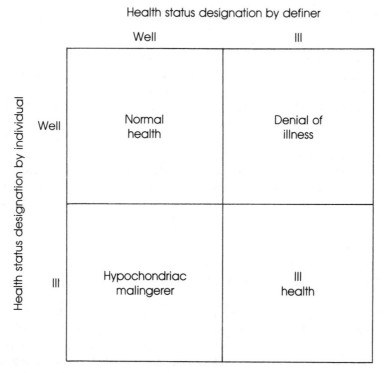

**FIGURE 2-3.** Interaction of health assessment by individual and health definer.
*(Reprinted with permission from Twaddle, A.C. The concept of health status. Social Science and Medicine, 8. Copyright © 1974, Pergamon Press, Ltd.)*

behavior. Health was viewed as maintenance of the level of stability necessary for human survival and some degree of creature comfort.

The last definition of health to be presented in this section is that of Grossman, an economist. This definition, although emphasizing balance, stands out as markedly different from the others. Grossman defined health as:

> . . . *a durable commodity to be purchased, an investment to be made. The end goal is an economic balance between the money and time spent in health behaviors, health services, health supporting products, health-related services and the level of health achieved by an individual, family or society.*[28]

Grossman proposed that individuals inherit an initial "stock" of health that depreciates over time and can be increased by investment. Death occurs when the stock falls below a specified level. A novel feature of the economic model of health is that it proposes that an individual can choose to some extent the length of life or the amount of health desired during any given period of life by the investments that are made. Examples of direct investments in the stock of health include time, medical care, diet, exercise, and housing. Grossman believes that health is being demanded increasingly by consumers for two major reasons: (1) As a commodity, health enters consumer preference profiles, and (2) sick days are a source of loss or disutility.

Since depreciation of health occurs at an increasing rate after a certain point in the life span, more money must be spent to produce less health. Throughout life, time is as important as medical care in health investment. Grossman has combined both qualitative and quantitative variables in his definition. For instance, measurement of the initial stock of health is a subjective estimate on one's part of the actual state of one's health. The annual amount spent on health care represents a quantitative variable.

Economists have been giving increasing attention to the question of whether mathematical functions can be constructed to define health. Such functions are seen as potentially useful in more precise quantification of data for cost/benefit analysis as a basis for economic decisions relevant to health.

## DEFINITIONS OF HEALTH FOCUSING ON BOTH ACTUALIZATION AND STABILITY

The definitions of health presented in this section represent mixed models. That is, the definitions take into account both the need for growth and actualization and the need for stability and balance. The definitions presented here recognize that man seeks actively to transcend those conditions that surround him in meaningful and innovative ways as well as to adapt to his environment in an orderly and effective fashion.

Wu has described health as a state characterized by optimal performance, physiologic homeostasis, and behavior stability. Health is not the absence of conflict but the manner in which frustrating or anxiety-producing situations are handled. Wu defined health as:

> . . . *a feeling of well-being, a capactiy to perform to the best of one's ability, and the flexibility to adapt and adjust to varying situations created by the subsystems of man or the suprasystems in which he exists.*[29]

Wu has proposed that wellness and illness represent distinct entities with a repertory of behaviors for each. Within this frame of reference, both wellness (health) and illness can exist simultaneously. Evaluation of both are critical to comprehensive health assessment.

Imogene King proposed a definition of health emphasizing both actualization and stability. She defined health as:

> *A dynamic state in the life cycle of an organism which implies continuous adaptation to stresses in the internal and external environment through optimum use of one's resources to achieve maximum potential for daily living.*[30]

King described health as a process of growth and development that is futuristic in orientation while at the same time avoiding major deviations in basic human functions or those functions characteristic of a given culture.

Oelbaum identified 26 functions or behaviors of adults in optimum health.[31] The behaviors that she identified can be categorized under the two dimensions of actualization and stabilization as illustrated in Table 2-1. Behaviors under the heading of actualization reflect self-direction and initiative, while behaviors under the heading of stabilization represent reactive adjustment and adaptation responses.

Oelbaum has suggested a four-point ordinal scale that could be used with the 26 descriptive statements to assess specific levels of health attained by individuals:

• 4 points — self-reliance and proficiency in carrying out the function or behavior
• 3 points — ordinarily performs the task on one's own fairly well
• 2 points — usually reliant on others or performs the task poorly
• 1 point — total dependence on others for performance of the task or complete avoidance of the task[32]

While the criteria proposed by Oelbaum for assessing wellness would need considerable empirical investigation to yield a health index that was reliable, valid, sensitive, and widely applicable to a variety of age groups, the criteria provide a conceptualization of health on which to build further research efforts.

The following definition of health has been proposed by the author. It emphasizes both actualizing and stabilizing tendencies:

## TABLE 2-1　FUNCTIONS OF ADULTS IN OPTIMUM HEALTH

| Actualization | Stability |
|---|---|
| 1. Provides for own comfort and relaxation | 1. Performs activities of daily living |
| 2. Obtains and maintains an environment conducive to well-being | 2. Has a stable body image perceived as being socially acceptable |
| 3. Maintains optimum motor function | 3. Efficiently disposes of metabolic wastes |
| 4. Obtains, digests, and metabolizes appropriate amounts of food that promote optimal nutrition | 4. Has an appropriate intake and healthy distribution of excretion of fluids and electrolytes |
| 5. Builds and maintains meaningful interpersonal relationships, is comfortable with interdependence | 5. Guards self against overwhelming changes; regulatory and defense systems intact and helpful |
| 6. Accumulates knowledge and skills that bring one success in one's chosen life roles | 6. Maintains good hygiene |
| 7. Demonstrates personality growth and creative expression appropriate to one's developmental level and prized by one's culture | 7. Juxtaposes the tasks of various life roles with minimal conflict while keeping in touch with own needs |
| 8. Demonstrates high quality cerebral functioning | 8. Holds expectations and makes decisions reflecting understanding of his own limitations and situational realities |
| 9. Is a team member of own prevention/rehabilitation team; has sufficient understanding, initiative, self-control, and financial resources to maintain health | 9. Efficiently uses oxygen |
| 10. Recognizes and cherishes the uniqueness of own identity and the uniqueness of each other person | 10. May have symptoms, but they are yielding to prescribed therapy; uses therapies to help carry out own wellness work |
| 11. Humanistically expresses love and respect for all life and the quality of that life | 11. Receives and recognizes sensory input |
| 12. Mobilizes resources to meet own needs; begins by expressing needs freely to another person | 12. Demonstrates functional verbal and nonverbal communication |
| 13. Demonstrates a zeal for living | 13. Attains healthful balance of productive work and rest |

Copyright © 1974, American Journal of Nursing Company. Adapted from *American Journal of Nursing*, September 1974, *74*(9), p 1623.

---

### TABLE 2-2.  PROPOSED CRITERIA FOR EVALUATING HEALTH

1. Exhibits personal growth and positive change over time
2. Identifies long-term and short-term goals that guide behavior
3. Prioritizes identified goals
4. Exhibits awareness of alternative behavioral options to accomplish goals
5. Perceives optimum health as a primary life purpose
6. Engages in interpersonal relationships that are satisfying and fulfilling
7. Actively seeks new experiences that expand knowledge or increase competencies for personal care
8. Displays a high tolerance for new and unusual situations or experiences
9. Derives satisfaction from the experience of daily living
10. Expends more energy in acting on the environment than in reacting to it
11. Recognizes barriers to growth and deals constructively in removing or ameliorating them
12. Uses self-monitoring and feedback from others to determine personal and social effectiveness
13. Maintains conditions of internal stability compatible with continuing existence
14. Anticipates internal and external threats to stability and takes preventive actions

---

> *Health is the actualization of inherent and acquired human potential through satisfying relationships with others, goal directed behavior, and competent personal care while adjustments are made as needed to maintain stability and structural integrity.*[33]

Criteria for evaluating health based on the above definition appear in Table 2-2.

According to this definition and related criteria, individuals in optimum health actively seek new information relevant to the attainment of life goals, derive pleasure from experiences of personal and environmental mastery, and exhibit a high tolerance for new and unusual internal and external stimuli. Health reflects a process of development characterized by frequent experiences of challenge, achievement, and satisfaction.

## HEALTH AND ILLNESS: DISTINCT OR OPPOSITE ENDS OF A CONTINUUM

The issue of whether health and disease are separate entities or opposite ends of a continuum has fascinated scientists for some time. Are health and illness quantitatively or qualitatively different?

Theorists presenting health and illness as a continuum usually identify possible reference points, such as (1) optimal health, (2) suboptimal health or incipient illness, (3) overt illness and disability, and (4) very serious illness or approaching death.[34] This scale has only one point representing health while three points on the scale represent varying states of illness. Dunn proposed a more balanced continuum with death representing one end of the scale and peak wellness representing the opposite end.[35] The continuum described by Dunn allows the differentiation of varying levels of health as well as varying levels of illness. When health and illness are assumed to represent a single continuum, it is difficult to discuss healthy aspects of the ill individual. The presence of illness ascribes the "sick role," and the individual is expected to direct all energies toward finding the cause of the illness and engaging in behaviors that will result in a return to health as soon as possible.

Manifestations of health in the presence of illness have lead some theorists to propose separate but parallel continuums for health and illness. Sorochan has commented that everyone free from disease is not equally healthy. He proposed gradations of health separate from gradations of illness, which would allow individuals to be at any stage of health regardless of their position on the illness continuum.[36] Oelbaum stresses the interrelationship of health and illness, even though she considers the concepts to be separate entities rather than opposite ends of a continuum. She states that apathy toward the work of wellness is the precursor of disease. The particular health behaviors or functions that are poorly performed will influence the type of disease, disorder, or damage that will follow.[37]

Increasing acceptance of the premise that health is more than the mere absence of disease has added support to the belief that health and illness are qualitatively different and should be studied as separate but related concepts. In Figure 2-4, differing levels of health are depicted in interaction with the experience of

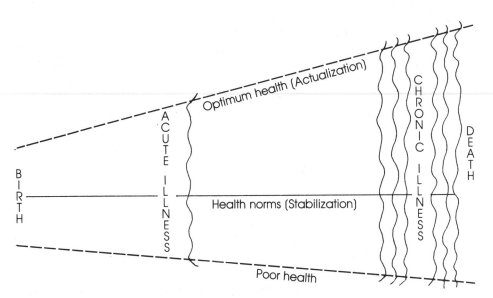

**FIGURE 2-4.** The health continuum throughout the life span.

---

### TABLE 2-3   TYPOLOGY OF HEALTH CRITERIA

---

I. Health as a physiologic process or state (biologic orientation)
   A. Medicine — absence of disease
   B. Physiology — predictability and integrity of system processes
   C. Anatomy — integrity of cellular structures
   D. Microbiology — absence of abnormal microbial activity
II. Health as a feeling state (psychologic orientation)
   A. Psychiatry — absence of cognitive, affective, and psychomotor disorders
   B. Psychology — continuing behavioral adjustment to changing environmental contingencies and the ongoing development of human personality
III. Health as a capacity to function (sociologic orientation)
   A. Sociology — performance of roles and tasks within society appropriate for a given level of growth and development
   B. Social work — effective implementation of occupational and familial roles resulting in economic solvency and societal efficiency
IV. Health as a holistic process (biopsychosocial orientation)
   Nursing — actualization of human potential through purposeful self-initiated behavior, satisfying relationships with others, and competent personal care

---

illness. Illness is diagrammed as representing discrete events throughout the life process that can serve as barriers to one's continuing quest for health. However, poor health can exist without specific covert or overt illness.

## CONCLUSION

In summary, a typology of major health criteria espoused by various disciplines is presented in Table 2-3. The table is an attempt to contrast and compare prevailing definitions of health within the various disciplines. Nursing is identified as the major group of health professionals ascribing to a holistic definition of health.

## REFERENCES

1. Oelbaum, C.H. Hallmarks of adult wellness. *American Journal of Nursing,* 1974, *74,*1623.
2. Balinsky, W., & Berger, R. A review of the research on general health status indexes. *Medical Care,* 1975, *13,*283–293.
3. Sorochan, W. Health concepts as a basis for orthobiosis. In Hart E., & Sechrist, W. (Eds.), *The dynamics of wellness.* Belmont, Calif.; Wadsworth, 1970, p. 3.
4. Dolfman, M.L. The concept of health: An historic and analytic examination. *Journal of School Health,* 1973, *43,*493.

5. Wylie, C.M. The definition and measurement of health and disease. *Public Health Reports,* February 1970, *85,*100–104.
6. Temkin, O. What is health? Looking back and ahead. In Galdston, I. (Ed.), *Epidemiology of health.* New York: Academy of Medicine, Health Education Council, 1953, p. 21.
7. Wylie, *op. cit.,* p. 100.
8. Dunn, H.L. What high-level wellness means. *Canadian Journal of Public Health,* November 1959, p. 447.
9. Dunn, H.L. High-level wellness for man and society. *AJPH,* June 1959, *49,*789.
10. Dunn, H.L. Points of attack for raising the levels of wellness. *Journal of the National Medical Association,* July 1975, *49,*233–235.
11. Dunn, H.L. *High Level Wellness.* Thorofare, N.J.: Charles B. Slack, 1980, p. 4.
12. Hoyman, H.S. Our modern concept of health. *Journal of School Health,* September 1962, p. 253.
13. Bauer, W.W., & Schaller, W.E. *Your health today.* New York: Harper & Row, 1965, p. 15.
14. Bermosk, L.S., Porter, S.E. *Women's health and human wholeness.* New York: Appleton, 1979, p. 11.
15. Hanchett, E. *Community health assessment.* New York: Wiley, 1979, p. 162.
16. Beeson, G. The health-illness spectrum. *American Journal of Public Health,* November 1967, *57,*1904.
17. Dubos, R. *Man adapting.* New Haven: Yale University Press, 1965, p. 349.
18. Aubrey, L. Health as a social concept. *British Journal of Sociology,* June 1953, *4,*115.
19. Ryle, J. The meaning of normal. *Lancet,* 1947, *252:*4.
20. Parsons, T. Definitions of health and illness in the light of American values and social structure. In Jaco, E.G. (Ed.), *Patients, physicians and illness.* New York, Free Press, 1958, p. 176.
21. *Ibid.,* p. 178.
22. Patrick, D.L., Bush, J.W., & Chen, M.M. Toward an operational definition of health. *Journal of Health and Social Behavior,* 1973, *14,*6.
23. *Ibid.*
24. Twaddle, A.C. The concept of health status. *Social Science and Medicine,* January 1974, *8,*35.
25. *Ibid.*
26. Hadley, B.J. Current concepts of wellness and illness: Their relevance for nursing. *Image,* 1974, *6,*24.
27. Murray, R. & Zentner, J. *Nursing concepts for health promotion.* Englewood Cliffs, N.J.: Prentice-Hall, 1975, p. 7.
28. Grossman, M. *The demand for health: A theoretical and empirical investigation.* New York: Columbia University Press, 1972, pp. 1–8.
29. Wu, R. *Behavior and illness.* Englewood Cliffs, N.J.: Prentice-Hall, 1973, p. 112.
30. King, I.M. *Toward a theory of nursing.* New York: Wiley, 1971, p. 24.
31. Oelbaum, *op. cit.,* p. 1623.
32. Oelbaum, *ibid.,* p. 1624.
33. Pender, N.J. Presentation, Conference on Health Promotion. New Jersey State Nurses' Association, Newark, New Jersey, 1975.
34. Sorochan, *op. cit.,* p. 5.
35. Dunn, 1980, *op. cit.,* p. 5.
36. Sorochan, *op. cit.,* p. 4.
37. Oelbaum, *op. cit.,* p. 1623.

# CHAPTER 3
# Health-Protecting (Preventive) Behavior

In many instances, the need for care in illness represents a lack of care directed toward prevention earlier in the life span of individuals. Absence of such care may result from the solely curative orientation of health professionals, limited competence on the part of individuals for self-care, or the lack of knowledge about preventive strategies. Since illness frequently serves as a barrier to optimum growth and the realization of personal potential, maintaining an illness-free state through preventive efforts is highly desirable. Freedom from the energy demands of illness allows individuals to direct greater energies toward self-actualization.

Nurses at the forefront of professional practice are assuming an increasingly important role in health protection (prevention). The primary goal of health-protecting behaviors is the removal or avoidance of encumbrances to growth, maturation, fulfillment, and self-actualization throughout the life cycle. Encumbrances may be personal illness, disturbances in interpersonal relationships, or social disruption. Individuals need assistance from health professionals in establishing an effective plan of health protection that is flexible, individually tailored, and periodically revised as needed to fit the changing goals of the client. A plan for preventive care throughout the life span is as important as a plan for care in illness within the hospital setting.

## LEVELS OF PREVENTION

Prevention has been described as consisting of three levels: primary, secondary, and tertiary.[1,2] Each level of prevention occurs at a distinct point in time relative to the occurrence of disease processes and requires specific nursing interventions. The three levels of prevention as traditionally defined in public health are presented below.

- Primary prevention—includes generalized health promotion as well as specific protection against disease.
- Secondary prevention—emphasizes early diagnosis and prompt intervention to halt the pathologic process, thereby shortening its duration and severity and

**41**

enabling the individual to regain normal function at the earliest possible point.
• Tertiary prevention—comes into play when a defect or disability is fixed, stabilized, or irreversible. Rehabilitation, the goal of tertiary prevention, is more
  than halting the disease process itself; it is the restoring of the individual to an
  optimum level of functioning within the constraints of the disability.

While the above definitions are widely accepted, the author believes that
greater clarity could be achieved by differentiating between "health promotion"
and "specific protection against disease," rather than using primary prevention
as a concept that encompasses both types of activities. Therefore, the following
two definitions are proposed to replace the single definition of primary prevention:

• Health promotion—activities directed toward *sustaining* or *increasing* the level
  of well-being, self-actualization, and personal fulfillment of a given individual
  or group.
• Primary prevention—activities directed toward *decreasing* the probability of
  encountering illness, including active protection of the body against unnecessary
  stressors.

This differentiation is consistent with current theoretical and research efforts to
explicate health as a positive state in its own right, rather than simply the opposite
of a negative state (illness).

Health promotion can be described as maintaining current health status or
moving to a more desirable level of health. Movement is always toward a positively
valued state of existence, rather than away from a negatively valued one. On the
other hand, prevention is a defensive posture or set of actions taken to ward off
specific illness or their sequelae that may threaten the quality of life or longevity.
Prevention is better described by the term *health-protecting behavior* because of
its emphasis on guarding or defending the body from injury. This term was first
introduced into the literature by Harris and Guten,[3] who used it as a synonym for
both illness prevention and health promotion. To the author's knowledge, use of
the term specifically for preventive actions is original in this book. Thus, it is
proposed that there are three levels of prevention or health-protecting behavior,
and a distinctly different category of activity, health promotion. The motivation
and goals for health protection and health promotion are related but distinctly
different.

The three levels of prevention will be described below. Health promotion will
be discussed in detail in Chapter 4.

**Primary Prevention**
Providing specific protection against disease to prevent its occurrence is the most
desirable form of prevention. Primary preventive efforts spare the client the cost,
discomfort, and threat to the quality of life that illness poses or, at the least, delay
the onset of illness. Early breakthroughs in primary prevention centered on control
of acute disease and resulted in mass immunization efforts for childhood health

problems such as diphtheria, pertussis, and smallpox. Effective measures for producing artificial active immunity to polio, measles, mumps, and influenza were developed later. Immunization clinics within health departments, mandatory immunization requirements for school admission, and mass media have been used to promote a high level of immunization against acute diseases among children.

Primary prevention of chronic health problems presents a different kind of challenge for health care professionals. Preventive measures for such illnesses generally consist of counseling, education, and adoption of specific health practices or changes in lifestyle by the client. Examples of counseling and educative efforts directed toward primary prevention include weight control to prevent the onset of diabetes, nutrition education (low-sodium diet) to maintain normal systolic and diastolic blood pressure, smoking cessation programs for prevention of cancer of the lung and cardiovascular disorders, and education concerning the danger of overexposure to direct sunlight as a risk factor for skin cancer. Primary prevention also encompasses counseling and education of women of child-bearing age to prevent birth defects that may result from use of drugs, alcohol, or tobacco during pregnancy. Accident-prevention programs, use of protective equipment to prevent blindness or deafness, and self-care education to prevent frequent colds or respiratory disorders that may lead to chronic lung disease also represent forms of primary prevention for chronic health problems. Referral of the school-age child with a possible streptococcal infection to the physician for prompt throat culture and treatment represents primary prevention for rheumatic fever.

Primary prevention is also important in the area of mental health. Counseling individuals and families to help them recognize, avoid, or deal constructively with problems or situations that may pose a threat to mental health is an important preventive measure. Family/individual counseling by the nurse or use of peer support groups are two ways in which clients can learn to manage life stress or cope successfully with specific life crises.

Another approach to primary prevention that the nurse must be concerned about is that of environmental control. While individual protective measures to avoid illness are increasingly available for a number of health problems, control of air, water, and noise pollution represent complementary approaches to disease control. Minimizing contamination of the work or general environment by asbestos dust, silicone dust, smoke, chemical pollutants, and excessive noise represents a critical organizational/political approach to primary prevention of acute and chronic illness.

**Secondary Prevention**
Secondary prevention consists of organized, direct screening efforts or education of the public to promote early case finding of individuals with disease so that prompt intervention can be instituted to halt pathologic processes and limit disability. Early diagnosis of a health problem can decrease the catastrophic effects that might otherwise result for the individual and family from advanced illness and its many complications. Public education to promote breast self-examination,

use of home kits for the detection of occult blood in stool specimens, and familiarity with the seven cancer danger signals are all directed toward identification of signs of possible illness by individuals in order to promote prompt use of health services for early detection. Screening programs for hypertension, diabetes, uterine cancer (pap smear), breast cancer (examination and mammography), glaucoma, and sexually transmitted diseases are continuing public health efforts for secondary prevention. Vision and hearing screening, scoliosis screening, and assessment of children for developmental delays or disabilities are preventive programs frequently carried out within the school setting. Careful and systematic observation of children and adolescents for malnutrition (undernutrition or overnutrition), neurologic disorders (seizures, tics, and other abnormal behaviors), drug abuse, alcohol abuse, and other behavioral problems also constitute important secondary prevention efforts.

While individuals are often the initial focus of secondary prevention, such efforts may also be extended to families or significant others. The early identification of syphilis or gonorrhea should prompt the investigation of contacts and their treatment, while detection of hypertension or diabetes should result in further exploration of family history and screening of other family members that could potentially have the same illness. Secondary preventive efforts in the area of mental health may consist of assisting family members to deal with the stress of mental illness or the anxiety and stigma of hospitalization of a family member for a mental health problem. Such efforts are directed toward enhancing the ability of families to cope with the current crisis and decreasing the possible after-effects of highly stressful experiences.

Where primary prevention is not available, secondary prevention (early diagnosis and treatment) represents the first line of defense against disease. In other situations, primary preventive measures may be available but not used, resulting in the need for secondary-level intervention. In either case, organized screening programs and public education efforts will continue to be critical for the detection of health problems in their early phases.

### Tertiary Prevention

Tertiary prevention begins early in the period of recovery from illness and consists of such activities as consistent and appropriate administration of medications to optimize therapeutic effects, moving and positioning to prevent complications of immobility, and passive and active exercises to prevent disability. Continuing health supervision during rehabilitation to restore an individual to an optimal level of functioning is an important role of the professional nurse. Minimizing residual disability and helping the client learn to live productively with disabilities that cannot be cured are the goals of tertiary prevention. Tertiary preventive measures are appropriate for clients of all ages: the child with cerebral palsy or cystic fibrosis and the adult following a stroke or other neurologic insult are examples.

Rehabilitation programs are frequently offered during the posthospitalization phase of illness and provide an intensive period of restorative care. Often the nurse must assist the client and family in dealing with feelings of hopelessness about the illness, interpret the rationale for rehabilitation, and teach client and family self-care and rehabilitation measures.[4] Cardiac rehabilitation programs following myocardial infarction or cardiovascular surgery are excellent examples of tertiary prevention services. Emphasis in such programs is on meeting the physical and emotional needs of clients and promoting lifestyle changes, e.g., dietary and exercise habits, or environmental modifications, e.g., decreased stress, that minimize the probability of recurrence of the problem.

Follow-up of client and family after the intensive phase of rehabilitation is critical to maintain the health level or benefits achieved during the initial phase. The dynamic nature of chronic illness mandates continuity of care and support of the client over time to insure stability and/or progress. When deterioration and increasing disability is inevitable over time, slowing the pace of progressive disability and maintaining the optimum level of health of the client is vital to continuing self-actualization and personal fulfillment. As negative forces (exacerbations and social visibility of illness) that disrupt health increase, positive actions to thwart movement to lower levels of health and functioning must increase through health-promotion efforts (see Chapter 4).

The ultimate goal of tertiary prevention is to help clients live full and productive lives, managing the problems of chronicity successfully.[5] In chronic illness, clients are in most instances their own primary resource for self-care. The responsibility for continuing preventive efforts must be assumed by the client with assistance and support from family, health professionals, and other community resources.

In summary, prevention is an important responsibility of nurses in all care settings. Minimizing the occurrence of disease and its complications as well as promoting optimum restoration can greatly enhance the quality of life for individuals of all ages. Examples of primary, secondary, and tertiary preventive measures are presented in Table 3-1.

## MOTIVATION OF HEALTH-PROTECTING (PREVENTIVE) BEHAVIOR

A gap exists currently between the knowledge that all behavior is motivated and the ability to predict sources of motivation for specific health behaviors. While demographic charactertistics of clients and dimensions of preventive behaviors (type, duration, complexity) have been examined and sometimes linked with predisposition to take preventive actions, knowing these parameters is far from understanding the complex interplay of factors that enter prevention decisions. Developing hypotheses concerning potential sources of motivation for preventive behavior, testing hypotheses, and integrating the findings in an explanative/predictive model or framework demands considerable investigative effort. While a number of different models have been proposed, the one selected for presentation in this chapter is the Health Belief Model.[6] This model has had the most empirical support from studies conducted to date. The evolution and dimensions of the model will be discussed and research supportive of the model presented.

## TABLE 3-1   EXAMPLES OF PREVENTIVE MEASURES

| Disease or Condition | Before Disease or Condition Occurs: Measures of Primary Prevention | After Disease or Condition Occurs: Measures of Secondary and Tertiary Prevention |
|---|---|---|
| Pertussis Diphtheria Tetanus Smallpox Poliomyelitis Measles German measles Mumps | For each of these diseases there are safe, specific, effective measures to produce artificial active immunity. | Early diagnosis and prompt treatment, isolation of contacts where indicated, prevention and/or treatment of complications, restorative and rehabilitative measures. |
| Rheumatic fever | Maintenance of good general health and nutrition, treatment of predisposing streptococcal infections, prophylactic treatment of contacts. | Early diagnosis and prompt treatment to prevent cardiovascular-renal complications, nutrition counseling, health teaching regarding activities of daily living, postoperative rehabilitation (if heart surgery performed). |
| Diabetes | Genetic counseling, weight control, control of stressful situations. | Early diagnosis, prompt treatment, instructions for administering insulin, nutrition counseling, prevention of infections, care of skin and toenails, self-management in altered lifestyle, emotional support for good mental hygiene. |

### The Health Belief Model

The Health Belief Model was developed in the early 1950s by Rosenstock,[7] Hochbaum,[8] and Kegeles[9] to provide a paradigm for exploring actions taken by individuals not currently suffering specific illness but offered measures to avoid illness. At that time, the major concern of the U.S. Public Health Service was the widespread failure of individuals to accept screening, early detection, and other preventive measures that were generally free or provided at nominal charge. The model was addressed to the very practical problem of predicting those individuals who would or would not use preventive measures.

The model is derived from psychologic theory. Salient dimensions of the model are goal setting based on perceived consequences, subjective estimates of

**TABLE 3-1  (continued)**

| Disease or Condition | Before Disease or Condition Occurs: Measures of Primary Prevention | After Disease or Condition Occurs: Measures of Secondary and Tertiary Prevention |
| --- | --- | --- |
| Hypertension | Nutrition education, control of stress, regular medical check-up, avoidance of smoking. | Early diagnosis and treatment, antihypertensive medication where indicated, self-management in altered lifestyle, adherence to prescribed dietary regimen, restorative and rehabilitative measures for late manifestations and complications. |
| Syphilis | Health education, family living and sex education, treatment of pregnant syphilitic women to prevent congenital syphilis, investigation of contacts with treatment where necessary. | Early diagnosis and prompt treatment, case finding and follow-up of patients and contacts, prevention and/or treatment of manifestations of late syphilis (e.g., blindness, heart disease, central nervous system involvement), rehabilitation of patient with late symptomatic syphilis. |

From Benson, E.R., & McDevitt, J.C. *Community health and nursing practice.* Englewood Cliffs, N.J., Prentice-Hall, 1976, with permission.

desired outcomes, and decision making under uncertainty. As a decision model, the health belief approach reflects social learning theory, Atkinson's views of risk-taking behavior and achievement motivation, and Edwards' behavioral decision theory.[10] This approach to predicting behavior is often referred to as "value expectancy" since the determinants of behavior include (1) the value placed on a particular outcome or goal by a given individual and (2) the individual's expectation that a particular action will produce the desired outcome.[11] Considering the centrality of individual decision making in preventive behavior and understanding the perceptual, motivational, and social factors behind such decisions are instrumental to successful professional intervention to promote preventive actions.

A major problem with psychologic explanations of behavior that emphasize decision-making processes is the lack of correspondence in many studies between attitudes/beliefs, intentions, and overt actions. One approach taken to resolve such discrepancies has been to study very specific actions to be performed at identified points in time.[12] The more specific the action focus, the more likely attitudes, beliefs, and intentions are to correspond with behavioral outcomes.

The Health Belief Model focuses on specific preventive behaviors for particular diseases. It is disease-specific and action-specific. The first problems on which the model was tested were programs for the prevention of tuberculosis, polio, and dental disease and for early detection of cervical cancer. These problems represent major health threats for which immunization, screening, or other preventive health measures are available. Results of early studies partially supported the predictive potential of the model and provided the impetus for continued testing.[13] The Health Belief Model as modified by Becker[14] is presented in Figure 3-1. Components of the model are divided into individual perceptions, modifying factors, and variables that affect the likelihood of initiating action. Individual perceptions directly affect predisposition to take action, while demographic, sociopsychologic, and structural variables act as modifying factors that only indirectly affect action tendencies.

## Individual Perceptions

*Perceived Susceptibility.* An individual's own estimated subjective probability that he or she will encounter a specific health problem constitutes perceived susceptibility.[15] Any individual falls somewhere on a continuum from high to low in estimating personal degree of risk for developing a specific illness. A person may deny any possibility of contracting a particular illness, accept a slight statistical possibility but consider the chances slight, or be strongly convinced that at some point in his or her lifetime the illness will occur. A number of studies have clearly supported the importance of perceived susceptibility as a predictor of preventive behavior.[16] Relatively high subjective estimates of susceptibility have been shown to be correlated with obtaining screening for cervical cancer, breast cancer, cardiovascular disorders, tuberculosis, Tay-Sachs disease, and dental problems. In addition, obtaining immunizations and acceptance of accident prevention measures have also been shown to be correlated with perceived susceptibility.[17]

Hochbaum[18] conducted one of the earliest studies on the role of perceived susceptibility in preventive behavior. He studied 1200 adults in an attempt to determine the key factors underlying the decision to obtain an x-ray for the detection of tuberculosis. In the group with high perceived susceptibility, 82 percent had obtained a chest x-ray during a specified period of time prior to the interviews, while only 21 percent of the individuals with low perceived susceptibility had obtained an x-ray.

Because of the limitations of retrospective studies, Kegeles[19] conducted a prospective study in which beliefs concerning susceptibility to dental disease were measured initially and use of preventive dental services was determined at a later time. He found that perception of susceptibility was correlated with subsequent number of dental visits. Fifty-eight percent of those believing themselves highly susceptible to dental disease made visits, while only 42 percent of those with low perceived susceptibility made such visits. Haefner and Kirscht[20] conducted an experimental study in which attempts were made to increase readiness to engage in preventive behaviors among the study population through communications about specific health problems. The messages were intended to increase beliefs

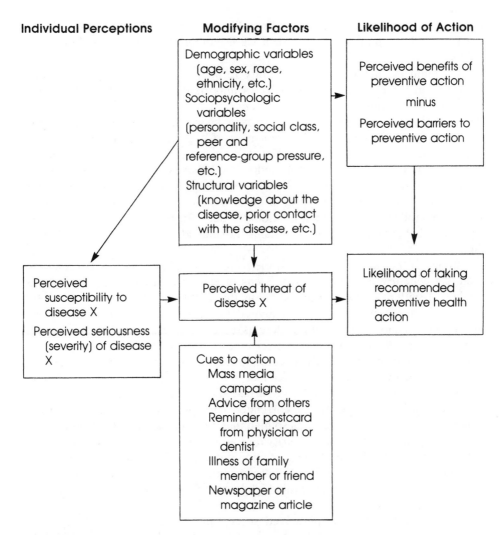

**Individual Perceptions**     **Modifying Factors**     **Likelihood of Action**

**FIGURE 3-1.** The Health Belief Model. *(From Becker, M.H., Haefner, D.P., Kasl, S.V., et al. Selected psychosocial models and correlates of individual health-related behaviors. Medical Care, 1977, 15, 27–46, with permission.)*

in susceptibility, seriousness, and benefits of preventive behavior. Manipulation of the three variables resulted in a significantly greater number of physician visits for routine check-ups in the experimental group, as opposed to the control group following the intervention.

Extending the concept of susceptibility to include resusceptibility to illness previously experienced, Elling *et al.*[21] found that mothers' beliefs in the probability of their children contracting rheumatic fever a second time correlated highly with prophylactic administration of penicillin and keeping clinic appointments. Becker *et al.*[22] found that mothers who believed that their children were highly susceptible to the recurrence of otitis media were more likely to give medication appropriately and keep follow-up appointments than were mothers who did not exhibit such beliefs.

In summary, perceived susceptibility to acute or chronic illness has been supported in the research literature as an important determinant of preventive behavior. In addition, augmenting perceived susceptibility as an experimental variable has resulted in significant increases in the incidence of preventive actions. *Perceived Seriousness.* Perceived seriousness of a given health problem can be judged either by the degree of emotional arousal created by the thought of the disease or by the difficulties that an individual believes a given health condition would create for him. Perceived seriousness may include the broad implications of the illness for work, family life, or social relationships and commitments. A number of studies have shown a relationship between perceived seriousness and preventive behaviors, while a few studies have failed to support such a relationship.[23]

In one of the supporting studies, the relationship of perceived seriousness to obtaining genetic screening for Tay-Sachs disease was studied. The study was conducted within a Jewish population in the Baltimore–Washington area. Indivduals from the population were invited to participate in screening, and all adults who appeared for screening were asked to complete a brief questionnaire. Approximately 500 participants were selected at random for study, and questionnaires were sent to a randomly selected group of 500 nonparticipants. Severity was measured by the reported impact of learning of being a carrier on family planning in the future. Interestingly, participation in the screening program was negatively rather than positively correlated with perceived seriousness. It appeared that perceived severity was so high that it became an inhibiting rather than a facilitating factor for action. Severity appeared to produce overwhelming threat and subsequent avoidance of the screening program.[24] This finding is consistent with other studies that have shown that very low levels of perceived seriousness are not sufficiently motivating, while high levels of perceived seriousness thwart constructive actions.[25]

According to Becker,[26] perceived susceptibility and perceived seriousness combine to determine the total perceived threat of an illness to a specific individual. Theoretically, the extent of threat represents the negative valence of the illness and predisposition for avoidance. A number of studies have explored the impact of these factors in combination. Fink *et al.*[27] found that perception of personal susceptibility to breast cancer and belief in the serious nature of the disease determined participation versus nonparticipation in a cancer-screening program for detection of breast abnormalities. Tash *et al.*[28] in exploring the relationship between attitudes and use of preventive dental visits found a significant negative relationship between perceived susceptibility to dental problems and dental visits and a significant positive correlation between perceived seriousness of dental disease and visits. The negative relationship was explained as reflecting the low level of perceived susceptibility to dental disease as a result of frequent preventive visits. While initial beliefs in susceptibility may have been high, repeated visits decreased such beliefs because appropriate preventive measures had been taken.

While both perceived susceptibility and perceived seriousness have received some support from completed research for their role in motivating preventive behavior, susceptibility has been most frequently supported as a motivational factor. Evidence for the role of perceived seriousness in motivating preventive behavior is less clear. In some studies perceived seriousness has been positively related; in others, negatively related; and in still other studies, no relationship has been evident at all. Further research is needed to clarify the contribution of perceived seriousness to motivation to engage in specific preventive behaviors.

### Modifying Factors
Modifying factors proposed in the Health Belief Model as affecting predisposition to take preventive action include a variety of demographic, sociopsychologic, and structural factors. However, they have had little specific testing in research based on the model.

*Demographic Factors.* While some demographic factors, such as sex, age, income, and education, have been clearly shown to be correlated with use of health services, their relationship to the use of preventive services in the absence of symptoms is much less clear. Sex is the demographic variable most predictive of preventive behaviors, and women exhibit a predisposition to engage in those behaviors more frequently than men. Education as a determining factor is supported by some studies in which the level of formal education correlated positively with the frequency of preventive actions. In other studies, years of formal education does not emerge as a significant predictor variable. Race and ethnicity appear to be factors in use of preventive services only when they are associated with socioeconomic level. Socioeconomic status appears to exert an effect only when significant cost or time is required to carry out preventive actions. Further exploration of demographic variables can yield information about users of preventive services and identify low-use populations for special motivational or programmatic efforts. However, such information provides little assistance to health professionals in structuring meaningful interventions to increase the incidence of health-protecting actions.

*Sociopsychologic Variables.* Social pressure or social influence appear to play a role in stimulating appropriate health actions even when low levels of individual motivation exist. Reference groups can affect health behavior by changing attitudes and beliefs or by forcing conformity with group behavior norms. Bond[29] found that women involved in discussion groups regarding techniques for early detection of breast cancer (breast self-examination) were more likely to report continued use of early detection measures than women who were taught breast self-examination in lecture sessions with little opportunity for peer interaction. It appeared that group support and pressure provided motivation to adopt the new health practice.

In another study, Lambert[30] noted the importance of support and encouragement from family members and friends in use of dental clinics offered by public health personnel within the community. Endorsement of dental services by significant others and "word of mouth" advertising affected incidence of use by individuals of differing age, ethnicity, and socioeconomic background.

The importance of normative beliefs (expectations of significant others) concerning health-related behaviors has been further supported by the work of Ajzen and Fishbein.[31,32] Normative beliefs are defined as the perceived behavioral expectations of others and motivation to comply with those expectations.[33] In predicting intentions to participate in an influenza immunization program, normative beliefs (expectations of others) emerged as a meaningful variable. However, it is important to note that the impact of expectations of significant others was weak compared to the effects of beliefs about possible outcomes or consequences of the target behaviors.

In studying the incidence of polio vaccinations among children, Gray *et al.*[34] found that expectations of friends were powerful sources of motivation for parents to obtain immunizations for their children. Parents appeared to seek polio vaccination for their children not only to prevent the occurrence of disease but also to fulfill the expectations of friends and family members concerning what "good parents should do." Meeting the behavioral norms of important reference groups appeared to play a significant role in this study in promoting use of preventive measures.

*Structural Variables.* Two such variables presumed by the model to influence preventive behavior include knowledge about the target disease and prior contact with it. Few studies address these variables. In one study, Heinzelmann[35] found that continuation of penicillin prophylaxis among college students was directly related to the history of past bouts of rheumatic fever and expectations of recurrence. Becker[36] found higher compliance rates with the treatment regimen for otitis media when mothers reported that their child was often ill and that illness was a major threat to their child. Becker *et al.*[37] also found that the number of asthma attacks that children had experienced previously affected mothers' compliance with a medical regimen for control of asthmatic symptoms. Further research is needed to clarify the extent to which knowledge about a disease or previous experience with it contribute to motivation for preventive actions.

*Cues to Action.* Cues, while proposed as affecting the incidence of health behavior by triggering appropriate overt actions, have not been systematically studied. This may be due to the transient nature of cues and the difficulties of retrospectively recalling stimuli that initiated specific behaviors.[38] The intensity of cues needed to trigger preventive actions given a certain level of readiness to engage in such activities is unknown. The general assumption is made that the higher the level of readiness to act, the lower the intensity of the cue needed to trigger behavior. In other words, a negative relationship is postulated between intensity of cue and level of readiness to engage in preventive actions. Cues can be either internal or external. Examples of internal cues include uncomfortable symptoms, feelings of fatigue, or recall of the condition of affected individuals to whom the individual is close. External cues include, for example, mass media, advice from others, posters, billboards, newspaper or magazine articles, or a reminder postcard from health professionals who have previously provided services. While the need for cues to initiate behavior is logical in light of what is known about operant conditioning, the role of cues in triggering preventive health actions is not well defined. There is a need for further research that addresses the relationship between cue configurations, cue intensity, cue-use patterns, and health-related behaviors.

### Likelihood of Action

Two additional factors identified in the model as affecting the probability of action are perceived benefits and perceived barriers. In the model, it is proposed that benefits minus barriers determine the likelihood of taking recommended preventive health actions.[39] At least six studies have shown a significant positive relationship between perceived benefits and preventive behavior, while in a smaller number of studies a significant positive relationship has not been shown. In several studies where an attempt was made to measure the effect of perceived barriers on preventive actions, the majority showed a significant relationship, with greater barriers resulting in fewer preventive actions.[40]

*Perceived Benefits.* Beliefs about the effectiveness of recommended preventive actions appear to be important determinants of health-protecting behavior. Kegeles,[41] in a field experiment to identify factors associated with participation in a screening program for cervical cancer, found that women who obtained a pap smear were more likely than nonparticipants to believe that the test could detect cervical cancer, that such a test could reveal cancer prior to the occurrence of symptoms, and that early detection would lead to a more favorable prognosis. Other studies also support the relationship between beliefs in benefits and use of cancer-screening programs. Haefner and Kirscht[42] found a higher incidence of physician visits for routine check-ups to detect cancer and other health problems by a group exposed to a communication that addressed the benefits of early detection than by a group not exposed to the communication. In another study, belief that accidents could be prevented among sugarcane field workers by use of a protective glove resulted in greater frequency of use of the glove as a safety device.[43]

Battistella[44] reported that "perceived chances of recovery" (that is, perceived benefits from medical care) were inversely related to the length of delay before seeking care. The lower the perceived chances of recovery, the longer individuals waited before seeking medical attention. In a study of follow-up care of school-age children referred for a medical problem, Gabrielson *et al.*[45] found that belief in the effectiveness or potential success of follow-up care was positively associated with the frequency with which parents complied with follow-up recommendations.

*Perceived Barriers.* The barriers to obtaining preventive care can take many forms and be perceived or real. Cost, inconvenience, unpleasantness, or extent of life change required are only a few of the possible blocks to engaging in preventive behaviors. Perceptions of inability to follow through with health recommendations may be an imagined or real barrier to taking preventive actions. Fear of pain or discomfort from dental procedures and anticipated costs for such care have been shown to be negatively related to the frequency of obtaining preventive dental services.[46,47] A study by Antonovsky and Kats[48] indicated that the expense of preventive dental care was a significant factor in frequency of use.

Barriers to action have seldom been studied in a systematic fashion in research based on the Health Beliefs Model. With emphasis on lifestyle change for the prevention of chronic disease, it appears critical to examine the extent to which duration, complexity, and degree of change required in health practices serve as barriers to adoption of specific prevention measures. Research efforts must not only be directed toward the identification of barriers but also toward identifying effective strategies for decreasing such blocks to action. Interactions between level of readiness, cue intensity, and barriers must be studied systematically to determine quantitative and qualitative relationships.

## PROPOSED MODIFICATIONS OF THE HEALTH BELIEF MODEL

Modifications of the Health Belief Model have been proposed by Pender[49] and will be addressed in this section. The modified model is presented in Figure 3-2. Suggested changes are based on research to date concerning the determinants of preventive behavior. However, the integrated model needs empirical testing before reliable conclusions can be drawn concerning the contribution of each addition to the model's prediction potential.

For greater clarity concerning the point of maximum impact of various factors within the model on preventive behavior, individual perceptions and modifying factors have been placed within the decision-making phase, while perceived barriers and behavioral cues have been placed within the action phase. It is the belief of the author that perceived benefits and perceived value of early detection are important considerations early in the decision-making phase, rather than serving as a balancing factor with perceived barriers to affect the likelihood of taking action. Consumers increasingly demand accurate information about the efficacy of medical treatments and preventive measures. Consideration of such information appears to be an important part of the decision-making phase regarding specific preventive actions to undertake. Clients must be convinced of the personal benefits of preventive measures before adopting and/or integrating health-protecting behaviors as part of a continuing lifestyle. While barriers are placed as a primary consideration in the action phase, consideration of potential barriers and plans to minimize their impact should be an integral part of decision-making activities.

### Individual Perceptions
Two variables have been added to the model as individual perceptions that appear to affect predisposition to engage in preventive behavior: the importance of health and perceived control. Each of these variables will be described and a rationale presented for its inclusion within the Health Belief Model.

*Importance of Health.* While the importance (salience) of health or health concern has been identified as a factor to be considered in a number of studies exploring determinants of preventive behavior, the variable has not been explicitly included

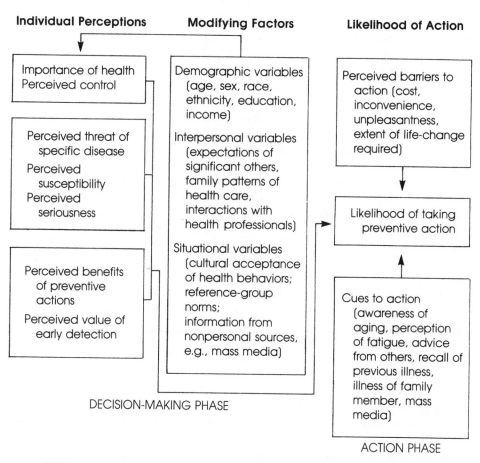

**Individual Perceptions**  **Modifying Factors**  **Likelihood of Action**

Importance of health
Perceived control

Perceived threat of
specific disease
Perceived
susceptibility
Perceived
seriousness

Perceived benefits
of preventive
actions
Perceived value of
early detection

Demographic variables
(age, sex, race,
ethnicity, education,
income)

Interpersonal variables
(expectations of
significant others,
family patterns of
health care,
interactions with
health professionals)

Situational variables
(cultural acceptance
of health behaviors;
reference-group
norms;
information from
nonpersonal sources,
e.g., mass media)

Perceived barriers to
action (cost,
inconvenience,
unpleasantness,
extent of life-change
required)

Likelihood of taking
preventive action

Cues to action
(awareness of
aging, perception
of fatigue, advice
from others, recall of
previous illness,
illness of family
member, mass
media)

DECISION-MAKING PHASE

ACTION PHASE

**FIGURE 3-2.** Pender's Proposed modifications of the Health Belief Model.

in recent formulations of the Health Belief Model. Several studies indicate that inclusion of the variables "importance of health" might strengthen the potential of the model for explaining health behaviors. Becker, Drachman, and Kirscht,[50] in their study of mothers' compliance with medical regimen for children being treated for pharyngitis or otitis media, found that measures of general health concern consistently predicted giving-medication (penicillin) and keeping-appointments. General health concern was measured by (1) agreement with the statement, "I worry a lot about my children's health," (2) whether parents took their child to the doctor right away for a set of designated symptoms, (3) whether they gave their children vitamins and special foods to keep them well, and (4) ownership of a fever thermometer.

Antonovsky and Kats[51] included "salience of dental health" as a possible predisposing motivational factor in a study of the determinants of preventive dental visits. They found that individuals who believed that it was worth spending considerable out-of-pocket money on preventive dental measures were more likely to make prevention-oriented dental visits than those who placed less monetary value on dental care. Suchman,[52] in looking at preventive behavior, also found that worry or concern about health was positively correlated with taking actions to protect health.

Two other studies lend support to the "importance of health" in motivating preventive behavior. Radius et al.,[53] in studying adolescent perspectives on health and illness, analyzed interviews with 112 white youths between the ages of 12 and 18 years in Washtenaw County, Michigan. Health emerged as a major concern of adolescents, with the findings consistent across all sex and age groups. Of the males, 45.4 percent stated that they worried about their health, while 43.5 percent of the females had similar concerns. Of those admitting worry about health, at least 63 percent stated that they worried somewhat or a lot about health. Despite the fact that more than 50 percent of males and females were not worried about their health, it is encouraging that concern was as high as reported during the adolescent years, when individuals are least likely to experience overt threats to well-being.

Kirscht et al.[54] in studying public response to various types of written communications to participate in a multiphasic screening program found that a positive communication emphasizing the importance of health was more effective in promoting participation than a neutral message or one containing threat. The group receiving the positive health message was superior in the number of appointments made and kept for screening services.

In the above studies, concern about protecting health emerged as an important predictor of preventive behavior. While contradictory findings have been reported,[55] a number of studies appear to support "importance of health" as a meaningful variable in determining health-protection actions. This may well reflect the increasing general orientation of the American public toward prevention rather than primarily toward the treatment of disease.

*Perceived Control.* The public's beliefs about the relationship between individual behavior and health have received increased attention as health promotion and prevention of chronic illness have emerged as national health initiatives. It has been stated that our present health care system creates dependency and little initiative among its users for assuming active responsibility for personal health.

The concept of "locus of control" from social learning theory[56,57] offers an explanation for perceived control of health. One of the most significant areas of exploration within the domain of locus of control in recent years has been "health locus of control."[58] Investigations within this area have focused on the relationship between beliefs about internal–external control and physical health and well-being. The importance of this field of study was noted by Rosenstock[59] at a 1975 National Heart and Lung Institute Working Conference on Health Behavior. In discussing individual responsibility for health maintenance, Rosenstock raised the question as to whether perceptions of internal-external control of health could be changed in adults, and if so, how such changes might be accomplished. He commented:

*Ongoing research suggests that external control, alienation or powerlessness are associated with higher rates of morbidity, lower rates of compliance, lower health motivation, reduced tendency to seek behaviorally relevant information, reduced utilization of health care services, and reduced ability to control weight, smoking and use of alcohol and other drugs.[60]*

Whether perceptions of control are mediated by ethnic background, socioeconomic status, or patterns of child-rearing has not yet been determined, but it appears that further exploration of "control phenomenon" is critical to understanding predisposition to engage in preventive behavior.

A number of studies have been reported that support the importance of perceived control in predicting the occurrence of preventive behaviors. Kirscht,[61] in exploring the relationships between locus of control, perceived susceptibility to illness, and perceived benefits of preventive actions found that those who were internally controlled viewed themselves as less susceptible to illness and identified preventive measures as more efficacious than did externally controlled individuals. Age was significantly correlated with perceptions of control, with younger individuals believing that they exerted more control over health than did older persons. Women believed that they had more control over health than did men.

In studies of smoking behavior, James, Woodruff, and Werner[62] found that nonsmokers were more likely to be internal in locus of control orientation than were smokers. In addition, they found that persons who believed in the health-damaging effects of smoking and had quit were more internal than were individuals who believed that smoking was hazardous to health but did not quit. In another study, Platt[63] found internally controlled individuals able to change smoking behavior to a greater extent than were externally controlled individuals. Williams[64] found a greater incidence of smoking behavior among external-control ninth grade adolescents than among those who were internally controlled. In a study of 35 participants in a smoking cessation program, health locus of control and health values emerged as important variables in predicting smoking reduction.[65] Individuals who held internally oriented health locus of control beliefs and who valued health highly were more successful in achieving changes in their smoking behavior than were externally controlled individuals.

While the above studies support the importance of locus of control as a determinant of smoking behavior, some studies have failed to show this association.[66] Further research is needed to clarify the relationship between smoking behavior and locus of control, since smoking represents one of the most prevalent risk factors for cancer and cardiovascular disorders among adolescents and adults.

Locus of control has also been explored in relation to weight and weight loss. O'Bryan[67] found overweight women to be more externally controlled than women near normal weight. Balch and Ross[68] in using a self-control weight-reduction program found significant correlations between internality and completion of the program and internality and success of the program (achievement of weight loss higher than the median). These findings would suggest not only that locus of control may be an important factor in predicting health behaviors but that it should also be taken into consideration in tailoring preventive measures to individual orientations. The importance of health locus of control has also been supported in studies of use of birth control, seat-belt use, preventive dental care, and the likelihood of obtaining immunizations for influenza.

In further exploring the effects of perceived control on health behaviors, caution must be taken to avoid confusing motivation for control and expectancy of control. Kirscht[69] differentiated between these "control" phenomenon. Studies of the two dimensions of control may yield interesting findings concerning their singular or combined effects on the frequency of preventive actions.

## Modifying Factors

Specific interpersonal variables suggested for inclusion in the model as modifying factors are family patterns of health care and interactions with health professionals. These variables appear to act indirectly on preventive health behaviors by encouraging or discouraging individuals to act according to their individual perceptions concerning the value of preventive behaviors.

*Family Patterns of Health Care.* Rosenstock,[70] in the Working Conference on Health Behavior sponsored by the Heart and Lung Institute, emphasized the importance of socialization of the child in the nuclear family in determining lifelong health care patterns. Children learn through their own health care experiences and through the health care patterns observed in significant adults. Tyroler *et al.*,[71] in studying families' participation in an oral polio vaccine program, found similarity of health behavior within families in both upper and lower socioeconomic groups. Similarity between preventive behavior of mother and child was high, between wife and husband intermediate, and between father and child relatively low. High maternal influence on preventive behavior has also been reported by Steele and McBroom,[72] who found that the level of education of the dominant female within the household correlated highly with the degree of preventive behavior.

Becker and Green[73] have reviewed family-level influences on health behaviors. It is apparent that for children, parents (particularly mothers) exert considerable influence on use of preventive measures. It also appears that when families are experiencing internal problems in communication and relationships, they are less likely to adopt preventive behaviors that require major changes in health practices and lifestyle. Antonovsky and Kats[74] found that individuals who talked with family and friends about dental problems were more likely to obtain preventive dental visits than those who reported no such interactions.

It is possible that the extent of impact of family or significant others on health behaviors interacts with locus of control. Saltzer[75] identified 116 undergraduate university students, ranging in age from 17 to 51 years, as either internal or external locus of control, based on a Weight Locus of Control Scale developed for purposes of the study. Individuals who were internals and highly valued health, physical appearance, or both were more likely to be influenced by their personal beliefs about the consequences of weight loss than by the expectations of significant others. Individuals who were externals and highly valued health and personal appearance or both were more likely to be influenced by the expectations of others than by beliefs about outcomes in their intentions to lose weight. These findings would imply that individuals who are internally oriented may even in early years be less likely to be influenced by family patterns of health care than externally controlled individuals who may respond more readily to the expectations of others and role modeling in developing preventive health behaviors.

### Interactions with Health Professionals

The nature of interactions with health professionals has been shown in a number of studies to affect the incidence and consistency of health-protecting behaviors. For this reason, it is suggested as an interpersonal variable to be specifically included in the model.

Maiman et al.[76] studied the impact of interpersonal similarity between nurse and client and positive written appeals on learning self-care measures to prevent the occurrence of asthmatic attacks and decrease related emergency room visits. The condition of interpersonal similarity was created by selecting a nurse for the educational sessions that was also an asthmatic and comparing her impact on clients with that of nonasthmatic emergency room nurses. Results of the study indicated that whether the nurse who was an asthmatic did or did not overtly identify that point of interpersonal similarity to the client, her interventions were more effective than those of other nurses in lowering emergency room use. This effect occurred irrespective of whether positive written appeals concerning control of asthmatic attacks were given to clients. Perceived similarity between client and health professional may well have enhanced the effectiveness of educational sessions.

Perceptions of the level of expertise of health care professionals may also affect predispositions to engage in recommended preventive behaviors. At least two studies have shown that the greater the credibility of an information source, the more persuasive the motivational message. In contrast, when an information source was perceived as lacking expertise, persons not only reacted negatively against the recommended behavior but actively avoided the behavior advocated.[77,78]

A number of studies that address the impact of interaction with health professionals on health-related behavior have focused on compliance with medical regimens. While findings concerning compliance cannot be generalized to use of preventive measures, several studies will be cited to indicate the potential impact of "interactions with health professionals" on client behaviors.

In studying compliance behavior, Becker et al.[79] measured medical motivation (willingness to accept physician's advice), belief in diagnosis, and continuity of care. He found that belief and trust in the physician as well as a continuing relationship with the same physician facilitated mothers' compliance with a treatment regimen for pharyngitis and otitis media in their child. Charney et al.[80] found that mothers were more likely to adhere to medical regimens for their child if the child was examined by the regular family physician rather than a substitute or fellow physician. Francis et al.[81] in examining mothers' compliance with medical regimens for their children found that compliance was better if mothers were satisfied with their original contacts with the physician, that is, if they found the physician friendly, understanding, warm, and readily willing to share information about the child's diagnosis and aspects of medical treatment. Gouldner[82] noted that lack of compliance with medical care regimens was more likely if little interaction and discussion took place between client and care provider and if the rationale for treatment was not explained to the client. These findings support the importance of exploring various dimensions of the relationship between the client and the health care provider in terms of its impact on preventive behavior. It is possible that clients' perceptions of expertise, humanness, empathy, and care in interactions with health professionals as well as continuity of relationships will impact on the extent to which clients engage in preventive actions. Such findings would have major implications for the current health system where health care is often fragmented with a number of different health professionals providing services to the same clients.

## SUMMARY

Within this chapter, the Health Belief Model has been presented as an important paradigm for predicting and explaining the occurrence of health protecting (preventive) behaviors. In addition, suggestions for modifications in the model have been proposed by the author. While the suggestions for changes in the model are based on empirical research, testing of the modified model is imperative to determine the differential contribution of the various factors to accurate prediction of the occurrence of preventive behaviors. By and large, the Health Belief Model has been tested on preventive measures requiring single acts of compliance. More attention must be given to the adequacy of the model in predicting and explaining participation in lifelong monitoring activities (i.e., blood pressure checks, breast self-examination) and major lifestyle modifications for prevention of specific disorders (i.e., adoption of low-sodium diet for prevention of hypertension). Carefully planned prospective studies will provide greater insight into the applicability of the model to prevention of chronic disorders.

Both the Health Belief Model and the Modified Health Belief Model are based on the notion of "value expectancy." Decisions are made under conditions of uncertainty in order to avoid negatively valued outcomes or personal threat, e.g., illness, disability, nonproductivity, discomfort, and death. The Health Belief Model has a clearcut avoidance orientation and is disease specific. Rosenstock[83] has questioned the extent to which a preventive model with an avoidance orientation is adequate to explain positive health actions directed toward the achievement of higher levels of health, self-actualization and fulfillment. It is the premise of the author that while the Health Belief Model has predictive potential for preventive behavior, it is inadequate to explain behavior directed toward health promotion. Therefore, a model for health promotion will be presented in the next chapter.

## REFERENCES

1. Shamansky, S.L., & Clausen, C.L. Levels of prevention: Examination of the concept. *Nursing Outlook,* February 1980, *28,*104–108.
2. Archer, S.E., & Fleshman, R. *Community health nursing: Patterns and practice.* North Scituate, Mass.: Duxbury Press, 1975.
3. Harris, D.M., & Guten, S. Health-protective behavior: An exploratory study. *Journal of Health and Social Behavior,* 1979, *20,*17–29.
4. Robischon, P. Prevention and chronic illness. In Spradley, B.W. (Ed.), *Contemporary community health nursing.* Boston: Little, Brown, 1975, pp. 39–40.
5. Strauss, A.L. *Chronic illness and the quality of life.* St. Louis: Mosby, 1975, p. 133.
6. Becker, M.H. (Ed.) *The Health Belief Model and personal health behavior.* Thorofare, N.J.: Charles B. Slack, 1974.
7. Rosenstock, I.M. Why people use health services. *Milbank Memorial Fund Quarterly,* July 1966, *44,*94–127.
8. Hochbaum, G.M. Public participation in medical screening programs: A sociopsychological study. *Public Health Service Publication (No. 572).* Washington, D.C.: U.S. Government Printing Office, 1958.
9. Kegeles, S.S., Kirscht, J.P., Haefner, D.P., *et al.* Survey of beliefs about cancer detection and taking Papanicolaou tests. *Public Health Report,* September 1965, *80,*815–823.
10. Maiman, L.A., & Becker, M.H. The health belief model: Origins and correlates in psychological theory. In Becker, M.H. (Ed.), *The Health Belief Model and personal health behavior.* Thorofare, N.J.: Charles B. Slack, 1974, pp. 9–26.
11. *Ibid.,* p. 10.
12. Fishbein, M., & Ajzen, I. *Belief, attitude, intention and behavior: An introduction to theory and research.* Reading, Mass.: Addison-Wesley, 1975.
13. Rosenstock, I.M. Historical origins of the Health Belief Model. In Becker, M.H. (Ed.), *The Health Belief Model and personal health behavior.* Thorofare, N.J.: Charles B. Slack, 1974, pp. 1–8.
14. Becker, M.H., Haefner, D.P., Kasl, S.V., *et al.* Selected psychosocial models and correlates of individual health-related behaviors. *Medical Care,* May 1977, *15,*27–46.
15. Rosenstock, 1966, *op. cit.,* p. 104.
16. Becker, 1977, *op. cit.,* p. 35.
17. Becker, M.H., & Maiman, B.A. Sociobehavioral determinants of compliance with health and medical care recommendations. *Medical Care,* January 1975, *13,*10–24.
18. Hochbaum, G.M. Why people seek diagnostic x-rays. *Public Health Reports,* 1956, *71,*377.
19. Kegeles, S.S. Why people seek dental care: A test of a conceptual formulation. *Journal of Health and Human Behavior,* 1963, *4,*166 ff.
20. Haefner, D.P., & Kirscht, J.P. Motivational and behavioral effects of modifying health beliefs. *Public Health Reports,* 1970, *85,*478.
21. Elling, R., Whittemore, R., & Green, M. Patient participation in a pediatric program. *Journal of Health and Human Behavior,* 1960, *1,*183.
22. Becker, M.H., Drachman, R.H., & Kirscht, J.P. A new approach to explaining sick-role behavior in low income populations. *American Journal of Public Health,* 1974, *64,*205–216.
23. Becker, 1977, *op. cit.*
24. Becker, M.H., Kaback, M.M., Rosenstock, I.M., & Ruth, M.V. Some influences on program participation in a genetic screening program. *Journal of Community Health,* 1975, *1,*3.
25. Leventhal, H. Fear communications in the acceptance of preventive health practices. *Bulletin of the New York Academy of Medicine,* 1965, *41,*1144 ff.

26. Becker *et al.,* 1977, *op. cit.,* p. 30.

27. Fink, R., Shapiro, S., & Roester, R. Impact of efforts to increase participation in repetitive screenings for early breast cancer detection. *American Journal of Public Health,* 1972, *62,*328 ff.

28. Tash, R.H., O'Shea, R.M., & Cohen, L.K. Testing a preventive-symptomatic theory of dental health behavior. *American Journal of Public Health,* 1969, *59,*514.

29. Bond, B.W. *Group discussion-decision: An appraisal of its use in health education.* Minneapolis, Minn.: Department of Health, 1965.

30. Lambert, C., Jr. Interpersonal factors associated with the utilization of a public health dental clinic (Doctoral dissertation, Brandeis University, 1962). *Dissertation Abstracts International,* 1962, *23,*609–610. (University Microfilms No. 62-3071).

31. Ajzen, I., & Fishbein, M. The prediction of behavior from attitudinal and normative variables. *Journal of Experimental Social Psychology,* 1970, *6,*466–487.

32. Ajzen, I., & Fishbein, M. Attitudinal and normative variables as predictors of specific behaviors. *Journal of Personality and Social Psychology,* 1973, *27,*41–57.

33. Fishbein & Ajzen, 1975, *op. cit.,* p. 302.

34. Gray, R.M., Kesler, J.P., & Moody, P.M. The effects of social class and friends' expectations on oral polio vaccination participation. *American Journal of Public Health,* December 1966, *56,*2028–2032.

35. Heinzelman, F. Factors in prophylaxis behavior in treating rheumatic fever: An exploratory study. *Journal of Health and Human Behavior,* 1962, *2,*73.

36. Becker, M.H., Drachman, R.H., & Kirscht, J.P. Predicting mothers' compliance with pediatric medical regimens. *Journal of Pediatrics,* 1972, *81,*843–854.

37. Becker, M.H., Radius, S.M., Rosenstock, I.M., *et al.* Compliance with a medical regimen for asthma: A test of the Health Relief Model. *Public Health Reports,* May–June 1978, *93,*268–277.

38. Rosenstock, I.M. Historical origins of the health belief model. In Becker, M.H. (Ed.), *The Health Belief Model and personal health behavior.* Thorofare, N.J.: Charles B. Slack, 1974, p. 5.

39. *Ibid.,* p. 4.

40. Becker *et al.* 1977, *op. cit.,* p. 35.

41. Kegeles, S.S. A field experiment attempt to change beliefs and behavior of women in an urban ghetto. *Journal of Health and Social Behavior,* 1969, *10,*115.

42. Haefner & Kirscht, *op. cit.*

43. Suchman, E.A. Preventive health behavior: A model for research on community health campaigns. *Journal of Health and Social Behavior,* 1967, *8,*197.

44. Battistella, R.M. Factors associated with delay in the initiation of physicians' care among late adulthood persons. *American Journal of Public Health,* 1971, *61,*1348.

45. Gabrielson, I.W., Levin, L.S., & Ellison, M.D. Factors affecting school health follow-up. *American Journal of Public Health,* 1967, *57,*48.

46. Tash *et al., op. cit.*

47. Kegeles, *op. cit.*

48. Antonovsky, A., & Kats, R. The model dental patient: An empirical study of preventive health behavior. *Social Science and Medicine,* 1970, *4,*367.

49. Pender, N.J. A conceptual model for preventive health behavior. *Nursing Outlook,* June 1975, *23,*385–390.

50. Becker *et al., op. cit.*

51. Antonovsky & Kats, *op. cit.*

52. Suchman, *op. cit.*

53. Radius, S.M., Dillman, T.E., Becker, M.H., Rosenstock, I.M., & Horvath, W.J. Adolescent perspectives on health and illness. *Adolescence,* Summer 1980, *15,*375–383.

54. Kirscht, J.P., Haefner, D.P., & Eveland, J.D. Public response to various written appeals to participate in health screening. *Public Health Reports,* November–December 1975, *90,*539–543.
55. Gordis, L., Markowitz, M., & Lilienfeld, A.M. Why patients don't follow medical advice: A study of children on long-term antistreptococcal prophylaxis. *Journal of Pediatrics,* 1969, *75,*957.
56. Rotter, J.B. *Social learning and clinical psychology.* Englewood Cliffs, N.J.: Prentice-Hall, 1954.
57. Rotter, J.B. Some problems and misconceptions related to the construct of internal versus external control of reinforcement. *Journal of Consulting Clinical Psychology,* 1975, *43,*56–67.
58. Wallston, K.A., & Wallston, B.S. Health locus of control. *Health Education Monographs,* Spring 1978, *6*(2).
59. Rosenstock, I.M. Individual responsibility for health maintenance. In Weiss, S.M. (Ed.), *Proceedings of the National Heart and Lung Institute Working Conference on Health Behavior* (DHEW Pub. No. NIH 76-868). Bethesda, Md.: Public Health Service, 1975.
60. *Ibid.,* p. 135.
61. Kirscht, J.P. Perceptions of control and health beliefs. *Canadian Journal of Behavioral Science,* March 1972, *4,*225–237.
62. James, W.H., Woodruff, A.B., & Werner, W. Effect of internal and external control upon changes in smoking behavior. *Journal of Consulting Psychology,* 1965, *29,* 184–186.
63. Platt, E.S. Internal-external control and changes in expected utility as predictions of the change in cigarette smoking following role-playing. Paper presented at the Eastern Psychological Association, Philadelphia, 1969.
64. Williams, A.F. Personality and other characteristics associated with cigarette smoking among young teenagers. Unpublished research. Boston: The Medical Foundation, Inc., 1972.
65. Kaplan, G.D., & Cowles, A. Health locus of control and health value in the prediction of smoking reduction. *Health Education Monographs,* Spring 1978, *6,*129–137.
66. Best, J.A., & Steffy, R.A. Smoking modification tailored to subject characteristics. *Behavior Therapy,* 1971, *2,*177–191.
67. O'Bryan, G.G. The relationship between an individual's I-E orientation and information-seeking learning and use of weight control relevant information. (Doctoral dissertation, University of Nevada, 1972). *Dissertation Abstracts International,* 1972, *33B,*447B. (University Microfilms No. 72-19,541).
68. Balch, P., & Ross, A.W. Predicting success in weight reduction as a function of locus of control: A unidimensional and multidimensional approach. *Journal of Consulting Clinical Psychology,* 1975, *43,*119.
69. Kirscht, *op. cit.*
70. Rosenstock, 1975, *op. cit.,* p. 135.
71. Tyroler, H.A., Johnson, A.L., & Fulton, J.T. Patterns of preventive health behavior in populatons. *Journal of Health and Human Behavior,* Fall 1965, *6,*128–140.
72. Steele, J.L., & McBroom, W.H. Conceptual and empirical dimensions of health behavior. *Journal of Health and Social Behavior,* December 1972, *13,*382–392.
73. Becker, M.H., & Green, L.W. A family approach to compliance with medical treatment: A selected review of the literature. *International Journal of Health Education,* 1975, *18,*173.
74. Antonovsky & Kats, *op. cit.*
75. Saltzer, E.B. Locus of control and the intention to lose weight. *Health Education Monographs,* Spring 1978, *6,*118–128.

76. Maiman, L.A., Green, L.W., Gibson, G., & MacKenzie, E.J. Education for self-care by adult asthmatics. *JAMA,* May 4, 1979, *241,* 1919–1922.
77. Hewgill, M.A., & Miller, G.R. Source credibility and response to fear-arousing communications. *Speech Monographs,* June 1965, *32,*95–101.
78. Powell, E.A., & Miller, G.R. Social approval and disapproval cues in anxiety-arousing communications. *Speech Monographs,* June 1967, *34,*152–159.
79. Becker, Drachman, & Kirscht, *op. cit.*
80. Charney, E., Bynum, R., Eldredge, D., *et al.* How well do patients take oral penicillin? A collaborative study in private practice. *Pediatrics,* 1967, *40,*188.
81. Francis, V., Korsch, B.M., Morris, M.J. Gaps in doctor–patient communication: Patients' response to medical advice. *New England Journal of Medicine,* 1969, *280,*535.
82. Gouldner, A.W. The norm of reciprocity: A preliminary statement. *American Sociological Review,* 1960, *25,*161.
83. Rosenstock, I.M. Historical origins of the Health Belief Model. In Becker, M.H. (Ed.), *The Health Belief Model and personal health behavior.* Thorofare, N.J.: Charles B. Slack, 1974, pp. 6–8.

# CHAPTER 4
# A Proposed Model for Health-Promoting Behavior

In the previous chapter, two models that describe the determinants of health-protecting behavior were presented: the Health Belief Model and the Modified Health Belief Model. Health-protecting behaviors are directed toward *decreasing* the probability of encountering illness by active protection of the body against unnecessary stressors or detection of illness at an early stage. In contrast, health-promoting behaviors are directed toward *sustaining* or *increasing* the level of well-being, self-actualization, and fulfillment of a given individual or group. The Health Promotion Model proposed in this chapter is a complementary counterpart to models of health-protecting behavior. Health promotion focuses on movement of the individual toward a positively valenced state of increased health and well-being. Health threats (negatively valenced states) that are relevant to health-protecting behavior have little conceptual significance in health promotion. Growth, maturation, and expression of inherent and acquired human potential are some of the goals toward which health promotive behaviors are directed.

Components of the Health Promotion Model presented in Fig. 4-1 are based on a synthesis of the literature on health promotion and wellness to date. While the number of research studies focused on health is limited, the model presented in this chapter is offered as an organizing framework for research efforts and for health-promoting interventions. A major requirement of a theoretical model is that it is consistent with knowledge to date but remains flexible and subject to change as hypotheses derived from the model are empirically tested.

Health-promoting behaviors almost without exception are continuing activities that must be an integral part of an individual's lifestyle. Some examples of such behaviors are physical exercise, maintenance of optimum nutrition, and development of social support systems. Frequently, old patterns of behavior must be extinguished and new patterns of behavior learned.

Health-promoting behaviors are an expression of the actualizing tendency. The individual behaves in ways that maximize positive arousal, such as increased self-awareness, delight, enjoyment, and pleasure. As an example, jogging is almost always a health-promoting behavior for the child or young adult. Jogging is motivated by actualizing tendencies, the goals being increased physical endurance, greater psychomotor competence, enhanced physical energy, and improved per-

**65**

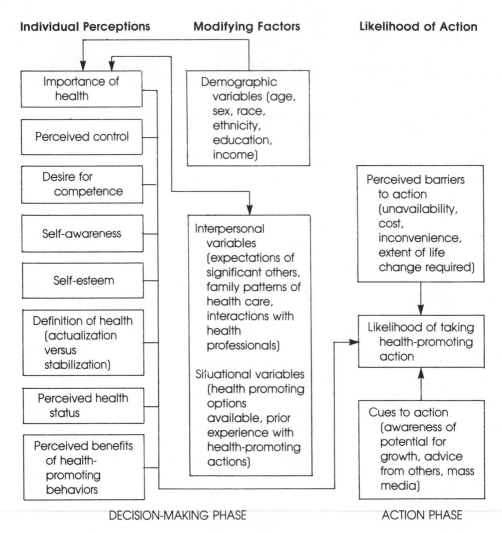

**Individual Perceptions**  **Modifying Factors**  **Likelihood of Action**

DECISION-MAKING PHASE  ACTION PHASE

**FIGURE 4-1.** Proposed Health Promotion Model.

sonal appearance. Seldom do children or adolescents run primarily to avoid the risk of cardiovascular problems in middle age, even though they may be aware that a relationship exists between exercise and the incidence of illness. While many middle-aged or elderly adults may begin jogging because they are ''at risk'' for cardiovascular disorders (avoidance motives), as the internal sensations and feelings engendered by running become more salient, approach tendencies often assume greater dominance in the motivation of behavior. Thus, jogging, which began as a preventive effort, serves both health-protecting and health-promoting functions.

Health-promoting behaviors represent man *acting* on his environment as he moves toward higher levels of health rather than *reacting* to external influences or threats posed by the environment. Man seeks to increase the complexity, intensity, variation, and meaningfulness of stimuli within his environment in order to increase positive tensions that promote change.[1]

## THE HEALTH PROMOTION MODEL

The Health Promotion Model is organized similarly to the Health Belief Model and the Modified Health Belief Model. That is, determinants of health-promoting behavior are categorized into individual perceptions, modifying factors, and variables affecting likelihood of action. Health-promoting behavior is also similar to health-protecting behavior because it consists of a decision-making phase and an action phase. Components of the proposed Health Promotion Model will be presented and discussed sequentially in this chapter.

### Individual Perceptions

Personal factors that facilitate or sustain health-promoting behavior have been identified within the model as (1) the importance of health, (2) perceived control, (3) desire for competence, (4) self-awareness, (5) self-esteem, (6) definition of health, (7) perceived health status, and (8) perceived benefits of health-promoting behaviors. Each factor is hypothesized to have motivational significance.

*The Importance of Health.* In a pilot study conducted by the author,[2] using the Health Values Scale developed by Wallston, Maides, and Wallston,[3] 78 percent of the 98 adults between 28 and 64 years of age completing the scale identified health as an important value or goal by placing it in first to fourth place. Health was ranked in fifth to tenth place by 22 percent of the respondents and appeared to be viewed by this group as an enabling state to be attained in order to facilitate the pursuit of higher-priority goals.

The impact of valuing health on the frequency of health-promoting behaviors received support from a study of 88 college students conducted by Wallston, Maides, and Wallston.[4] They found that individuals who held a high health value, that is, ranked health within the top four out of ten value positions, chose more health-related pamphlets to read when they were made available to them than did individuals with a low health value. The data support the notion that placing a high value on health results in information-seeking behavior directed toward becoming more knowledgeable on health and health-related topics.

*Perceived Control.* The effect of perceived personal control on health behavior has been supported in a number of studies. Williams[5] found that individuals who were internally controlled reported more frequent use of seat belts than individuals who were externally controlled. James, Woodruff, and Werner[6] found that nonsmokers were more likely to be internally controlled than smokers, although this finding has been questioned as a result of additional research.[7]

Wallston *et al.*[8] found that success in weight loss depended on structuring the weight-loss program according to each student's locus of control, either internal or external. Individuals who were externally controlled achieved greater weight loss than internally controlled persons in a group program relying on social pressures as motivation. Internals achieved greater weight loss than externally controlled individuals in a self-directed program. Perceived control of health status not only can make a difference in successful performance of health-promoting behaviors but in the effectiveness of differing strategies for inducing or facilitating continuing practice of such behaviors.

Desire for control of health versus perceived probability of control of health status need to be conceptually and empirically differentiated. Kirscht's[9] work attempted to clarify this distinction. Perceiving to be in control as well as having a strong desire for control should result in overt health-promoting behaviors. However, having a strong desire for control but little perceived probability of control may result in helplessness, frustration, and behavioral inhibition.

*Desire for Competence.* Competence represents the ability to interact or transact effectively with the environment.[10] Motivation toward competence and mastery of the internal and external environments reflects the inherent tendency of the central nervous system toward spontaneous activity.[11] The activities of young children are often directed toward environmental mastery. Active efforts are made by competence-seeking individuals to subordinate the forces of the physical and social environment to personal influence in order to promote continuing self-actualization.

Desire for competence and mastery emerge repeatedly between episodes of homeostatic crisis.[12] Satisfaction appears to lie in arousal, positive states of tension, and effective interactions with the environment, rather than in inactivity or passivity. As individuals become increasingly complex, the desire for competence can be differentiated into motives such as mastery, achievement, power, and autonomy.

The desire for competence in self-care appears to serve as a motivational force toward the acquisition of knowledge, resources, and skills that enhance health status. Self-determination in health has only recently received major attention from the public and health professionals. The public is slowly being resocialized to expect greater mastery of factors within the external and internal environments that impinge on personal health. Self-initiated activity rather than passivity represents a new emphasis in health care delivery.

*Self-awareness.* The need for greater self-awareness was repeatedly stressed in the literature of the 1970s. Sensitivity training, consciousness raising, values clarification, analysis of biologic rhythms, and biofeedback represent different approaches to increased self-awareness.

Glasser,[13] in describing the process of positive addiction to health-promoting behaviors, such as running and meditation, focused on the importance of self-awareness. Almost all runners whom he studied reported increased awareness of muscle movement, gliding or floating sensations, rhythmic breathing, and pleasurable experiences of motion. Meditators reported increased awareness of self, increased sensitivity to inner resources, and feelings of synchrony in body functions. A state was described by both groups in which there was decreased awareness of surroundings and increased awareness of the internal environment. This state was highly desirable and addictive in a positive way. The experience of increased self-awareness appeared to play an important role in motivating continued practice of health-promoting behavior.

The importance of self-awareness in effectively managing stress is supported by much of the literature on biofeedback.[14–16] Through increased awareness of autonomic processes, such as heart rate, blood pressure, and brain waves, these functions can be favorably modified toward healthier and more pleasant states. Levels of muscle tension can be markedly decreased and neuroendocrine functioning modified. The health-promoting potential of increased self-awareness has received considerable support in the literature.

*Self-esteem.* The inclusion of self-esteem as a motivational factor in health promotion is based on the assumption that individuals who regard themselves highly are more likely than persons with low self-esteem to set aside time for involvement in health-promoting behaviors. Belief in personal worth allows individuals to spend time on self-improvement, free from feelings of selfishness or guilt. In a study of 221 adolescents and young adults, Sonstroem[17] found that self-esteem was significantly correlated with level of perceived physical ability (0.05) and subsequently with actual physical performance. Interestingly, the measured level of physical fitness and self-esteem were not significantly correlated. Regardless of actual level of fitness, higher self-esteem resulted in better physical performance.

In a study of 42 individuals over 65 years of age participating in supervised physical training, Sidney and Shephard[18] found significant improvements in perceived body image (a component of self-esteem) in those individuals who trained hardest. They made greater movement toward closing the gap between perceived and desired body image than did individuals who trained less frequently and less intensively. Improved body image may well have served as reinforcement and motivation for continuing the training program.

Hanson and Nedde[19] conducted a study of sedentary, middle-aged women who participated in a long-term physical-training program. Self-concept was significantly improved after training. Barry *et al.*,[20] in a study of elderly individuals participating in a physical conditioning program, failed to find any changes in self-concept after training. While neither of the above studies addressed the relationship between initial self-concept and extent of participation in the respective programs, the results indicate the need for further exploration of the relationship between self-esteem and participation in health-promoting behaviors.

*Definition of Health.* The definition of health to which an individual subscribes is likely to influence the extent to which he engages in health behaviors. Defining health as adaptation or stability would predispose individuals toward health-protecting behaviors as opposed to health-promoting behaviors. Thus, behavior would be directed toward avoiding illness and disease, which represent deviations from normal. Defining health primarily as actualization should result in self-initiated activities directed toward attaining higher levels of health, self-direction, change, and growth. Since how goals are defined determines the means used to achieve them, differences in definitions of health would predict differing patterns of health-related behaviors.

The prevailing definition of health within the medical community has been "an absence of illness." As the public redefines health as a positive construct rather than a negative one, the nature of behaviors directed toward maintaining health should also change.

*Perceived Health Status.* Perceived health status appears to play a role in the frequency and intensity of health-promoting behaviors. Sidney and Shephard[21] in studying a group of elderly men and women engaged in physical training classes for 14 weeks found that individuals who exhibited more physical complaints or symptoms on the Cornell Medical Index Health Questionnaire had a lower frequency and lower intensity of participation in the exercise program than individuals reporting few symptoms on the index. All individuals had been examined by a physician prior to the program, and any overt clinical symptoms of illness had been ruled out. The prolonged experience of uncomfortable symptoms even in the absence of identifiable illness may represent a threat, induce fear and avoidance, and reduce personal capacity to engage in positive health behaviors. "Feeling good" may be a source of motivation for taking actions that increase personal health status.

Kaplan and Cowles[22] have suggested that an appropriate approach for smoking cessation may be to encourage initially other health-promoting behaviors, e.g., exercise, through which individuals experience rapid and noticeable changes in well-being. Experiences of increased well-being and improved health status can then be used to reinforce the value of good health and promote more extensive changes in lifestyle that individuals perceive as difficult.

In a study of 502 individuals between 45 and 69 years of age, Palmore and Luikart[23] analyzed the impact of perceived health, activity level, sociopsychologic, and socioeconomic variables on life satisfaction in middle age. They found that self-rated health correlated higher with life satisfaction than did any of the other variables included in the study, such as organizational or social activity, productivity, or career anchorage. Either individuals who are healthy perceive themselves as more satisfied, or self-perceptions of health result in behaviors directed toward achieving increased satisfaction.

*Benefits of Health-Promoting Behaviors.* In comparing 30 middle-aged males with low-frequency participation in a program of physical activity with 30 males with high-frequency participation, Brunner[24] found marked differences in perceived personal benefits. High-frequency participants ranked keeping fit physically as the most important benefit, while low-frequency participants ranked keeping physically fit fifth in importance. The low-frequency participants ranked the short-term benefit of relaxation at the end of the day as the major benefit of the physical-activity program.

When the 60 male participants in Brunner's study were queried as to whether the exercise program had instilled a desire for continued participation in physical activity, 47 percent of the high-frequency group responded affirmatively, while only 27 percent of the low-frequency group gave a similar response. The data suggest that the perception of long-term benefits rather than short-term benefits from health-promoting behavior may determine frequency of participation and predisposition to continue the target behaviors.

Sidney and Shephard,[25] in studying 42 elderly men and women participating in supervised physical training, found that individuals who participated more frequently and more intensively than others showed greater awareness of the importance of health and fitness as a benefit and greater appreciation of physical activity as an esthetic experience. The group participating most frequently and most intensively in the program also showed more favorable attitudes toward physical activity than did low-frequency participants. Perception of benefits from health-promoting behavior appeared to facilitate continued practice of newly acquired bebaviors. In addition, repetition of the behavior itself appeared to reinforce and strengthen beliefs about benefits.

*Summary.* In summary, individual perceptions that are proposed as affecting the decision-making phase of health-promoting behavior include importance of health, perceived control, desire for competence, self-awareness, self-esteem, definition of health, perceived health status, and perceived benefits. According to the literature cited, each factor appears to influence readiness to engage in health-promoting behaviors. Further research is needed to determine the extent to which each factor contributes to readiness in differing populations and groups.

## Modifying Factors

*Demographic Factors.* Characteristics such as age, sex, race, ethnicity, education, and income serve as modifying factors for health behavior. Table 4-1 illustrates the differences between men and women in perceived benefits from a planned exercise program. Both sexes believed that improved fitness was a major benefit of the program; only women identified psychologic well-being as an important outcome. In the same study, sex also affected level of perceived health. While 61 percent of the men considered their health above average, only 43 percent of the women rated their health as better than average.[26]

When the elderly individuals in the Sidney and Shephard study were compared to high school students[27] and middle-aged individuals[28] on the perceived value of exercise, the older subjects valued exercise significantly more as a means of maintaining physical fitness and as an esthetic experience than did the students or younger adults. A closer look at demographic variables and their impact on health-promoting behaviors will most likely result in the identification of critical differences between age, sex, or ethnic groups that must be considered in structuring appropriate health-promotion programs.

*Interpersonal Factors.* Interpersonal factors within the model that are proposed as modifying influences on health-promoting behaviors include expectations of sig-

TABLE 4-1   PERCEIVED MOTIVATION FOR JOINING A PHYSICAL-ACTIVITY
PROGRAM

| Perceived Motive | Men | | Women | |
| --- | --- | --- | --- | --- |
| | SCORE | RANK | SCORE | RANK |
| Physical health | | | | |
| Improve fitness or health | 18 | 1 | 37 | 1 |
| Body appearance, weight control | 5 | | 8 | |
| Medical advice | 0 | | 0 | |
| Psychologic well-being | | | | |
| Increased vigor, alertness | 0 | | 13 | 3 |
| Relief of tension, anxiety, | | | | |
| aggression, relaxation | 0 | | 0 | |
| Social | | | | |
| To socialize, make friends | 0 | | 2 | 6 |
| Pressure to join from others | 0 | | 3 | |
| Recreational/hedonistic | | | | |
| Fun, curiosity | 7 | 4 | 7 | 5 |
| Program and facilities | | | | |
| Exercise instruction by professional | 14 | 2 | 27 | 2 |
| Exercise testing | 5 | | 12 | |
| Altruism | | | | |
| To assist science | 9 | 3 | 12 | 4 |

From Sidney, K.H., and Shephard, R.J. Attitudes toward health and physical activity in the elderly.
Effects of a physical training program. *Medicine and Science in Sports,* 1976, *8,* 246–252, with
permission.

nificant others, family patterns of health care, and interactions with health professionals. The impact of these factors on health behaviors has been supported in
reported research.

In studying the responses of 239 men to a physical-exercise program, Heinzelmann[29] found that the expectations of significant others, in this case, the spouse,
were important in continuing participation in the program. Although few men
reported joining the program primarily as a result of pressure from their wives,
positive attitudes toward the program on the part of their wives was critical to
continuing participation and program adherence. Eighty percent of those men
with wives exhibiting positive attitudes toward the program had excellent or good
adherence patterns. Only 40 percent of men with wives exhibiting neutral or
negative attitudes had excellent or good adherence. In the same study, social
aspects were seldom mentioned as a reason for joining the program. However,

as supportive relationships formed among members of the group, they became important to each other. Consequently, at the end of the program 26 percent of the participants felt that group camaraderie was a critical factor in developing a sense of commitment to stay in the program.

In an interview study of 400 individuals conducted by the author to determine the effects of personal attitudes and expectations of others on selected health behaviors, exercising regularly was significantly influenced by both factors. Expectations of others had less effect than did personal attitudes on maintaining weight within recommended limits, openly expressing feelings, avoiding high-stress situations, and preparing for major life crises.[30]

Families provide the setting in which many patterns of behavior are learned. Family patterns of health care influence the emerging values and lifestyles of offsprings. Tyroler,[31] in studying health-protecting behavior (polio immunization), found a high correlation between the behavior of mothers and children, moderate correlation between the behavior of husbands and wives, and a very low correlation between the health behaviors of fathers and children. Steele and McBroom[32] found that the level of education of the dominant female within the household correlated highly with the frequency of health behavior. Mothers appear to function as important decision makers and role models for behavior in the area of health. The development of health-promoting lifestyles during childhood may avoid the more difficult task of changing stabilized and resistant health-damaging behaviors in adults.

Interactions with health professionals can serve as an important factor in the decision to engage in specific health behavior. In studying compliance behavior of mothers to pediatric regimens, Becker, Drachman, and Kirscht[33] found that willingness to accept a physician's advice was related to the mother's belief in the accuracy of the diagnosis, the continuity of care that she believed she had received previously, and the existence of a continuing relationship with the same physician. While these findings cannot be generalized to the practice of health-promoting behaviors, the results would suggest that certain dimensions of the client–health professional relationship play a critical role in the impact of the health care provider on the behaviors of the client.

Sidney and Shephard[34] found that an important reason for participation of the 42 adults that they studied in a physical-activity program was that the instruction and guidance of health professionals was readily available. In fact, competent direction of the program by health professionals ranked second in the reasons for participation. The results of this study reinforce the need for direction of health-promotion programs by competent and appropriately prepared health personnel.

*Situational Factors.* Important situational determinants of health-promoting behavior appear to include health-promoting options available and prior experience with health-promoting actions. The availability of a range of behavioral options increases the opportunity to make responsible choices after considering all the alternatives. For example, if low-cholesterol, low-calorie, or low-sodium meals are not available when one is dining out, there is little opportunity in that situation to behave in a healthful way. Also, if vending machines are stocked with foods high in refined sugars and low in nutritional value, options for healthy behavior by school-age children, industrial workers, and office personnel are limited. Individuals may wish to behave in ways that promote health, but situational constraints can prevent them from selecting healthful options.

Previous experience with health-promoting actions increases feelings of competence in following through with appropriate behavior. Some of the cognitive and psychomotor skills necessary to plan nutritious meals, maintain an exercise program, and deal with stress may have been learned previously from participation in similar activities. Feelings of comfort with required knowledge and skills will facilitate the implementation of health-promoting behaviors.

**Likelihood of Action**

The two factors proposed as being particularly salient during the action phase of health-promoting behavior are perceived barriers to action and cues that trigger activity. Barriers to health-promoting behavior may be imagined or real. Barriers are often individual perceptions about the unavailability, inconvenience, or difficulty of a particular health-promoting option. In a pilot interview study conducted by the author of 100 residents in a moderate-sized town in northern Illinois, individuals reported perceptions of both positive and negative consequences of specific health behaviors. For instance, while the respondents perceived that maintaining weight within recommended limits would improve health, enhance psychologic well-being, improve body image, and improve appearance, negative consequences were also identified, such as being deprived of favorite foods and experiencing negative changes in personality. The challenge for health professionals is in assisting individuals to overcome barriers to health-promoting behaviors. This can be accomplished by removing actual barriers, increasing the salience of positive consequences of desired behaviors, or by decreasing the frequency or intensity of negative consequences.

Cues that trigger health-promoting actions may be internal or external. Personal awareness of the potential for growth may serve as an important internal cue for behavior. It also appears that "feeling good" as a result of initial experiences with health activities can serve as a cue for continuing behavior. Conversations with others regarding their patterns of exercise, nutrition habits, rest and relaxation, management of stress, and interpersonal relationships can serve as external cues for health promotion. In addition, mass media can provide cues for action through programs about personal health, family health, and environmental concerns. The intensity of the cue needed to trigger action will depend on the level of readiness of the individual to engage in health-promoting activity.

**SUMMARY**

The Health Promotion Model presented in this chapter is offered as an organizing framework for research and practice. Literature supporting the inclusion of various factors in the model has been reported. While the model is divided into two phases, the decision-making phase and the action phase, movement of individuals back and forth between both phases in a cyclical fashion more accurately describes the health-promotion process.

Christiansen,[35] in a recent study of the determinants of health-promoting behavior, found that importance of health, perceived control, and perceived health status were significant predictors of health behaviors. While the predictive equation used for the study was not intended as a test of the Health Promotion Model, support for three components of the model resulted. The importance of demographic variables, e.g., education, occupation, household size, age, and religion in predicting health behaviors was also supported by the study. Additional research is needed to test the usefulness of the model in explaining and predicting health-promoting behaviors.

## REFERENCES

1. White, R.W. Motivation reconsidered: The concept of competence. *Psychological Review,* 1959, *66,*297–333.
2. Pender, N.J. Unpublished report of pilot study on health as a personal value, 1978.
3. Wallston, K.A., Maides, S., & Wallston, B.S. Health-related information seeking as a function of health-related locus of control and health value. *Journal of Research in Personality,* 1976, *10,*215–222.
4. *Ibid.*
5. Williams, A.F. Factors associated with seat belt use in families. *Journal of Safety Research,* 1972, *4,*133–138.
6. James, W.H., Woodruff, A.B., & Werner, W. Effect of internal and external control upon changes in smoking behavior. *Journal of Consulting Psychology,* 1965, *29,* 184–186.
7. Best, J.A., & Steffy, R.A. Smoking modification tailored to subject characteristics. *Behavior Therapy,* 1971, *2,*177–191.
8. Wallston, B.S., Wallston, K.A., Kaplan, G.D., & Maides, S.A. Development and validation of the health locus of control (HLC) scale. *Journal of Consulting Clinical Psychology,* 1976, *44,*580–585.
9. Kirscht, J.P. Perceptions of control and health beliefs. *Canadian Journal of Behavioral Science,* 1972, *4,*225–237.
10. White, *op. cit.,* p. 321.
11. *Ibid.,* p. 321.
12. *Ibid.,* p. 322.
13. Glasser, W. *Positive addiction.* New York: Harper & Row, 1976.
14. Girdano, D., & Everly, G. *Controlling stress and tension: A holistic approach.* Englewood Cliffs, N.J.: Prentice-Hall, 1979.
15. Brown, B.B. *Stress and the art of biofeedback.* New York: Harper & Row, 1977.
16. Fuller, G.D. *Biofeedback: Methods and procedures in clinical practice.* San Francisco, Calif.: Biofeedback Press, 1977.
17. Sonstroem, R.J. Physical estimation and attraction scales: Rationale and research. *Medicine and Science in Sports,* 1978, *10,*97–102.
18. Sidney, K.H., & Shephard, R.J. Attitudes toward health and physical activity in the elderly. Effects of a physical training program. *Medicine and Science in Sports,* 1976, *8,*246–252.

19.  Hanson, J.S., & Nedde, W.H. Long-term physical training effect in sedentary females. *Journal of Applied Physiology,* 1974, *37,*112–116.
20.  Barry, A.J., Steinmetz, J.R., Page, H.F., & Rodahl, K. The effects of physical conditioning in older subjects. II. Motor performance and cognitive function. *Journal of Gerontology,* 1966, *21,*192–199.
21.  Sidney & Shephard, *op. cit.*
22.  Kaplan, G.D., & Cowles, M.A. Health locus of control and health value in the prediction of smoking reduction. *Health Education Monographs,* Spring 1978, *6,* 129–137.
23.  Palmore, E., & Luikart, C. Health and social factors related to life satisfaction. *Journal of Health and Social Behavior,* March 1972, *13,*68–80.
24.  Brunner, B.C. Personality and motivational factors influencing adult participation in vigorous physical activity. *Research Quarterly,* 1969, *40,*464–469.
25.  Sidney & Shephard, *op. cit.,* pp. 250–252.
26.  *Ibid.,* pp. 247–249.
27.  Kenyon, G.S. Values held for physical activity by selected urban secondary school students in Canada, Australia, England and the United States. University of Wisconsin, U.S. Office of Education, Contract S-376, 1968.
28.  Massie, J.F., & Shephard R.J. Physiological and psychological effects of training. *Medicine and Science in Sports,* 1971, *3,*110–117.
29.  Heinzelmann, F., & Bagley, R.W. Response to physical activity programs and their effects on health behavior. *Public Health Reports,* 1970, *85,*905–911.
30.  Pender, N.J. Effects of personal attitudes and expectations of others on the frequency of health-promoting behaviors among adults. Unpublished manuscript.
31.  Tyroler, H.A., Johnson, A.L., & Fulton, J.T.: Patterns of preventive health behavior in populations. *Journal of Health and Human Behavior,* Fall 1965, *6,*128–140.
32.  Steele, J.L., & McBroom, W.H. Conceptual and empirical dimensions of health behavior. *Journal of Health and Social Behavior,* December 1972, *13,*382–392.
33.  Becker, M.H., Drachman, R.H., & Kirscht, J.P. Predicting mother's compliance with pediatric medical regimens. *Medical Care,* 1972, *81,*843–854.
34.  Sidney & Shephard, *op. cit.* N.B.
35.  Christiansen, K.E. The determinants of health promoting behavior. Doctoral dissertation, College of Nursing, Rush University, October 1981.

# Part II
# STRATEGIES FOR PREVENTION AND HEALTH PROMOTION: THE DECISION-MAKING PHASE

The purpose of this section is to assist nurses in identifying appropriate interventions to be used with clients during the decision-making phase of health behavior. Specific strategies described include health assessment, values clarification, health education for self-care, and the development of a health-protection/promotion plan. In Chapter 5 a comprehensive approach to health assessment is described. Nurses or students of nursing are encouraged to select those aspects of the assessment that are appropriate for their practice setting. In Chapter 6 numerous approaches to values clarification, an important part of health counseling, are presented. The importance of clients understanding personal values and priorities as a basis for health care planning cannot be stressed too strongly. Health education for self-care is discussed in Chapter 7, and a format for a health-protection/ promotion plan is presented in Chapter 8. As a whole, Part II offers practical and innovative ideas to nurses concerned with the delivery of prevention and health promotion services to individuals, families, and community groups.

# CHAPTER 5
# Health Assessment

The basis for competent professional care to protect and promote health is a thorough assessment of client health status. Such an assessment not only includes comprehensive evaluation of current health but appraisal of those health problems for which clients are at risk, review of present lifestyle, and identification of health and health-related beliefs. Comprehensive assessment provides information critical to (1) developing a plan of care that enhances personal health status, (2) decreasing the probability or severity of chronic disease, and (3) assisting clients in gaining increased control over their own health through competent self-care. Personal health habits, lifestyle, and the environment in which clients live have major impact on the quality of life experienced and on longevity.

The components of health assessment discussed in this chapter are the health history, physical examination, physical-fitness evaluation, nutritional assessment, risk appraisal, life-stress review, lifestyle and health habits assessment, and health beliefs review. Each component except the physical examination will be discussed in detail to provide a practical framework for the nurse to use in conducting assessment of individual clients. Where descriptive detail is limited, the reader will be referred to other sources for expanded explanations and illustrations of that aspect of the assessment process.

## CREATING A CLIMATE FOR COMPREHENSIVE ASSESSMENT

Obtaining a thorough health assessment is one of the most critical dimensions of preventive/promotive care. Without personal data on which to base nursing interventions, much valuable time can be lost for both client and nurse. Since a considerable amount of time is required for comprehensive assessment, this time should be distributed over several visits. During initial client contact, the nurse should provide the client with an overview of those areas of health to be assessed during subsequent appointments. This allows the client to be prepared better to provide specific information.

A number of contacts with the client and family may be required before the nurse–client relationship is developed to the point where the client feels comfortable in sharing information about personal health habits and lifestyle. The client must be convinced that the nurse will maintain the confidentiality of information and use it solely for the purpose of promoting the personal health and welfare of the client.

The home of the client provides a nonthreatening environment in which to conduct the health assessment. Even physical examination and physical-fitness evaluation generally conducted in the clinic or laboratory setting can be successfully completed in the home. Use of the home setting for assessment permits the nurse to observe the family and physical environment as well as the individual client.

An important feeling to create during the health assessment is one of unconditional acceptance of the client by the nurse. An empathetic, supportive, non-judgmental attitude on the part of the nurse creates an open climate for interaction. If the client believes that he or she is being personally judged by the nurse during the assessment process, the information provided by the client may be what is deemed socially acceptable rather than an accurate description of health status and personal health practices. Such distorted information thwarts meaningful health evaluation and planning and subsequent preventive/promotive care.

## HEALTH HISTORY

The assessment of current health status is obtained in part through a complete health history. In a study of 104 asymptomatic freshmen at Pennsylvania State University School of Medicine, the history was the best case-finding method for existing disease. It was the unit of the comprehensive health screen that was most cost effective. Anemias and infections uncovered by laboratory tests could have been detected by following up on clues in the health history.[1]

A suggested format for the adult health history is presented in Figure 5-1. This topical outline has been developed by the author based on review of the literature and personal experience in conducting health histories. The reader is also referred to guidelines for both adult and pediatric health histories in *A Guide to Physical Examination,* by Barbara Bates.[2] Learning to collect a meaningful history is an important part of the assessment of clients of all ages.

After completing the health history, a physical examination provides additional information concerning the client's physical and mental status. Since a comprehensive review of the physical examination procedure is beyond the scope of this book, the reader is referred to several excellent texts for explicit guidelines on the physical examination process.[3-6]

The history and physical examination provide the basis for early detection of any abnormalities that may exist. If further evaluation, laboratory tests or treatment are needed, clients may be referred to their private physician or appropriate clinic for further work-up and differential diagnosis. If the client has no existing source of medical care, the nurse can function as an advocate for the client in obtaining appropriate services.

Name of client _____

Address _____

Phone number _____

Private physician _____

Place of employment _____

Demographic data on client (age, occupation, marital status, education, religion, and race)
Source of referral, if any
Date of history
Source of history (client or relative)
Chief complaint, if any. Nature and duration of health problem, in client's own words
Present illness, if any. Chronologic narrative on current health problem: initial onset, setting in which it occurred, whether it recurred or was exacerbated, feelings and symptoms, treatments, response to treatments, meaning of illness to patient. Each symptom should be described by location, quality, severity, onset, duration, frequency, and factors that relieve or aggravate it. Relevant risk factors or family history should be included
Past medical history
     General state of health (client's perception)
     Childhood illnesses
     Immunizations (tetanus, pertussis, diphtheria, polio, measles, German measles, mumps, flu, pneumonia)
     Major adult illnesses
     Operations (report complications or sequelae)
     Injuries
     Emergency room visits
     Hospitalizations, not already described
     Obstetrical history (women)
     Current medications being used, including home remedies
     Use of coffee, alcohol, other drugs, and tobacco
     Allergies or drug sensitivities
Family and genetic history
     Age and health or cause of death of immediate family members, i.e., parents, siblings, spouse, children, and grandparents, if known
     Occurrence of chronic health conditions in members of immediate family, such as diabetes, tuberculosis, heart disease, high blood pressure, stroke, renal disease, cancer, arthritis, anemia, headaches, nervous disorders, mental illness, or symptoms like those of the patient
Psychosocial history
     Birth date and places of residence
     Family structure
     Educational history

**FIGURE 5-1.**   Adult health history (continued on next page).

Significant experiences during childhood and adolescence
Marital history
Current lifestyle
Home situation
Significant others and support systems
Religious and cultural beliefs that affect perceptions of health, illness, and
health care
Job history
Travel and military history
Use of leisure time
Financial status
Sources of satisfaction and distress
Typical day (physical activity, diet, sleep, recreation, and social activities)
*(Psychosocial factors are further assessed in the lifestyle and health-habits
assessment)*
Review of systems
General: usual weight, recent weight change, weakness, fatigue, fever, chills,
dizziness, sweating, anorexia
Skin: rashes, lumps, itching, dryness, color changes, changes in pigmented
areas or changes in hair and nails, bruising or bleeding
Head: headache, head injury, syncope
Eyes: vision, glasses or contact lenses, date of last eye examination, pain,
redness, excessive tearing, double vision, halos around lights, color blind-
ness, night blindness, photophobia
Ears: hearing, tinnitus, vertigo, earaches, infection, discharge, itching
Nose and sinuses: frequent colds, nasal stuffiness, chronic discharge, obstruc-
tion, hayfever, nosebleeds, sinus pain
Mouth and throat: condition of teeth and gums, last dental examination, sore
tongue, frequent sore throats, hoarseness, halatosis
Neck: lumps in neck, swollen glands, goiter, restricted motion
Breasts: self-examination, lumps, pain, nipple discharge, swelling, asymmetry,
dimpling, trauma
Respiratory: cough, excessive sputum, hemoptysis, wheezing, asthma, bron-
chitis, emphysema, tuberculosis, tuberculin test, last chest x-ray film
Cardiovascular: palpitations, chest pain, heart murmurs, dyspnea, orthopnea,
paroxysmal dyspnea, peripheral edema, cyanosis, hypertension, varicose
veins, intermittent claudication, thrombophlebitis
Gastrointestinal: trouble swallowing, heartburn, belching, bloating, food in-
tolerance, nausea, vomiting, hematemesis, indigestion, change in bowel
habits, rectal bleeding or black tarry stools, constipation, diarrhea, abdominal pain, hemorrhoids, jaundice, liver or gallbladder trouble, hepatitis
Urinary: frequency of urination, polyuria, nocturia, dysuria, hematuria, urgency,
hesitancy, incontinence, penile discharge (male), force of stream, passage
of stones or gravel
Genitoreproductive
Male: hernias, scrotal pain or masses, frequency of intercourse, impotence,
premature ejaculation, history of venereal disease

**FIGURE 5-1** (continued).

Female: age at onset of menstruation, regularity, frequency, length of periods, amount of bleeding, bleeding between periods or after intercourse, last menstrual period, dysmenorrhea, amenorrhea, age of menopause, postmenopausal difficulties (if any) last pap smear, frequency of intercourse, birth-control methods, itching or discharge, frigidity or orgasmic dysfunction.

Musculoskeletal: limitation of movement, trauma, pain, heat, redness, tenderness, swelling or crepitus of joints, backache, muscle pains or cramps

Neurologic: fainting, incoordination, seizures, paralysis, local weakness, numbness, tingling, tremors, pain, unusual reactions to heat and cold

Lymph nodes: enlargement, pain

Endocrine: goiter, exophthalmia, excessive sweating, excessive thirst, excessive hunger, polyuria, glycosuria, changes in secondary sex characteristics

Psychiatric: depression, hostility, apathy, phobias, nervousness

**FIGURE 5-1**   (continued).

The congruency between the findings of the nurse and client's perception of health status should be determined. Dubos[7] has indicated that all too often, although laboratory tests and physical-examination findings are normal, the client continues to insist that something is wrong. Both objective and subjective data from the health history and physical examination should be carefully reviewed, since human health transcends physiologic normalcy. A holistic approach to evaluation of health status also includes assessment of how individuals feel, how they view themselves, and their ability to achieve important goals. Comparable views of client health status on the part of the nurse and client provide a solid base for collaborative health planning.

**PHYSICAL-FITNESS EVALUATION**

Physical fitness is an important part of personal health status. Methods and procedures have been developed, primarily in physical education, that can be used by the nurse to assess the level of physical fitness of children and adults. As adults continue to stay active into their later years, the need to assess the physical fitness of elderly clients as a basis for recommending appropriate physical activity will increase.

From the physical examination and laboratory tests, the nurse should have available information about the client's height, weight, resting heart rate (beats per minute), resting blood pressure (mm Hg), cholesterol, triglycerides, glucose, and high-density lipoproteins. Additional information to be collected as a basis for fitness evaluation is identified in the *adult physical-fitness evaluation* format presented in Figure 5-2. The form is an adaptation of the approach to fitness evaluation developed by Leroy Getchell, director of physical fitness programs at the Human Performance Laboratory, Ball State University, Muncie, Indiana.[8] The importance of physical-fitness evaluation skills for the nurse is stressed by

Name of Client _____ Date _____

Sex _____ Age _____ Physician _____

Body Composition:

Height _____ inches _____ cm

Weight _____ lbs _____ kg
(1 lb = 0.453 kg; 1 kg = 2.205 lbs)

Percentage Body Fat _____ percent

Lean Body Weight _____ lbs _____ kg

Fat Weight _____ lbs _____ kg

Skinfolds (mm)

Triceps _____ _____ _____ _____
Average

Subscapular _____ _____ _____ _____
Average

Midaxillary _____ _____ _____ _____
Average

Suprailiac _____ _____ _____ _____
Average

Abdominal _____ _____ _____ _____
Average

Thigh _____ _____ _____ _____
Average

Girth Measurements (cm)

Chest _____ Thigh _____ Biceps
(flexed) _____

Abdomen _____ Calf _____ Biceps
(at waist) _____ (relaxed) _____

Hips _____ Ankle _____ Wrist _____
(1 cm = 0.394 in; 2.54 cm = 1 in)

Step Test:

Number of Minutes _____ Stepping Rate _____

Bench Height _____ inches

**FIGURE 5-2.** Adult physical fitness evaluation. (*Adapted from Getchell, L.*, Adult Physical Fitness Evaluation. *Muncie, Ind.: Human Performance Laboratory, Ball State University, 1981. With permission.*)

Recoveries (beats)

1–1½ min _____

2–2½ min _____

3–3½ min _____

Total _____
        (Recovery Index)

Field Tests:

Bent-Knee Situps _____        (1 min for females, 2 min for males)

Toe Touch Point in Inches _____

**FIGURE 5-2**  (continued).

Borgman[9] in her discussion of the nurse's role in structuring an exercise and health-maintenance program.

### Measuring Percentage of Body Fat

An important part of measuring body density and percentage of body fat is the accurate measurement of skinfolds. A skinfold caliper is used on the right side of the body. The skinfold (two layers of skin and subcutaneous fat, not muscle) should be grasped between the thumb and forefinger. The calipers should be applied approximately 1 cm below the skinfold grasped and at a depth equal to the thickness of the fold. Skinfolds are picked up in the vertical plane, except for the subscapular and suprailiac, which are picked up at a slight angle. Each skinfold should be measured three times by regrasping the fold. The average value of the two closest readings should be used as the actual measure.[10] The skinfold sites are illustrated in Figure 5-3.

The first step for calculating the percentage body fat is the calculation of body density. This can be done in the following way for men and women:[11]

Men: body density (gm/cc) = 1.1043 − (0.00131 × subscapula measure in mm) − (0.001327 × thigh measure in mm)

Women: body density (gm/cc) = 1.0764 − (0.00088 × tricep measure in mm) − (0.00081 × suprailiac measure in mm)

The computation for the percentage of body fat is as follows:

Percentage body fat = (4.570/body density − 4.142) × 100

The following formula can be used to calculate lean body weight:

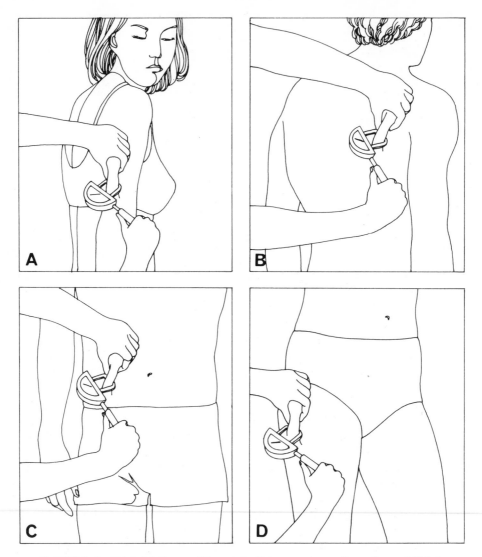

**FIGURE 5-3.** Skinfold sites. **a.** Triceps. **b.** Subscapula. **c.** Suprailiac. **d.** Thigh.

$$\text{Fat weight} = \text{body weight*} \times \frac{\%\ \text{body fat}}{100}$$

$$\text{Lean body weight} = \text{body weight} - \text{fat weight}$$

Men: desired weight = lean weight/0.88 (12% body fat)

Women: desired weight = lean weight/0.82 (18% body fat)

*1 lb = 0.45 kg; kilogram units should be used for body weight.

**Girth Measurements**
Girth measurements that represent norms serve as rough guidelines for appropriate body proportions:

Women
• Bust and hips: same
• Abdomen (at waist): 25 to 26 cm less than bust and hips
• Thigh: 15 cm less than waist
• Calf: 15 to 18 cm less than thigh
• Ankle: 13 to 15 cm less than calf
• Biceps (upper arm): relaxed, 2 times the size of the wrist

Men
• Chest and hips: same
• Abdomen (at waist): 13 to 18 cm less than chest and hips
• Thigh: 20 to 25 cm less than abdomen
• Calf: 18 to 20 cm less than thigh
• Ankle: 15 to 18 cm less than calf
• Biceps (upper arm): relaxed, 2 times the size of the wrist

**The Step Test**
The step test is a field version of the laboratory stress test and can be performed when appropriate monitoring equipment and personnel are not available for stress testing. If the step test is conducted in a clinic setting, the electrocardiogram may be monitored. The availability of a physician for emergency back-up is suggested if the client is over 40 years of age, obese, or has a history of cardiovascular difficulties. The step test is not as physiologically stressful as the laboratory stress test, but caution should be exercised in testing individuals with high-risk profiles for cardiovascular disease. While the risk of step testing has not been reported, in a study of 170,000 laboratory stress tests, the mortality rate was 1 per 10,000 and the morbidity rate 2.4 per 10,000.[12]

For the step test, a step 17 to 18 inches high is recommended. The step rate should be 30 steps per minute for men and 24 steps per minute for women. Each step consists of the following sequence: left foot up; right foot up; left foot down; right foot down. Pulse rates are measured after stepping for 3 minutes at the prescribed cadence. Either apical or carotid pulse may be used. Radial pulse may also be checked along with one of the above. With the client comfortably seated in a chair following step testing, pulse rates are counted for 30 seconds at the following intervals:[13]

• 1 to 1½ minutes after cessation of exercise
• 2 to 2½ minutes after cessation of exercise
• 3 to 3½ minutes after cessation of exercise

The sum of the three 30-second pulses is the recovery index. Normative values for recovery for men and women are presented in Table 5-1.

**TABLE 5-1   THREE-MINUTE STEP-TEST
RECOVERY INDEX**

|  | Cumulated Pulse Rate | |
| --- | --- | --- |
|  | MEN | WOMEN |
| Excellent | 132 or less | 135 or less |
| Good | 150–133 | 155–136 |
| Average | 165–149 | 170–154 |
| Fair | 180–164 | 190–171 |
| Poor | Above 180 | Above 190 |

Adapted from Getchell, B. *Physical fitness: A way of life* (2nd ed.). New York: Wiley, 1979, pp. 72–73. With permission.

**Testing Muscle Strength and Endurance**

As a test of muscular strength and endurance, bent knee sit-ups, as illustrated in Figure 5-4 can be used. For females, the number of sit-ups per minute is counted, while for males, the number of sit-ups in 2 minutes is calculated. Older subjects or those with cardiovascular disorders must be observed carefully for fatigue during strength and endurance testing. Sit-ups should be terminated if signs of distress occur in the client. Normative data for sit-ups for men and women are presented in Table 5-2. For additional tests of strength and endurance, the reader should consult Getchell[14] or other physical-fitness and health-education references.[15,16]

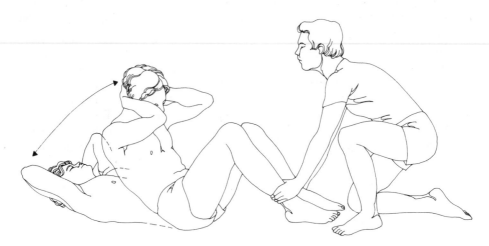

**FIGURE 5-4.** Bent-knee sit-ups.

## TABLE 5-2   EVALUATION OF BENT-KNEE SIT-UPS

|  | Women:<br>Number of Sit-ups,<br>1 min | Men:<br>Number of Sit-ups,<br>2 min |
|---|---|---|
| Excellent | 33 or above | 69 or above |
| Good | 27–32 | 60–68 |
| Average | 26–20 | 59–52 |
| Fair | 16–21 | 51–42 |
| Poor | 16 or fewer | 41 or fewer |

Adapted from Getchell, B. *Physical fitness: A Way of Life* (2nd ed.). New York: Wiley, 1979, pp. 56–57. With permission.

### Evaluating Flexibility

Flexibility is also an important component of physical fitness. It is the ability to move muscles and joints through their maximum range of motion. Flexibility may decrease with age or as a result of chronic illness. The lack of ability to flex or extend muscles or joints often reflects poor health habits, such as sedentary lifestyle, inappropriate posture, and/or faulty body mechanics. Loss of flexibility greatly decreases the client's ability to move about with ease and comfort.

As a quick test of flexibility, have the client bend over, keeping legs straight, and touch his or her toes. The continuum that can be used for evaluating extent of flexibility is presented in Table 5-3. Another test of flexibility, trunk flexion, is illustrated in Figure 5-5. Trunk flexion measures the ability of the client to stretch back and thigh muscles. The client sits on the floor with legs fully extended and feet flat against a box extending outward from the wall. Arms and hands are extended forward as far as possible and held for a count of three. With a ruler,

## TABLE 5-3   EVALUATION OF FLEXIBILITY

|  | Touch Point (in) |
|---|---|
| Excellent | +9 or more |
| Good | + 4 to 8 |
| Average | +1 to 3 |
| Fair | −2 to 0 |
| Poor | −12 to −2 |

+ indicates in front of toes
− indicates above toes
0  indicates at toes

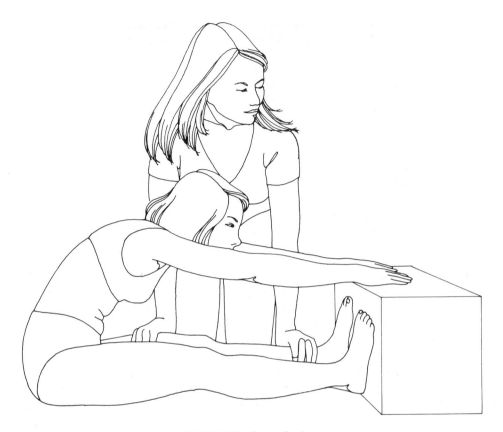

**FIGURE 5-5.** Trunk flexion.

the distance that the client can reach beyond the proximal edge of the box can be measured in inches. If the client cannot reach the edge, the distance of the fingertips from the edge is measured and reported as a negative number. Norms for trunk flexion for men and women are presented in Table 5-4.

In summary, body composition, girth measurements, cardiovascular status, muscle strength/endurance, and flexibility are critical physiologic parameters to consider in a comprehensive fitness evaluation. The data collected during this phase of assessment can be used to assist the client in planning an appropriate exercise or physical-activity program. Chapter 10 discusses specific approaches to increase physical fitness of clients.

## NUTRITIONAL ASSESSMENT

Effective planning for health promotion requires evaluation of the nutritional status of clients. Current weight, the percentage of body fat, lean body weight,

---

### TABLE 5-4 NORMS FOR TRUNK FLEXION (inches)

|  | Women | Men |
|---|---|---|
| Range | −4 to +10 | −6 to +8 |
| Average (Mean) | +2 | +1 |
| Desired range | + 2 to + 6 | + 1 to + 5 |

From Getchell, B. *Physical fitness: A way of life* (2nd ed.). New York: Wiley, 1979, p. 59. With permission.

dietary patterns, and the nutrient composition of the diet should be assessed. Height and weight tables for adults and growth standards for boys and girls from birth to age 18 are presented in Tables 5-5 and 5-6. Height should be measured in 1-inch heels for men and 2-inch heels for women. Weight should be taken with light-weight clothing. In addition to body weight, skinfold measurements provide a simple criterion for obesity.[17] Triceps skinfold thicknesses indicative of obesity for children, adolescents, and men and women of differing age groups are pre-

### TABLE 5-5a WEIGHT TABLE FOR ADULT MALES, ACCORDING TO HEIGHT AND FRAME

| Height | | Weight in Pounds (Frame) | | |
|---|---|---|---|---|
| FEET | INCHES | SMALL | MEDIUM | LARGE |
| 5 | 2 | 112–120 | 118–129 | 126–141 |
| 5 | 3 | 115–123 | 121–133 | 129–144 |
| 5 | 4 | 118–126 | 124–136 | 132–148 |
| 5 | 5 | 121–129 | 127–139 | 135–152 |
| 5 | 6 | 124–133 | 130–143 | 138–156 |
| 5 | 7 | 128–137 | 134–147 | 142–161 |
| 5 | 8 | 132–141 | 138–152 | 147–166 |
| 5 | 9 | 136–145 | 142–156 | 151–170 |
| 5 | 10 | 140–150 | 146–160 | 155–174 |
| 5 | 11 | 144–154 | 150–165 | 159–179 |
| 6 | 0 | 148–158 | 154–170 | 164–184 |
| 6 | 1 | 152–162 | 158–175 | 168–189 |
| 6 | 2 | 156–167 | 162–180 | 173–194 |
| 6 | 3 | 160–171 | 167–185 | 178–199 |
| 6 | 4 | 164–175 | 172–190 | 182–204 |

From Metropolitan Life Insurance Company (1960). Derived from data of the Build and Blood Pressure Study, 1959.

**TABLE 5-5b   WEIGHT TABLE FOR ADULT FEMALES, ACCORDING TO HEIGHT AND FRAME**

| Height | | Weight in Pounds (Frame) | | |
|---|---|---|---|---|
| FEET | INCHES | SMALL | MEDIUM | LARGE |
| 4 | 10 | 92–98 | 96–107 | 104–119 |
| 4 | 11 | 94–101 | 98–110 | 106–122 |
| 5 | 0 | 96–104 | 101–113 | 109–125 |
| 5 | 1 | 99–107 | 104–116 | 112–128 |
| 5 | 2 | 102–110 | 107–119 | 115–131 |
| 5 | 3 | 105–113 | 110–122 | 118–134 |
| 5 | 4 | 108–116 | 113–126 | 121–138 |
| 5 | 5 | 111–119 | 116–130 | 125–142 |
| 5 | 6 | 114–123 | 120–135 | 129–146 |
| 5 | 7 | 118–127 | 124–139 | 133–150 |
| 5 | 8 | 122–131 | 128–143 | 137–154 |
| 5 | 9 | 126–135 | 132–147 | 141–158 |
| 5 | 10 | 130–140 | 136–151 | 145–163 |
| 5 | 11 | 134–144 | 140–155 | 149–168 |
| 6 | 0 | 138–148 | 144–159 | 153–174 |

From Metropolitan Life Insurance Company (1960). Derived from data of the Build and Blood Pressure Study, 1959.

sented in Table 5-7. Procedures for calculating the percentage of body fat and the lean body weight were presented in the previous section under physical-fitness evaluation. Deviations from any of the norms on the above measurements should be noted by the nurse and recorded as a part of the nutritional assessment.

Current dietary patterns of clients and percentage of types of nutrients in their usual diet should also be assessed. Clients should be instructed to keep a record of everything eaten for 5 to 7 days during the week prior to their clinic appointment or home visit. The record can be kept on a food diary form that allows the listing of the types of foods and amounts consumed during regular meals and snacks. A simple format for a food diary for one day is illustrated in Figure 5-6. When such a diary is kept accurately, average fat, protein, and carbohydrate intake can be calculated and compared with *Dietary Goals for the United States.*[18] In Figure 5-7, current dietary patterns and recommended dietary goals for adults are presented. The nurse should note that in the *Dietary Goals*, the major changes recommended are a decrease in fat consumption and an increase in consumption of complex carbohydrates and naturally occurring sugars.

In order to convert food intake for each day to grams of fat, protein, and carbohydrates and subsequently to the percentage of total daily diet, a food-consumption chart is needed comparable to the one presented in Suitor and

## TABLE 5-6a  GROWTH STANDARDS FOR BOYS, FROM BIRTH TO AGE 18

| Age | Height (in), Percentiles | | Weight (lb), Percentiles | |
|---|---|---|---|---|
| | 50th | 95th | 50th | 95th |
| Birth | 19.8 | 21.1 | 7.5 | 9.1 |
| 1 mo | 21.4 | 22.9 | 9.4 | 11.1 |
| 3 mo | 24.0 | 25.4 | 13.4 | 16.0 |
| 6 mo | 26.7 | 28.3 | 18.0 | 21.3 |
| 9 mo | 28.7 | 30.2 | 21.4 | 25.1 |
| 1 yr | 30.2 | 32.0 | 23.3 | 27.8 |
| 2 yr | 34.6 | 27.1 | 29.3 | 33.3 |
| 3 yr | 37.8 | 40.3 | 32.5 | 37.9 |
| 4 yr | 40.8 | 43.3 | 36.1 | 42.4 |
| 5 yr | 43.4 | 46.4 | 40.3 | 47.6 |
| 6 yr | 45.9 | 49.0 | 44.7 | 53.4 |
| 7 yr | 48.1 | 51.4 | 50.9 | 61.5 |
| 8 yr | 50.5 | 54.1 | 57.4 | 70.4 |
| 9 yr | 52.8 | 56.8 | 64.4 | 80.4 |
| 10 yr | 54.9 | 59.2 | 71.4 | 91.4 |
| 11 yr | 56.4 | 60.9 | 78.9 | 102.5 |
| 12 yr | 58.6 | 63.7 | 86.0 | 113.5 |
| 13 yr | 61.3 | 67.4 | 98.6 | 131.9 |
| 14 yr | 64.1 | 70.7 | 111.8 | 148.1 |
| 15 yr | 66.9 | 72.8 | 124.3 | 160.6 |
| 16 yr | 68.9 | 74.0 | 133.8 | 169.8 |
| 17 yr | 69.8 | 74.4 | 139.8 | 174.0 |
| 18 yr | 70.2 | 74.5 | 144.8 | 179.3 |

From Public Health Service, *Obesity and health* (Publ. 1485).

Hunter.[19] Computerized programs are also available. Once the average or usual dietary patterns of the client have been identified, the nurse can provide needed assistance to the client with nutrition and weight control, as described in Chapter 11.

Any signs of malnutrition should also be noted. Physical signs suggestive of malnutrition are described by Caliendo[20] and in other nutrition texts. Laboratory tests in addition to those for cholesterol, triglycerides, glucose, and high-density lipoproteins, providing additional information concerning nutritional status, include those for protein (creatinine index, serum protein, serum albumin, total lymphocyte count, blood urea nitrogen, and uric acid), those for serum or plasma vitamin levels (water-soluble, fat soluble), and those for minerals (calcium, sodium, chloride, potassium, iron, phosphorus, and magnesium).[21]

## TABLE 5-6b  GROWTH STANDARDS FOR GIRLS, FROM BIRTH TO AGE 18

| Age | Height (in), Percentiles | | Weight (lb), Percentiles | |
|---|---|---|---|---|
| | 50th | 95th | 50th | 95th |
| Birth | 19.5 | 20.7 | 7.3 | 8.8 |
| 1 mo | 21.0 | 22.5 | 8.3 | 9.8 |
| 3 mo | 23.6 | 25.0 | 12.4 | 14.4 |
| 6 mo | 26.1 | 27.6 | 16.7 | 19.8 |
| 9 mo | 27.9 | 29.5 | 19.8 | 24.1 |
| 1 yr | 29.4 | 31.2 | 21.7 | 26.0 |
| 2 yr | 33.8 | 36.0 | 27.1 | 31.9 |
| 3 yr | 37.5 | 39.7 | 32.3 | 38.3 |
| 4 yr | 40.7 | 43.3 | 36.1 | 43.4 |
| 5 yr | 43.4 | 46.2 | 40.9 | 49.6 |
| 6 yr | 45.9 | 49.0 | 45.7 | 55.9 |
| 7 yr | 47.8 | 51.1 | 51.0 | 63.7 |
| 8 yr | 50.0 | 53.6 | 57.2 | 72.4 |
| 9 yr | 52.2 | 56.2 | 63.6 | 82.1 |
| 10 yr | 54.5 | 59.1 | 71.0 | 95.0 |
| 11 yr | 57.0 | 62.1 | 82.0 | 108.6 |
| 12 yr | 59.5 | 64.9 | 94.4 | 124.9 |
| 13 yr | 62.2 | 66.8 | 105.5 | 138.2 |
| 14 yr | 63.1 | 67.7 | 113.0 | 144.0 |
| 15 yr | 63.8 | 68.1 | 120.0 | 150.5 |
| 16 yr | 64.1 | 68.4 | 123.0 | 150.1 |
| 17 yr | 64.2 | 68.3 | 125.8 | 153.7 |
| 18 yr | 64.4 | 68.7 | 126.2 | 156.4 |

From Public Health Service, *Obesity and health* (Publ. 1485).

## TABLE 5-7  TRICEPS SKINFOLD THICKNESS INDICATING OBESITY (mm)

| Age (yr) | Males | Females |
|---|---|---|
| 5 | ≥12 | ≥15 |
| 10 | ≥13 | ≥17 |
| 15 | ≥15 | ≥20 |
| 20 | ≥16 | ≥28 |
| 25 | ≥20 | ≥29 |
| 30 and above | ≥23 | ≥30 |

After Seltzer, C.C., & Mayer, J.A. Simple criterion of obesity. *Post graduate medicine*, 1965. Copyright © 1965, McGraw-Hill, Inc.

Record *all* foods and drinks that you had during the day and during the night.

Day of Week (Mon  Tues  Wed  Thurs  Fri  Sat  Sun)

<u>Breakfast</u>

Foods and Drinks                                    Amounts (cups, tbsps)

<u>Lunch</u>

Foods and Drinks                                    Amounts (cups, tbsps)

<u>Dinner</u>

Foods and Drinks                                    Amounts (cups, tbsps)

<u>Snacks</u>

Time        Foods or Drinks                         Amount (cups, tbsps)

Do you take vitamin or mineral supplements?         Yes _____  No _____
Please list kind and how many per day.

**FIGURE 5-6.**  Food diary form.

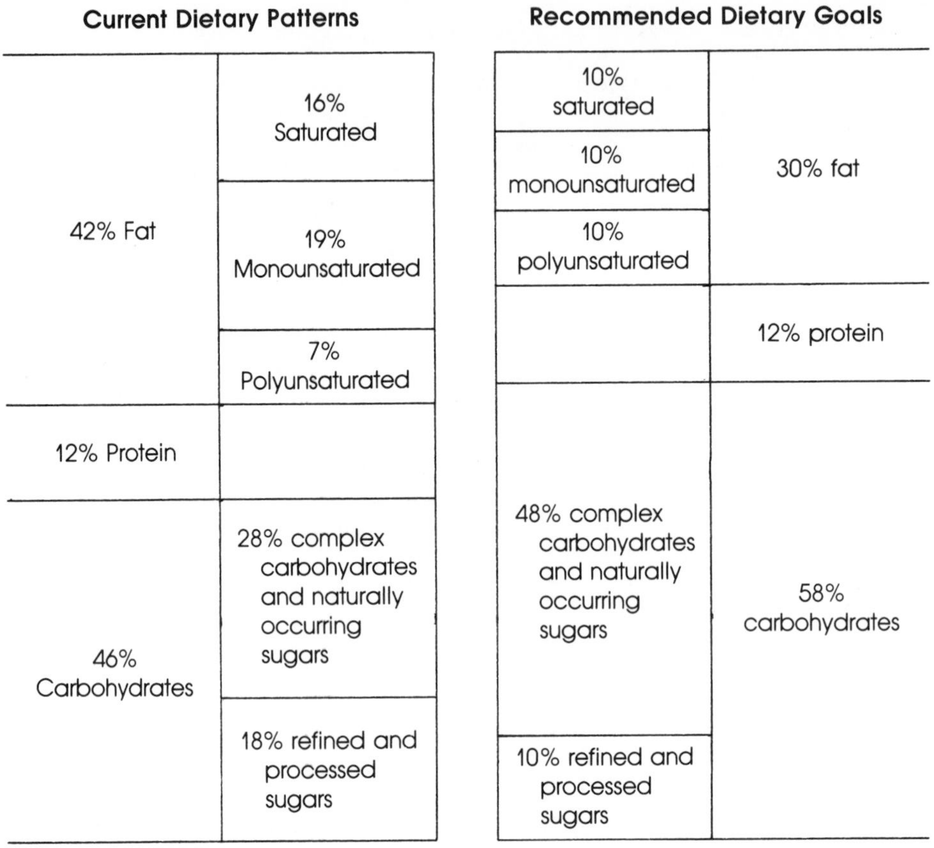

| Current Dietary Patterns | | Recommended Dietary Goals | |
|---|---|---|---|
| | 16% Saturated | 10% saturated | |
| | | 10% monounsaturated | 30% fat |
| 42% Fat | 19% Monounsaturated | 10% polyunsaturated | |
| | 7% Polyunsaturated | | 12% protein |
| 12% Protein | | | |
| 46% Carbohydrates | 28% complex carbohydrates and naturally occurring sugars | 48% complex carbohydrates and naturally occurring sugars | 58% carbohydrates |
| | 18% refined and processed sugars | 10% refined and processed sugars | |

**FIGURE 5-7.** Current dietary patterns and recommended dietary goals for adults in the United States. *(From Dietary Goals for the United States. U.S. Senate Select Committee on Nutrition and Human Needs, Washington, D.C.: Government Printing Office, December 1977.)*

Obesity and malnutrition occur in all socioeconomic classes. In addition, dietary risk factors are widespread in the American population. Therefore, assessment of nutritional status and dietary habits is an important part of holistic assessment.

## RISK APPRAISAL

Risk appraisal is a method for estimating individual risk for disease or death in which information from a client's medical history, physical examination, physical-fitness evaluation, and nutritional assessment are used with additional information to quantify personal risk factors. Risk is frequently estimated for the ensuing 5 or 10 years by using probability tables of death from specific causes.[22] The principle behind risk appraisal is that each person is faced with certain quantifiable health hazards as a member of a specific group and that average risks may be applied to a client if the health professional knows the client's characteristics and the mortality experience of a large group of cohorts with similar characteristics.

The usual format for risk appraisal is to collect data relevant to an individual and match those data against a data bank of actuarial statistics based on mortality rates by cause of death, from information gathered by the U.S. Public Health Service and insurance companies. Since the national data base presently available represents mortality alone, rather than mortality and morbidity statistics, the usefulness of risk appraisal is primarily limited to those diseases that have high resultant mortality rates.

Three important ideas relevant to risk appraisal have been presented by Steinbach:[23]

1. Each risk factor has an independent action of varying intensity.*
2. The total risk† for a given individual in developing any disease tends to increase with the number of risk factors present and the intensity of each risk factor.
3. Risk factors interact synergistically, according to rules not yet identified from scientific inquiry.

Risk factors may replace each other. For instance, a very high blood pressure and normal serum cholesterol may have the same atherogenic effects as a moderate blood pressure and hypercholesteremia. Much research needs to be completed before interaction and replacement rules for risk factors can be accurately identified. It appears that the actual risk from a single factor depends on the number and intensity of other coexisting factors in a given individual. As age advances, more factors accumulate and come into play, thus potentiating each other. This makes risk appraisal of the elderly an important nursing concern.

Risk factors can generally be classified according to the categories in Figure 5-8. The purpose of risk appraisal is to provide clients with a realistic evaluation of health threats to which they are particularly vulnerable prior to the development of signs and symptoms of disease. The approach to risk appraisal presented in Figures 5-9 and 5-10 has been developed by the author following extensive review of articles and materials in the field. The approach is practical and useful for the office or clinic setting. More detailed appraisal formats are available from several commercial sources for computerized analysis of individual risk based on comparison with national mortality data for selected health problems.[24-26]

---

*Threshold of risk* is the value of a risk factor below which the given factor no longer influences the total risk of a given individual for a specific disease. When all factors are at the threshold of risk, total risk should be at a minimum.
†*Total risk* is the cumulative effect of all risk factors or summed level of risk for a given individual for a specific disease.

While the level of risk for any given health problem generally increases with increasing number and intensity of factors, a word of caution is in order. Any single risk factor for which the client is at a high level may be so potent that by itself it may place the client at "high risk." Thus, the nurse should evaluate each risk factor for possible control through modification of health habits or lifestyle. Sennott[26a] has developed a difficulty index to assist clients in establishing priorities for behavior change. Use of the index in conjunction with risk data represents an interesting approach to individual risk-reduction counseling.

In using risk appraisal, health professionals must keep in mind that research is not conclusive on the extent of threat posed to health by each factor identified in the risk appraisal form. While all of the factors included are supported by considerable research, in some instances nonsupportive data can also be identified. Criteria used in risk appraisal must be modified as factors currently in use are shown to have little contribution to risk or new and more accurate predictors of risk are identified.

## LIFE STRESS REVIEW

The importance of stress in the direct or indirect causation of illness throughout the life span has been supported in numerous studies. The impact of stress on mental health and physical well-being has been evident in the work of Langer and Michael,[27] Holmes and Rahe,[28] and others. As a part of comprehensive health assessment, life stress review should include use of the following instruments: the Life-Change Index developed by Holmes and Rahe,[29] the State-Trait Anxiety Inventory developed by Spielberger,[30] the Signs of Distress developed by Everly and Girdano,[31] and Stress Charting developed at the Menninger Foundation by Walters.[32]

### Life-Change Index

Holmes and Rahe developed a tool to measure the extent of life change as a predictor of the probability of becoming ill. If enough changes occur within any given two-year period for the client, the chances of becoming ill are frequently

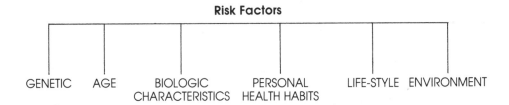

**FIGURE 5-8.** Categories of risk factors.

In each row, place a check in the box that best describes your current life situation or behavior.

**Risk for Cardiovascular Disease**

RISK FACTOR: ⟶ INCREASING RISK ⟶

| Sex and age: | | Female under 40 | Female 40–50 | Male 25–40 | Female after menopause | Male 40–60 | Male 61 or over |
|---|---|---|---|---|---|---|---|
| Family history (mother, father, brothers, sisters) | High blood pressure | No relatives with condition | | One relative | Two relatives | Three relatives | |
| | Heart attack | No relatives with condition | One relative with condition after 60 | Two relatives with condition after 60 | One relative with condition before 60 | Two relatives with condition before 60 | |
| | Diabetes | No relatives with condition | | One or more relatives with maturity onset diabetes | | One or more relatives with preadolescent or adolescent onset | |
| Blood pressure* | Systolic | 120 or below | 121–140 | 141–160 | 161–180 | 181–200 | above 200 |
| | Diastolic | 70 or below | 71–80 | 81–90 | 91–100 | 101–110 | above 110 |

*Indicates risk factors that can be fully or partially controlled.

**FIGURE 5-9.** Risk appraisal form (continued on next page).

In each row, place a check in the box that best describes your current life situation or behavior.

## Risk for Cardiovascular Disease

RISK FACTOR:

→ INCREASING RISK →

| RISK FACTOR | | | | | | | |
|---|---|---|---|---|---|---|---|
| Diabetes* | No diagnosis | Maturity onset, controlled | | Maturity onset, uncontrolled | Adolescent onset, controlled | Adolescent onset, uncontrolled | |
| Weight* | At or slightly below recommended weight | 10% overweight | 20% overweight | 30% overweight | 40% overweight | 50% overweight | |
| Cholesterol*† level (mg/100 ml) | Below 180 | 181–200 | 201–220 | 221–240 | 241–260 | 261–280 | Above 280 |
| Serum triglycerides* (mg/100 ml) fasting | 150 or below | | 151–400 | | 401–1000 | | Above 1000 |
| Percent of fat in diet* | 20–30% | | 31–40% | | 41–50% | | Above 50% |
| Frequency of exercise* — Recreational | Intensive recreational exertion (35–45 min at least 4 times/wk) | | Moderate recreational exertion | | Minimal recreational exertion | | No recreational exertion |
| Frequency of exercise* — Occupational | Intensive occupational exertion | | Moderate occupational exertion | | Minimal occupational exertion | | Sedentary occupation |

| Risk factor | | 7 or 8 hr sleep/night | | More than 8 hr sleep/night | | 4–6 hr sleep/night | |
|---|---|---|---|---|---|---|---|
| Sleep patterns* | | | | | | | |
| Cigarette smoking* | No./day | Nonsmoker | 1–10/day | 11–20/day | 21–30/day | 31–40/day | Over 40/day |
| | No. of yr smoked | Nonsmoker | Less than 10 yr | 11–15 yr | 16–20 yr | 21–30 yr | 31 yr or more |
| Stress* | Domestic | Minimal | | Moderate | High | Very high | |
| | Occupational | Minimal | | Moderate | High | Very high | |
| Behavior pattern* (particularly males) | | Type B — Relaxed, appropriately assertive, not time dependent, moderate to slow speech | | | Type A — Excessively competitive, aggressive, striving, hyperalert, time dependent, loud, explosive speech | | |
| Air pollution* | | Low | | | Moderate | High | |
| Use of oral contraceptives* (females) | | Do not use oral contraceptives | | Under 40 and use oral contraceptives | | Over 40 and use oral contraceptives | |

*Indicates risk factors that can be fully or partially controlled.
†Serum lipid analysis is also recommended to determine low-density (beta) and high-density (alpha) lipoprotein levels. Evidence suggests that high-density lipoprotein (HDL) carries cholesterol from tissues for metabolism and excretion. An inverse correlation appears to exist between HDL and coronary artery disease.

**FIGURE 5-9** (continued).

In each row, place a check in the box that best describes your current life situation or behavior.

## Risk for Malignant Diseases

RISK FACTOR:

INCREASING RISK →

| Risk Factor | | | | | | |
|---|---|---|---|---|---|---|
| **Breast Cancer (Women)** | | | | | | |
| Age | 20–29 | 30–39 | | 40–49 | 50 or over | |
| Race | Oriental | | Black | | Caucasian | |
| Family history (grandmother, mother, sister) | None | Mother, sister, or grandmother | | Mother and grandmother | Mother and sister | |
| Onset of menstruation | Over 12 yr of age | | | Under 12 yr of age | | |
| Pregnancy* — Time | First pregnancy before 25 | | First pregnancy after 25 | | No pregnancies | |
| Pregnancy* — No. | Three or more | | One or two | | None | |
| Weight* | 0–40% overweight | | | Above 40% overweight | | |
| Personal history | No evidence of dysplasia or previous breast cancer | | Breast dysplasia | | Previous breast cancer | |
| **Lung Cancer** | | | | | | |
| Cigarette smoking* — No./day | Nonsmoker | 1–10/day | 11–20/day | 21–30/day | 21–40/day | Over 40/day |
| Cigarette smoking* — No. of yr smoked | Nonsmoker | Less than 10 yr | 11–15 yr | 16–20 yr | 21–30 yr | 31 or more yr |

102

| Risk factor | Less than one yr | 1–5 yr | 6–10 yr | 11–15 yr | Over 15 yr |
|---|---|---|---|---|---|
| **Occupational exposure to toxic chemicals*‡** — Length of exposure | Less than one yr | 1–5 yr | 6–10 yr | 11–15 yr | Over 15 yr |
| Frequency and intensity of exposure | Low frequency and low intensity | Low frequency, moderate intensity (or vice versa) | Moderate frequency, moderate intensity | Moderate frequency, high intensity (or vice versa) | High frequency, high intensity |
| **Cervical Cancer** — Onset of sexual activity* | Before 16 yr of age | | 16–21 | 22–27 | After 28 yr of age |
| No. of sexual partners* | Two | | Three | | Four or more |
| Marital status* | Single | | | Married | |
| Sexual partner* | Circumcised | | | Uncircumcised | |
| **Colorectal Cancer** — Age | Below 45 yr of age | | | Above 45 yr of age | |
| Personal history | No history of ulcerative colitis | | Ulcerative colitis under 10 yr | Ulcerative colitis more than 10 yr | |
| Fiber content of diet* | High | | Moderate | Low | |
| Weight* (men) | Less than 40% overweight | | | More than 40% overweight | |
| Rectal bleeding or black bowel movement | Never | | Occasionally | Frequently | |

*Indicates risk factors that can be fully or partially controlled.
‡Chemicals such as asbestos, nickel, chromates, arsenic, chlormethyl ethers, radioactive dust, petroleum or coal products, and iron oxide.

**FIGURE 5-9** (continued).

In each row, place a check in the box that best describes your current life situation or behavior.

## Risk for Malignant Diseases

RISK FACTOR:

INCREASING RISK →

| Risk Factor | | | | |
|---|---|---|---|---|
| Uterine and Ovarian Cancer Age | Below 45 yr of age | Over 45 yr of age | | |
| Weight* | Less than 40% overweight | More than 40% overweight | | |
| Vaginal bleeding other than during menstrual period | Never | Occasionally | Frequently | |
| Skin Cancer Complexion | Dark | Medium | Fair | |
| Sun exposure (without protection) | Never or seldom | Occasionally | Frequently | |

## Risk for Auto Accidents

| Risk Factor | | | | | |
|---|---|---|---|---|---|
| Alcohol consumption* | Nondrinker | Occasionally small to moderate consumption | Frequently small to moderate consumption | Occasionally heavy consumption | Frequently heavy consumption |
| Mileage driven/yr* | Under 5000 miles/yr | 5001–10,000 miles/yr | 10,001–20,000 miles/yr | Over 20,000 miles/yr | |
| Use of seat belt* | Always | Usually | Occasionally | Never | |

| | Always | Usually | Occasionally | Never |
|---|---|---|---|---|
| Use of shoulder harness* | Always | Usually | Occasionally | Never |
| Use of drugs or medication that decrease alertness* | No use | Occasional use | Moderate use | Frequent use |

**Risk for Suicide**

| | | | | |
|---|---|---|---|---|
| Family history | No history | | One family member | Two or more family members |
| Personal history* | Seldom experience depression | Periodically experience mild depression | Frequently experience mild depression | Periodically experience deep depression | Frequently experience deep depression |
| Access to hypnotic medication* | No access | | Access to small or limited dosages | Unlimited access to large dosages |

**Risk for Diabetes**

| | | | | | |
|---|---|---|---|---|---|
| Weight* | Desired weight | 15% overweight | 30% overweight | 45% overweight | Above 45% overweight |
| Family history (parent or sibling) | None | | Either parent or sibling | Both parent and sibling |

*Indicates risk factors that can be fully or partially controlled.

**FIGURE 5-9** (continued).

| Health Problem | (1)<br>Total No.<br>Risk<br>Factors | (2)<br>No. for Which<br>Client Is in<br>Highest<br>Risk Level(s)* | (3)<br>Percent for Which<br>Client Is in Highest<br>Risk Level(s)<br>(Col. 2 ÷ Col. 1) |
|---|---|---|---|
| Cardiovascular<br>disease | 21† | _____ | _____ |
| Breast cancer | 8 | _____ | _____ |
| Lung cancer | 4 | _____ | _____ |
| Cervical cancer | 4 | _____ | _____ |
| Colorectal cancer | 5 | _____ | _____ |
| Uterine or ovarian<br>cancer | 3 | _____ | _____ |
| Skin cancer | 2 | _____ | _____ |
| Auto accidents | 5 | _____ | _____ |
| Suicide | 3 | _____ | _____ |
| Diabetes | 2 | _____ | _____ |

*High risk is risk within highest level of two to three levels within risk factor, or risk within highest two levels of four or more levels within risk factor.
†All subcategories under a given heading are counted individually. For example, Pregnancy—Time and Pregnancy–Number each count as a separate factor.

**FIGURE 5-10.** Profile of total risk.

increased. Stressful life events seem to precede many health problems such as tuberculosis, coronary heart disease, accidents, and possibly even malignant diseases. The Life-Change Index is presented in Figure 5-11. Modified forms of this index are available for different age and ethnic groups. The index can be administered to the client in a short period of time and scored by adding up the normative values for all life events checked. The extent of life stress can be evaluated using the scale for scoring presented in Table 5-8.

**State–Trait Anxiety Inventory**
A second instrument suggested for use as part of the life-stress review is the State–Trait Anxiety Inventory, which consists of 20 items pertaining to the amount of tension or anxiety the client feels at that moment (state), and 20 items concerning the way the client generally feels (trait). Sample questions from the inventory are presented in Figures 5-12 and 5-13. Clients respond by rating themselves on a 4-point scale for each item. The full-length test and test manual can be obtained by

Please check those life changes that you have experienced personally during the past *two years*.

| Life Event | Scale of Impact | |
| --- | :---: | --- |
| Death of Spouse | 100 | _____ |
| Divorce | 73 | _____ |
| Marital separation | 65 | _____ |
| Jail term | 63 | _____ |
| Death of close family member | 63 | _____ |
| Personal injury or illness | 53 | _____ |
| Marriage | 50 | _____ |
| Fired at work | 47 | _____ |
| Marital reconciliation | 45 | _____ |
| Retirement | 45 | _____ |
| Change in health of family member | 44 | _____ |
| Pregnancy | 40 | _____ |
| Sex difficulties | 39 | _____ |
| Gain of new family member | 39 | _____ |
| Business readjustment | 39 | _____ |
| Change in financial state | 38 | _____ |
| Death of close friend | 37 | _____ |
| Change to different line of work | 36 | _____ |
| Change in number of arguments with spouse | 35 | _____ |
| Mortgage over $20,000 | 31 | _____ |
| Foreclosure of mortgage or loan | 30 | _____ |
| Change in responsibilities at work | 29 | _____ |
| Son or daughter leaving home | 29 | _____ |
| Trouble with in-laws | 29 | _____ |
| Outstanding personal achievement | 28 | _____ |
| Spouse begins or stops work | 26 | _____ |

**FIGURE 5-11.** Life-change index (continued on next page). (*Reprinted with permission from Holmes, T., & Rahe, E., The social readjustment rating scale. Journal of Psychosomatic Research, 1967, 11, p. 213. Copyright © 1967, Pergamon Press, Ltd.*)

| Life Event | Scale of Impact | |
|---|---|---|
| Begin or end school | 26 | _____ |
| Change in living conditions | 25 | _____ |
| Revision of personal habits | 24 | _____ |
| Trouble with boss | 23 | _____ |
| Change in work hours or conditions | 20 | _____ |
| Change in residence | 20 | _____ |
| Change in schools | 20 | _____ |
| Change in recreation | 19 | _____ |
| Change in church activities | 19 | _____ |
| Change in social activities | 18 | _____ |
| Mortgage or loan less than $20,000 | 17 | _____ |
| Change in sleeping habits | 16 | _____ |
| Change in number of family get-togethers | 15 | _____ |
| Change in eating habits | 15 | _____ |
| Vacation | 13 | _____ |
| Christmas (if approaching) | 12 | _____ |
| Minor violations of the law | 11 | _____ |
| Total | | _____ |

**FIGURE 5-11** (continued).

contacting Consulting Psychologists Press, Inc., Palo Alto, California. The State–Trait Anxiety Inventory provides an efficient yet reliable means for assessing feelings of tension or stress experienced by clients. Test-retest reliability of the Trait Anxiety Inventory is reported as 0.73 for males and 0.77 for females.

**Signs of Distress**

In order to assist clients in understanding how they respond to stress, they must be made aware of the signs that provide personal feedback concerning an elevated stress level. Once clients are aware of their own biologic or behavioral responses to stress, they can use stress-management techniques presented in Chapter 12 more effectively. Signs of distress may be in terms of mood and disposition, muscles, bones and joints, or visceral organs. A check list for signs of distress is presented in Figure 5-14.

---

## TABLE 5-8 SCORING THE LIFE-CHANGE INDEX

| Score Range | Interpretation |
|---|---|
| 0–150 | No significant problems, low or tolerable life change |
| 150–199 | Mild life change (approximately 33% chance of illness) |
| 200–299 | Moderate life change (approximately 50% chance of illness) |
| 300 or over | Major life change (approximately 80% chance of illness) |

Reprinted with permission from Holmes, T., & Rahe, E. The social readjustment rating scale. *Journal of Psychosomatic Research,* 1967, *11,* p. 213. Copyright © 1967 Pergamon Press, Ltd.)

---

Directions: A number of statements which people have used to describe themselves are given below. Read each statement and then blacken in the appropriate circle to the right of the statement to indicate how you *feel* right now, that is, *at this moment*. There are no right or wrong answers. Do not spend too much time on any one statement but give the answer which seems to describe your present feelings best.

① = **Not at All;** ② = **Somewhat;**
③ = **Moderately So;** ④ = **Very Much So**

| | | | | |
|---|---|---|---|---|
| I feel at ease | ① | ② | ③ | ④ |
| I feel upset | ① | ② | ③ | ④ |
| I feel nervous | ① | ② | ③ | ④ |
| I am relaxed | ① | ② | ③ | ④ |
| I am worried | ① | ② | ③ | ④ |

**FIGURE 5-12.** Sample items from the self-evaluation questionnaire: State Anxiety Inventory. (*Reproduced by special permission from* The State–Trait Anxiety Inventory, *by Charles Spielberger, Richard Gorsuch, and Robert Lushene. Copyright © 1968, published by Consulting Psychologists Press, Inc., Palo Alto, Calif. 94306.*)

Directions: A number of statements that people have used to describe themselves are given below. Read each statement and then blacken in the appropriate circle to the right of the statement to indicate how you generally feel. There are no right or wrong answers. Do not spend too much time on any one statement, but give the answer that seems to describe how you generally feel.

① = **Not at All;** ② = **Somewhat;**
③ = **Moderately So;** ④ = **Very Much So**

| | | | | |
|---|---|---|---|---|
| I wish I could be as happy as others seem to be | ① | ② | ③ | ④ |
| I am "calm, cool, and collected" | ① | ② | ③ | ④ |
| I feel that difficulties are piling up so that I cannot overcome them | ① | ② | ③ | ④ |
| I am inclined to take things hard | ① | ② | ③ | ④ |
| I am content | ① | ② | ③ | ④ |

**FIGURE 5-13.**    Sample items from the self-evaluation questionnaire: Trait Anxiety Inventory. (*Reproduced by special permission from* The State–Trait Anxiety Inventory, *by Charles Spielberger, Richard Gorsuch, and Robert Lushene. Copyright © 1968, published by Consulting Psychologists Press, Inc., Palo Alto, Calif. 94306.*)

### Stress Charting

The Menninger Foundation Biofeedback Center in their stress management seminars use a stress-charting exercise that allows clients to list sources of stress. After listing as many stressors as possible, the client is instructed to write the number associated with each stressor in the section of the circle that describes the area of life in which the stressor occurs. If it is a stressor that is particularly troublesome, the client should place the number closer to the center of the circle. The center of the circle represents the client. The stress-charting exercise appears in Figure 5-15. Following completion of this portion of the life-stress review, the client should be aware of (1) the stresses that he or she is experiencing in daily living, (2) the areas of life in which multiple stressors are occurring, and (3) the personal closeness or distance of each stressor from the self.

Life-stress review provides the client with an understanding of personal sources of stress, level of stress, and specific responses to anxiety-producing life events. Increased self-awareness resulting from this component of health assessment facilitates the use of stress management and relaxation techniques described in Chapter 12.

## LIFESTYLE AND HEALTH-HABITS ASSESSMENT

Clients often have unreal expectations that physicians and nurses can undo the ill that clients have inflicted on themselves through health-damaging styles of living. While a healthy lifestyle does not guarantee freedom from chronic illness, much evidence indicates that there is a great deal that individuals can do to

**Mood and disposition signs**

_____ I become overexcited

_____ I worry

_____ I feel insecure

_____ I have difficulty sleeping at night

_____ I become easily confused and forgetful

_____ I become very uncomfortable and ill-at-ease

_____ I become nervous

**Musculoskeletal signs**

_____ My fingers and hands shake

_____ I can't sit or stand still

_____ I develop twitches

_____ My head begins to ache

_____ I feel my muscles become tense or stiff

_____ I stutter or stammer when I speak

_____ My neck becomes stiff

**Visceral signs**

_____ My stomach becomes upset

_____ I feel my heart pounding

_____ I sweat profusely

_____ My hands become moist

_____ I feel light-headed or faint

_____ I experience cold chills

_____ My face becomes "hot"

_____ My mouth becomes dry

_____ I experience ringing in my ears

_____ I get a sinking feeling in my stomach

**FIGURE 5-14.** Signs of Distress. (*From Girdano, D.A., & Everly, G.S.,* Controlling stress and tension: A holistic approach. *Bowie, Md.: Robert J. Brady, 1979, p. 137. With permission.*)

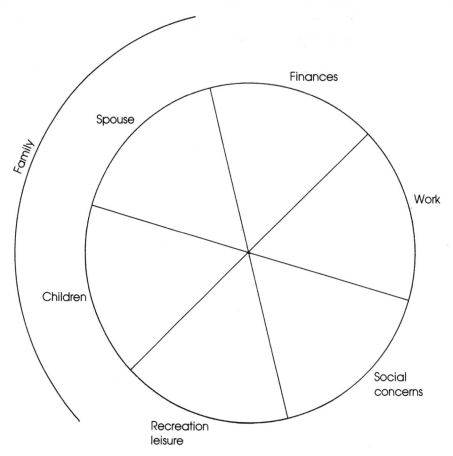

**FIGURE 5-15.**  Stress charting. *(Adapted with permission from Walters, D., Biofeedback Center, The Menninger Foundation, Topeka, Kan.)*

List of stressors:

| | |
|---|---|
| 1. | 9. |
| 2. | 10. |
| 3. | 11. |
| 4. | 12. |
| 5. | 13. |
| 6. | 14. |
| 7. | 15. |
| 8. | 16. |

maintain and enhance their health and prevent the early onset of disabling health problems. The Lifestyle and Health-Habits Assessment is intended to help the nurse assist the client in reviewing personal lifestyle in terms of its impact on health. A thoughtful review and follow-up counseling and education can greatly increase the motivation and competence of clients to care for themselves in a responsible manner.

The Lifestyle and Health-Habits Assessment is divided into ten sections: (1) competence in self-care, (2) nutritional practices, (3) physical or recreational activity, (4) sleep patterns, (5) stress management, (6) self-actualization, (7) sense of purpose, (8) relationships with others, (9) environmental control, and (10) use of health care system. Ideas used by the author in constructing the assessment guide have been drawn from many sources.[33-38] The Lifestyle and Health-Habits Assessment form is presented in Figure 5-16.

The rating in each category of the Lifestyle and Health-Habits Assessment can provide information useful in developing an individualized health-protection/

---

Please place an X before each statement that is true regarding your *present* way of life or personal habits. That is, what you generally do.

**General competence in self-care (14)**

_____ Take 12–15 deep breaths at least three times daily

_____ Drink 6–8 glasses of water each day in addition to other liquids

_____ Do not smoke

_____ Read articles or books about promoting health

_____ Know my body contours and physical sensations well

_____ Do not take laxative medications

_____ Know what my blood pressure and pulse readings should be

_____ Protect my skin from excessive sun exposure

_____ Know the seven danger signs of cancer

_____ Observe my body monthly for cancer danger signs

_____ Understand how to correctly examine my breasts (women only)

_____ Conduct monthly breast self-examination (women only)

_____ Use soft toothbrush regularly

_____ Dental floss regularly

Total number of items checked _____ Percent checked _____

**FIGURE 5-16.** Lifestyle and health habits assessment form (continued on next page).

**Nutritional practices (16)**

_____ Know about the "basic four" food groups

_____ Plan or select meals to meet nutritional needs

_____ Eat breakfast daily

_____ Eat three meals a day

_____ Avoid between meal snacks

_____ Drink only small amounts (no more than 3 cups/day) of caffeinated beverages (coffees, teas, or colas)

_____ Do not consume alcoholic beverages or do so in very limited amounts

_____ Limit intake of refined sugars (junk foods or deserts)

_____ Frequently use unprocessed foods or foods without preservatives or other additives

_____ Maintain adequate roughage (fiber) in diet (whole grains, raw fruits, raw vegetables)

_____ Read labels for nutrients in packaged food

_____ Eat more poultry and fish than red meats

_____ Chew foods thoroughly and eat slowly

_____ Add little or no salt to my food when cooking or during eating

_____ Keep weight within recommended limits for my height

_____ Avoid frequent consumption of charcoaled foods

Total number of items checked _____ Percent checked _____

**Physical or recreational activity (9)**

_____ Walk up stairs rather than riding the elevator

_____ Exercise vigorously for 30–40 minutes at least four times per week

_____ Regularly engage in recreational sports (swimming, soccer, bicycling)

_____ Perform stretching exercises at least four times per week to increase flexibility.

_____ Participate in individual sports for the pleasure of movement and physical fitness

**FIGURE 5-16**   (continued).

_____ Engage in competitive sports primarily for enjoyment rather than competition

_____ Maintain good posture when sitting or standing

_____ Often elevate my legs when sitting

_____ Seldom sit with legs crossed at knees

Total number of items checked _____ Percent checked _____

**Sleep patterns (9)**

_____ Get 7 hours of sleep per night (not $1\frac{1}{2}$ hours less or more)

_____ Wake up feeling fresh and relaxed

_____ Take some time for relaxation each day

_____ Fall asleep easily at night

_____ Sleep soundly

_____ Systematically relax voluntary muscles before sleep

_____ Sleep on a firm mattress

_____ Use a small pillow for sleep that maintains head and neck in a natural position

_____ Allow the thoughts and worries of the day to leave my mind, concentrating on passive but pleasant thoughts at bedtime

Total number of items checked _____ Percent checked _____

**Stress management (11)**

_____ Can laugh at myself

_____ Frequently laugh out loud with others

_____ Maintain adequate vitamin C intake when experiencing high stress

_____ Practice relaxation or meditation for 15–20 minutes daily

_____ Understand the relationship between stress and illness

_____ Create relaxed atmosphere at meal time

_____ Forget my problems and enjoy myself when immediate solutions are not possible

_____ Enjoy spending time in unstructured activities

**FIGURE 5-16** (continued).

| | |
|---|---|
| _____ | Consider it acceptable to cry, feel sad, angry, or afraid |
| _____ | Find constructive ways to express my feelings |
| _____ | Have attended training classes or biofeedback sessions to gain relaxation skills |

Total number of items checked _____ Percent checked _____

**Self-actualization (12)**

| | |
|---|---|
| _____ | Maintain an enthusiastic and optimistic outlook on life |
| _____ | Enjoy expressing myself in hobbies, the arts, exercise, or play |
| _____ | Like myself and enjoy occasional solitude |
| _____ | Continue to grow and change in positive directions |
| _____ | Am happy most of the time |
| _____ | Am a member of one or more community groups |
| _____ | Feel fulfilled in my work |
| _____ | Aware of personal strengths and weaknesses |
| _____ | Am proud of my body and my personality |
| _____ | Respect my own accomplishments |
| _____ | Find each day interesting and challenging |
| _____ | Look forward to the future |

Total number of items checked _____ Percent checked _____

**Sense of purpose (4)**

| | |
|---|---|
| _____ | Aware of what is important to me in life |
| _____ | Have identified short-term and long-term life goals |
| _____ | Am realistic about the goals that I set |
| _____ | Believe that my life has purpose |

Total number of items checked _____ Percent checked _____

**Relationships with others (11)**

| | |
|---|---|
| _____ | Have persons close to me with whom I can discuss personal problems and concerns |

**FIGURE 5-16**   (continued).

_____ Perceive myself as being well accepted by others

_____ Maintain meaningful and fulfilling interpersonal relationships

_____ Communicate easily with others

_____ Recognize accomplishments and praise other people easily

_____ Enjoy my neighbors

_____ Have a number of close friends

_____ Thoughtfully consider constructive criticism rather than reacting defensively

_____ Enjoy being touched and touching people close to me

_____ Find it easy to express concern, love, and warmth to others

_____ Enjoy meeting new people and getting to know them

Total number of items checked _____ Percent checked _____

**Environmental control (6)**

_____ When possible, prevent overwhelming changes in my environment

_____ Avoid purchasing aerosol sprays

_____ Seldom listen to loud rock music

_____ Do not permit smoking in my home or car

_____ Provide resources to meet my own personal needs

_____ Maintain safe living area free from fire or accident hazards

Total number of items checked _____ Percent checked _____

**Use of health care system (8)**

_____ Report any unusual signs or symptoms to a physician

_____ Question my physician or seek a second opinion when I do not agree with the recommended treatment

_____ Expect prompt, helpful, and courteous personalized service from health care personnel

_____ Discuss health care concerns or problems with the health professional most qualified to provide meaningful assistance

_____ Have breasts examined at least once a year by nurse or physician

_____ Have a pap smear at intervals recommended by my physician

**FIGURE 5-16**   (continued).

_____ Have a rectal examination at intervals recommended by my physician

_____ Attend educational classes on personal health care provided within the community

Total number of items checked _____ Percent checked _____

*Scoring:* Calculate the percentage of items checked in each category by dividing the number of items that you checked by the total number of items listed in the category (total number of items in each category is listed in parentheses by category title). Record below the percentage of items checked from each category.

| Category | Percentage of Items Checked | Rating (see below) |
|---|---|---|
| Competency in self-care | _____ | _____ |
| Nutritional practices | _____ | _____ |
| Physical or recreational activity | _____ | _____ |
| Sleep patterns | _____ | _____ |
| Stress management | _____ | _____ |
| Self-actualization | _____ | _____ |
| Sense of purpose | _____ | _____ |
| Relationships with others | _____ | _____ |
| Environmental control | _____ | _____ |
| Use of health care system | _____ | _____ |

For each category, the following scale may be used to evaluate the extent to which the client's lifestyle and health habits maintain or promote personal health.

| Rating | Percentage of Items Checked |
|---|---|
| Excellent | Greater than 85% |
| Good | 75–84% |
| Average | 65–74% |
| Fair | 55–64% |
| Poor | Below 55% |

**FIGURE 5-16**   (continued).

promotion program. Even though the percentage of behaviors performed in each category provides the basis for overall evaluation, the response to each behavior should be examined. For instance, if the client is a female and does not examine her own breasts monthly, then the response to that single item is important for educational and counseling follow-up. Through use of the comprehensive Lifestyle and Health-Habits Assessment, important data become available to the client for increasing self-awareness of personal patterns of living. Such information also facilitates nursing intervention.

A shorter lifestyle assessment form, the Wellness Index, consisting of 16 items has been developed by John Travis at the Wellness Resource Center in Mill Valley, California. This form provides an overall evaluation of wellness and lifestyle. The Wellness Index and instructions for evaluating the results appear in Figure 5-17. This form provides a less detailed assessment than the Lifestyle and Health-Habits Assessment but a graphically impressive one. It may be useful for initial assessment when client contact time is limited or the attention span of the client is short.

Through review of lifestyle and health habits, the client is assisted in systematically evaluating the extent to which personal behavior is supportive of health. This aspect of assessment is useful to the client as a basis for decisions concerning desired behavior and lifestyle change.

---

Circle the category that most closely answers the question.

1. I am conscious of the ingredients of the food I eat and their effect on me.     Rarely, Sometimes, Very Often   (R, S, VO)

2. I avoid overeating and abusing alcohol, caffeine, nicotine, and other drugs.     R, S, VO

3. I minimize my intake of refined carbohydrates and fats.     R, S, VO

4. My diet contains adequate amounts of vitamins, minerals, and fiber. R, S, VO

5. I am free from physical symptoms.     R, S, VO

6. I get aerobic cardiovascular exercise.     R, S, VO   (Very Often is at least 12–20 minutes 5 times per week vigorously running, swimming, or bike riding)

7. I practice yoga or some other form of limbering/stretching exercise. R, S, VO

8. I nurture myself.   R, S, VO   (Nurturing means pleasuring and taking care of oneself, for example, massages, long walks, buying presents for self, "doing nothing," sleeping late without feeling guilty, etc.)

---

**FIGURE 5-17.**   Wellness index (continued on next page). (*Used with permission from Travis, J.W., Wellness Workbook for Health Professionals. Mill Valley, Calif.: Wellness Resource Center, 1977.*)

9. I pay attention to changes occurring in my life and am aware of them as stress factors.     R, S, VO   (See Life-Change Index—a score of over 300 is considered very stressful)

10. I practice regular relaxation.     R, S, VO   (Suggested: 20 minutes a day "centering" or "letting go" of thoughts, worries, etc.)

11. I am without excess muscle tension.     R, S, VO

12. My hands are warm and dry.     R, S, VO

13. I am both productive and happy.     R, S, VO

14. I constructively express my emotions and creativity.     R, S, VO

15. I feel a sense of purpose in life and my life has meaning and direction.     R, S, VO

16. I believe I am fully responsible for my wellness or illness.     R, S, VO

Using your answers above to guide you, you can synthesize a graphic picture of your wellness. Each numbered pie-shaped segment of the circle below corresponds to the same numbered question on the preceding page. (They are divided into quarters representing four major dimensions of wellness.) Color in an amount of each segment corresponding to your answer to the question with the same number. The inner broken circle corresponds to "rarely," the next one to "sometimes," the third to "very often." You don't need to restrict yourself to these categories, however, and can fill in any amount in between. You may use different colors for each section if you like.

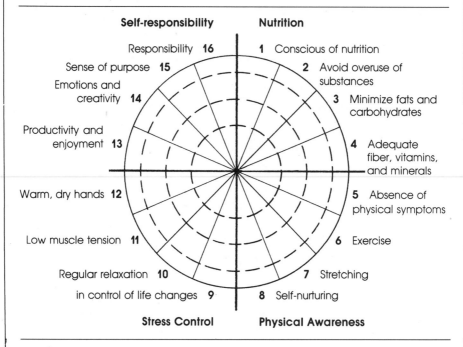

Now look at the shape of your index. Is it lopsided or balanced? This should provide beginning suggestions for improving your lifestyle and health habits.

**FIGURE 5-17**   (continued).

## HEALTH-BELIEFS REVIEW

In the last section of this chapter, a Health-Beliefs Review is included for use in clarifying the beliefs of the clients concerning personal control of their own health status. The Multidimensional Health Locus of Control (MHLC) Instrument developed by Wallston and Wallston[39-42] is recommended for assessing perceptions of health control. The two forms of the MHLC appear in Figures 5-18 and 5-19. Use of both forms yields more reliable data than use of either alone (one form only, reliability 0.67–0.77; two forms, reliability 0.83–0.86).

Three important subscales have been identified within the instrument. The three subscales and the items included in each are as follows for both forms A and B:

- Internal items: 1, 6, 8, 12, 13, 17
- Chance items: 2, 4, 9, 11, 15, 16
- Powerful-others items: 3, 5, 7, 10, 14, 18

---

This questionnaire is designed to determine the way in which different people view certain important health-related issues. Each item is a belief statement with which you may agree or disagree. Beside each statement is a scale that ranges from strongly disagree (1) to strongly agree (6). For each item we would like you to circle the number that represents the extent to which you disagree or agree with the statement. The more strongly you agree with a statement, the higher will be the number you circle. The more strongly you disagree with a statement, the lower will be the number you circle. Please make sure that you answer every item and that you circle *only one* number per item. This is a measure of your personal beliefs; obviously, there are no right or wrong answers.

Please answer these items carefully, but do not spend too much time on any one item. As much as you can, try to respond to each item independently. When making your choice, do not be influenced by your previous choices. It is important that you respond according to your actual beliefs and not according to how you feel you should believe or how you think we want you to believe.

**1 = Strongly Disagree; 2 = Moderately Disagree;**
**3 = Slightly Disagree; 4 = Slightly Agree;**
**5 = Moderately Agree; 6 = Strongly Agree.**

| | | | | | | |
|---|---|---|---|---|---|---|
| 1. If I get sick, it is my own behavior that determines how soon I get well again. | 1 | 2 | 3 | 4 | 5 | 6 |
| 2. No matter what I do, if I am going to get sick, I will get sick. | 1 | 2 | 3 | 4 | 5 | 6 |
| 3. Having regular contact with my physician is the best way for me to avoid illness. | 1 | 2 | 3 | 4 | 5 | 6 |

---

**FIGURE 5-18.** Multidimensional health locus of control scale, Form A (continued on next page). (*From Wallston, K.A., Wallston, B.S., & DeVellis, R. Development of the Multidimensional Health Locus of Control (MHLC) Scales.* Health Education Monographs, *Spring 1978, 6, 164–165. With permission.*)

| | | | | | | |
|---|---|---|---|---|---|---|
| 4. Most things that affect my health happen to me by accident. | 1 | 2 | 3 | 4 | 5 | 6 |
| 5. Whenever I don't feel well, I should consult a medically trained professional. | 1 | 2 | 3 | 4 | 5 | 6 |
| 6. I am in control of my health. | 1 | 2 | 3 | 4 | 5 | 6 |
| 7. My family has a lot to do with my becoming sick or staying healthy. | 1 | 2 | 3 | 4 | 5 | 6 |
| 8. When I get sick, I am to blame. | 1 | 2 | 3 | 4 | 5 | 6 |
| 9. Luck plays a big part in determining how soon I will recover from an illness. | 1 | 2 | 3 | 4 | 5 | 6 |
| 10. Health professionals control my health. | 1 | 2 | 3 | 4 | 5 | 6 |
| 11. My good health is largely a matter of good fortune. | 1 | 2 | 3 | 4 | 5 | 6 |
| 12. The main thing that affects my health is what I myself do. | 1 | 2 | 3 | 4 | 5 | 6 |
| 13. If I take care of myself, I can avoid illness. | 1 | 2 | 3 | 4 | 5 | 6 |
| 14. When I recover from an illness, it's usually because other people (for example, doctors, nurses, family, friends) have been taking good care of me. | 1 | 2 | 3 | 4 | 5 | 6 |
| 15. No matter what I do, I'm likely to get sick. | 1 | 2 | 3 | 4 | 5 | 6 |
| 16. If it's meant to be, I will stay healthy. | 1 | 2 | 3 | 4 | 5 | 6 |
| 17. If I take the right actions, I can stay healthy. | 1 | 2 | 3 | 4 | 5 | 6 |
| 18. Regarding my health, I can only do what my doctor tells me to do. | 1 | 2 | 3 | 4 | 5 | 6 |

**FIGURE 5-18** (continued).

The score on each subscale is the sum of the values circled for each item in that subscale. Scores within each subscale using both forms (A and B) can range from 12 to 72. The higher the score on the internal subscale, the more personal control clients believe that they exercise over their own health. The higher the scores on the chance subscale and powerful-others subscale, the higher the beliefs in the importance of chance and others respectively in controlling personal health. Normative means for adults on each subscale are as follows: internal, 50.4; chance, 31.0; power others, 40.9. The reader is referred to publications by Wallston and associates identified previously for more specific information on evaluating test results.

The information available to the nurse following completion of the MHLC

This questionnaire is designed to determine the way in which different people view certain important health-related issues. Each item is a belief statement with which you may agree or disagree. Beside each statement is a scale that ranges from strongly disagree (1) to strongly agree (6). For each item we would like you to circle the number that represents the extent to which you disagree or agree with the statement. The more strongly you agree with a statement, the higher will be the number you circle. The more strongly you disagree with a statement, the lower will be the number you circle. Please make sure that you answer every item and that you circle *only one* number per item. This is a measure of your personal beliefs; obviously, there are no right or wrong answers.

Please answer these items carefully, but do not spend too much time on any one item. As much as you can, try to respond to each item independently. When making your choice, do not be influenced by your previous choices. It is important that you respond according to your actual beliefs and not according to how you feel you should believe or how you think we want you to believe.

**1 = Strongly Disagree; 2 = Moderately Disagree;**
**3 = Slightly Disagree; 4 = Slightly Agree;**
**5 = Moderately Agree; 6 = Strongly Agree.**

1. If I become sick, I have the power to make myself well again.   1   2   3   4   5   6

2. Often I feel that no matter what I do, if I am going to get sick, I will get sick.   1   2   3   4   5   6

3. If I see an excellent doctor regularly, I am less likely to have health problems.   1   2   3   4   5   6

4. It seems that my health is greatly influenced by accidental happenings.   1   2   3   4   5   6

5. I can only maintain my health by consulting health professionals.   1   2   3   4   5   6

6. I am directly responsible for my health.   1   2   3   4   5   6

7. Other people play a big part in whether I stay healthy or become sick.   1   2   3   4   5   6

8. Whatever goes wrong with my health is my own fault.   1   2   3   4   5   6

9. When I am sick, I just have to let nature run its course.   1   2   3   4   5   6

10. Health professionals keep me healthy.   1   2   3   4   5   6

11. When I stay healthy, I'm just plain lucky.   1   2   3   4   5   6

12. My physical well-being depends on how well I take care of myself.   1   2   3   4   5   6

**FIGURE 5-19.** Multidimensional health locus of control scale, Form B (continued on next page). (*From Wallston, K.A., Wallston, B.S., & DeVellis, R., Development of the multidimensional health locus of control (MHLC) scales.* Health Education Monographs, *Spring 1978, 6, pp. 164–165. With permission.*)

| | | | | | | |
|---|---|---|---|---|---|---|
| 13. When I feel ill, I know it is because I have not been taking care of myself properly | 1 | 2 | 3 | 4 | 5 | 6 |
| 14. The type of care I receive from other people is what is responsible for how well I recover from an illness. | 1 | 2 | 3 | 4 | 5 | 6 |
| 15. Even when I take care of myself, it's easy to get sick. | 1 | 2 | 3 | 4 | 5 | 6 |
| 16. When I become ill, it's a matter of fate. | 1 | 2 | 3 | 4 | 5 | 6 |
| 17. I can pretty much stay healthy by taking good care of myself. | 1 | 2 | 3 | 4 | 5 | 6 |
| 18. Following doctor's orders to the letter is the best way for me to stay healthy. | 1 | 2 | 3 | 4 | 5 | 6 |

**FIGURE 5-19** (continued).

provides an indication of the extent to which clients believe that they can influence health through personal behaviors. If clients are low on internal control, perceptions of control may need to be changed. If clients are high on personal control, they exhibit an important aspect of readiness to learn about and engage in self-care.

## SUMMARY

The health assessment approach described in this chapter provides the nurse and client with important information to assist in developing individualized plans for protective/promotive care. Many of the tools presented are appropriate for use with children and adolescents as well as with adults. While nurses have assessed clients for many years, the need for additional assessment skills is apparent as nurses move toward greater autonomy in client care. In addition to the dimensions of assessment included in this chapter, the reader is encouraged to consult other sources for guidelines on assessment of human sexuality[43] and family structures.[44] Both of these areas, although beyond the scope of this book, are aspects of client experience that yield meaningful data for health planning.

## REFERENCES

1. Trautlein, J. *et al.* How much yield from a health screen? *Patient Care,* 1974, 65–69.
2. Bates, B. *A guide to physical examination.* Philadelphia: Lippincott, 1979.
3. *Ibid.*
4. Malasanos, L., Barkauskas, V., Moss, M., & Stoltenberg-Allen, K. *Health assessment.* St. Louis: Mosby, 1977.

5. Sauve, M.H., & Pecherer, A. *Concepts and skills in physical assessment.* Philadelphia: Saunders, 1977.
6. Frank-Stromborg, M., & Stromborg, P. *Primary care assessment and management skills for nurses: A self-assessment manual.* Philadelphia: Lippincott, 1979.
7. Dubos, R. Health and creative adaptation. *Human Nature,* 1978, *1,* 74–82.
8. Getchell, L. Adult physical fitness evaluation. Personal communication, April 1980.
9. Borgman M.F. Exercise and health maintenance. *Journal of Nursing Education,* 1977, *16,* 6–10.
10. Getchell, L. *Physical fitness: A way of life* (2nd ed.). New York: Wiley, 1979, pp. 78–79.
11. *Ibid.,* pp. 79–80.
12. Rochmis, P., & Blackburn, H. Exercise tests: A survey of procedures, safety and litagation experience in approximately 170,000 tests. *Journal of the American Medical Association,* 1971, *216,* 1061.
13. Getchell, *op. cit.,* pp. 70–73.
14. *Ibid.,* pp. 51–57.
15. Larsen, G.A., Malmboy, R.O.. *Coronary heart disease and physical fitness.* Baltimore: University Park Press, 1971.
16. Cooper, K.H. *The new aerobics.* New York: Evans, 1970.
17. Seltzer, C.C., & Mayer, J.A. Simple criterion of obesity. *Postgraduate Medicine,* 1965, *38,* A101.
18. U.S. Senate Select Committee on Nutrition and Human Needs. *Dietary goals for the United States.* Washington, D.C.: Government Printing Office, December 1977.
19. Suitor, C.W., & Hunter, M.F. *Nutrition: Principles and application in health promotion.* Philadelphia: Lippincott, 1980, Appendix 3, pp. 425–434.
20. Caliendo, M.A.. *Nutrition and preventive health care.* New York: Macmillan, 1981, Appendix I, pp. 648–655.
21. Suitor & Hunter, *op. cit.,* pp. 440–441.
22. LaDou, J., Sherwood, J.N., & Hughes, L. Health hazard appraisal in patient counseling (preventive medicine). *Western Journal of Medicine,* 1975, *122,* 177–180.
23. Steinbach, M. Risk factors and their interaction. *Revue Roumaine de Medecine Interne,* 1973, *10,* 355–363.
24. Robbins, L.C., & Hall, J.H. *How to practice prospective medicine.* Indianapolis: Slaymaker Enterprises, 1970.
25. Hall, J., & Zwemer, J: *Prospective medicine.* Indianapolis: Slaymaker Enterprises, 1979.
26. U.S. Department of Health and Human Services. Public Health Service. Office of Disease Prevention and Health Promotion. Office of Health Information, Health Promotion and Physical Fitness and Sports Medicine. Health Risk Appraisals: An Inventory. PHS Publication No. 81-50163 (June 1981).
26a. Sennott, L. Value-expectancy Theory and Health Behavior: An Exploration of Motivating Variables. Dissertation, University of Arizona, Tucson, 1980.
27. Langer, T., & Michael, S. *Life stress and mental health.* New York: Free Press, 1960.
28. Holmes, T., & Rahe, R: The social readjustment rating scale. *Journal of Psychosomatic Research,* 1967, *11,* 213.
29. *Ibid.*
30. Spielberger, C.D., Gorsach, R.L., & Lushene, R.E. *State-trait anxiety inventory manual.* Palo Alto, Calif.: Consulting Psychologists Press, 1970.
31. Everly, G.S., & Girdano, D.A. *The stress mess solution.* Bowie, Md.: Robert J. Brady, 1980.
32. Walters, D. Stress management seminar format. Personal Communication, Topeka, Kan., Menninger Foundation, 1980.
33. Larson, R. Thirty years of research on the subjective well-being of older Americans. *Journal of Gerontology,* 1978, *33,* 109–129.

34. Wan, T.T.W., & Livieratos, B. Interpreting a general index of subjective well-being. *Milbank Memorial Fund Quarterly/Health and Society,* 1978, *56,* 531–556.
35. Oelbaum, C.H. Hallmarks of adult wellness. *American Journal of Nursing,* 1974, *74,* 1623–1625.
36. Travis, J.W. *Wellness workbook for health professionals: A guide to attaining high level wellness.* Mill Valley, Calif.: Wellness Resource Center, 1977.
37. Kaplan, R.M., Bush, J.W., & Berry, C.C. Health status: Types of validity and the index of well-being. *Health Services Research,* Winter 1976, *11,* 478–507.
38. Belloc, N.B., & Breslow, L. Relationship of physical health status and health practices. *Preventive Medicine,* 1972, *1,* 409–421.
39. Wallston, B.S., & Wallston, K.A. Locus of control and health: A review of the literature. *Health Education Monographs,* 1978, *6,* 107–117.
40. Wallston, B.S., Wallston, K.A., Kaplan, G.D., & Maides, S.A. Development and validation of the Health Locus of Control (HLC) scale. *Journal of Consulting and Clinical Psychology,* 1976, *44,* 580–585.
41. Wallston, K.A., Maides, S., Wallston, B.S. Health-related information seeking as a function of health related locus of control and health value. *Journal of Research in Personality,* 1976, *10,* 215–222.
42. Wallston, K.A., Wallston, B.S., & DeVellis, R. Development of the Multidimensional Health Locus of Control (MHLC) scales. *Health Education Monographs,* 1978, *6,* 161–170.
43. Hogan, R. *Human sexuality: A nursing perspective.* New York: Appleton, 1980.
44. Friedman, M.M. *Family nursing: Theory and assessment.* New York: Appleton, 1981.

# CHAPTER 6
# Values Clarification

Advances in understanding human values have come about through the work of individuals in many disciplines, e.g., psychology, political science, philosophy, sociology, biology (bioethics), education, and communications. Exploration of the value concept in such diverse fields attests to the centrality of values in understanding human behavior. Values appear to be critical mediating variables in human actions or reactions to environmental stimuli. Values emerge over time as a result of development, personal experiences, interpersonal relations, and social circumstances. The importance of values in shaping health-protecting or health-promoting behaviors cannot be denied. In fact, both the Modified Health-Belief Model and the proposed Health-Promotion Model include importance (value) of health as a key motivational factor. The personal value placed on reducing the threat of illness and/or enhancing health status appears to affect the frequency and intensity with which health-protecting and health-promoting behaviors are practiced.

A *value* can be defined as an enduring belief that a specific mode of conduct or a particular end-state of existence is personally or socially preferable.[1] Values are organized into value systems that are relatively unchanging over time.[2] Individual value systems reflect personal needs, culture, society, and significant reference groups.[3] Because no two individuals have the same life experiences, no two personal value systems are exactly the same.

Rokeach,[4] in *The Nature of Human Values*, has identified five assumptions about values:

1. The total number of values that a person possesses is relatively small.
2. All persons everywhere possess the same values but to differing degrees.
3. Values are organized into value systems.
4. The antecedents of human values can be traced to culture, society, institutions and personality.
5. The consequences of human values will be manifested in virtually all phenomena that social scientists might consider worth investigating and understanding.

Two types of values are described by Rokeach: terminal values and instrumental values. Terminal values are concerned with desired end-states or goals, while instrumental values focus on desirable modes of conduct. A diagram of the two types of values is presented in Figure 6-1.

At the core of each personal value system is the self-concept. Changes in any part of the system affect the self-concept, other values, and subsequent behavior.[5] Shifts in human values have two possible outcomes: (a) greater consistency of values or among values, self-concept, and behavior and (b) increased value/value, value/self-concept, or value/behavior conflict.[6]

In the health care setting, values of the nurse, client, and society come together and interact. The outcomes of the interaction will depend on the level of self-awareness of the nurse and the extent to which the nurse can assist clients in clarifying their own values. At this point, a distinction must be made between *values clarification* and *values change:*

- Values clarification is the increased personal awareness of value priorities or degree of consistency between values and related attitudes and behavior.
- Values change is the reprioritization of values, abandonment of existing values, or acquisition of new values, and subsequent attitude and behavior change.

Values clarification will be discussed at length in this chapter. Values change will be covered in Chapter 9, under the topic of self-confrontation.

All behaviors express values in some way. Values determine the behaviors that will be enacted in order to adjust to the environment or to achieve higher levels of health and self-actualization.[7] The process of valuing has been described by Raths, Harmin, and Simon[8] as consisting of three phases and seven distinct steps. The valuing process is depicted in Table 6-1. From this process, specific values emerge in a hierarchical structure that serves as a guide to personal conduct, lifestyle, and interactions with others.

What should be the role of the nurse in values clarification as he or she works with children, adolescents, and adults in a variety of different health care settings? In the view of the author, the nurse plays a critical role in assisting clients to

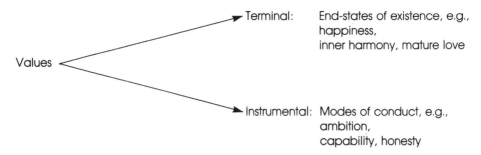

**FIGURE 6-1.** Types of values. *(From Rokeach, M. The nature of human values. New York: Free Press, 1973, with permission.)*

---

**TABLE 6-1   THE VALUING PROCESS**

| | |
|---|---|
| Choosing: | (1) Choosing values freely |
| | (2) Choosing from alternatives |
| | (3) Thoughtfully considering the consequences or outcomes of each alternative |
| Prizing: | (4) Cherishing, being happy with the choice |
| | (5) Willing to make values known to others |
| Acting: | (6) Doing something with the choice |
| | (7) Integrating values into life style |

From Raths, L.E., Harmin, M., & Simons, S.B. *Values and teaching: Working with values in the classroom.* Columbus, Ohio: Charles E. Merrill, 1966. With permission.

clarify personal values, make self-initiated changes in value hierarchies, reduce conflicts, and achieve greater consistency among values, attitudes, and behaviors in areas relevant to prevention and health promotion. In order to assist clients in this way, nurses must rely heavily on their counseling skills, seeking assistance as needed from nurse, counselor, or psychologist colleagues.

## STRATEGIES FOR VALUES CLARIFICATION

Modern life offers multiple choices that make selection a bewildering problem. While choices should set paths of action that individuals wish to follow, consistent behavior is required to "act out" the values that clients hold.[9,10] Values clarification can facilitate decision making and problem solving in the area of health by promoting behavior consistent with health-related values.[11] Values clarification can also serve as a consciousness-raising activity for clients by increasing awareness of personal priorities, identifying ambiguities or confusion in priorities, and determining what major value/behavior conflicts or inconsistencies exist. The notion behind values clarification is that awareness of ambiguities, conflicts, or inconsistencies will result in self-dissatisfaction (dissatisfaction with the self-concept). In an effort to enhance self-esteem, clients will make the changes necessary to decrease inconsistencies.

Many problems throughout the life span stem from not having adequately worked through value issues in the areas of work, school, leisure, religion, health, family, and friends at an early age. The aim of the values-clarifying process is not to impose a value, course of action, opinion, or solution on clients but to encourage them to look at alternatives and their consequences.[12] The nurse is encouraged to review the strategies presented in this chapter and carefully consider their usefulness for individual clients within his or her current caseload.

## EXAMINING VALUE HIERARCHIES

A number of instruments have been developed to determine the value hierarchies of individuals. One of the most frequently used instruments for measuring values is the Value Survey developed by Rokeach.[13] It is composed of two parts in which terminal values and instrumental values can be ranked. Wallston and Wallston adapted the Value Survey to include "health" as a value and developed the Health Value Scale.[14] Kavanagh[15] recently presented helpful reviews on six additional value instruments. He suggested use of the following tools for examining personal values in the counseling setting:

1. The Allport–Vernon–Lindzey Study of Values (SV)[16]
2. The Survey of Personal Values (SPV)[17]
3. The Survey of Interpersonal Values (SIV)[18]
4. The Differential Value Profile (DVP)[19]
5. The Personal Orientation Inventory (POI)[20,21]
6. Ways to Live[22]

Since review of each of the above instruments is beyond the scope of this book, the reader is referred to *The Mental Measurements Yearbook*[23] for further descriptive details. The *Yearbook* will provide information about the scope of the instruments, reliability, validity, qualifications for administration, and publishing scource. As examples of value-assessment tools available, the Value Survey and Health Value Scale will be presented and discussed.

### Value Survey[24]

The survey consists of two lists, each containing 18 values. The first list contains terminal values; the second list contains instrumental values. Test-retest reliability for the survey has been found to be between 0.69 and 0.80 on terminal values and between 0.61 and 0.72 on instrumental values. Reliability data are based primarily on college populations. The Value Survey uses gummed stickers on pressure-sensitive paper so that the stickers can be removed initially and arranged in the preferred order. They can also be rearranged until the client is sure that the order of ranking represents an accurate presentation of personal perceptions of values. This instrument provides information on 36 values and can be completed by the client in 15 to 20 minutes. The instructions and survey items appear in Figure 6-2.

A major limitation of the Value Survey for purposes of client counseling is that "health" is not included in the list of 18 terminal values. The author would suggest inclusion of "health" in the list for clinical use but cautions the reader that this change may alter the reliability and validity of the instrument.

The Health Value Scale presented next is a shortened version of Rokeach's Terminal Value Survey with "health" added as a value. The nurse as health counselor may choose to use the original Value Survey, adapt it by the inclusion of "health," or use the Health Value Scale.

Below are 18 values listed in alphabetical order. Your task is to arrange them in order of their importance to YOU, as guiding principles in YOUR life. Each value is printed on a gummed label that can be easily peeled off and pasted in the boxes on the left-hand side of the page. Study the list carefully and pick out the one value that is the most important for you. Peel it off and paste it in Box 1 on the left. Then pick out the value that is second-most important for you. Peel it off and paste it in Box 2. Then do the same for each of the remaining values. The value that is least important goes in Box 18. Work slowly and think carefully. If you change your mind, feel free to change your answers. The labels peel off easily and can be moved from place to place. The end result should truly show how you really feel.

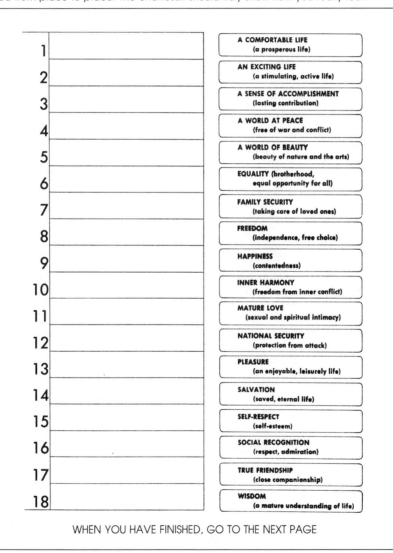

1
2
3
4
5
6
7
8
9
10
11
12
13
14
15
16
17
18

**A COMFORTABLE LIFE**
(a prosperous life)

**AN EXCITING LIFE**
(a stimulating, active life)

**A SENSE OF ACCOMPLISHMENT**
(lasting contribution)

**A WORLD AT PEACE**
(free of war and conflict)

**A WORLD OF BEAUTY**
(beauty of nature and the arts)

**EQUALITY** (brotherhood,
equal opportunity for all)

**FAMILY SECURITY**
(taking care of loved ones)

**FREEDOM**
(independence, free choice)

**HAPPINESS**
(contentedness)

**INNER HARMONY**
(freedom from inner conflict)

**MATURE LOVE**
(sexual and spiritual intimacy)

**NATIONAL SECURITY**
(protection from attack)

**PLEASURE**
(an enjoyable, leisurely life)

**SALVATION**
(saved, eternal life)

**SELF-RESPECT**
(self-esteem)

**SOCIAL RECOGNITION**
(respect, admiration)

**TRUE FRIENDSHIP**
(close companionship)

**WISDOM**
(a mature understanding of life)

WHEN YOU HAVE FINISHED, GO TO THE NEXT PAGE

**FIGURE 6-2.** Value survey (continued on next page). (*Distributed by Halgren Tests, 873 Persimmon Ave., Sunnyvale, California 94087. Reprinted from Rokeach, M. The nature of human values. New York: Free Press, 1973, pp. 357–361. With permission.*)

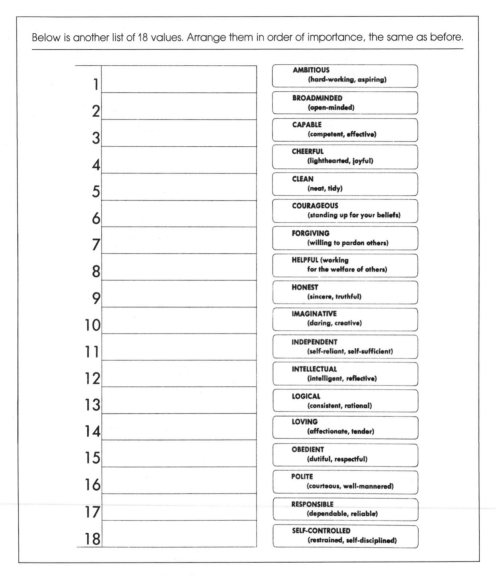

Below is another list of 18 values. Arrange them in order of importance, the same as before.

|  | |  |
|---|---|---|
| 1 | | **AMBITIOUS** (hard-working, aspiring) |
| 2 | | **BROADMINDED** (open-minded) |
| 3 | | **CAPABLE** (competent, effective) |
| 4 | | **CHEERFUL** (lighthearted, joyful) |
| 5 | | **CLEAN** (neat, tidy) |
| 6 | | **COURAGEOUS** (standing up for your beliefs) |
| 7 | | **FORGIVING** (willing to pardon others) |
| 8 | | **HELPFUL** (working for the welfare of others) |
| 9 | | **HONEST** (sincere, truthful) |
| 10 | | **IMAGINATIVE** (daring, creative) |
| 11 | | **INDEPENDENT** (self-reliant, self-sufficient) |
| 12 | | **INTELLECTUAL** (intelligent, reflective) |
| 13 | | **LOGICAL** (consistent, rational) |
| 14 | | **LOVING** (affectionate, tender) |
| 15 | | **OBEDIENT** (dutiful, respectful) |
| 16 | | **POLITE** (courteous, well-mannered) |
| 17 | | **RESPONSIBLE** (dependable, reliable) |
| 18 | | **SELF-CONTROLLED** (restrained, self-disciplined) |

**FIGURE 6-2** (continued).

**Health Value Scale[25]**

The Health Value Scale is an adaptation of Rokeach's Terminal Value Survey. The scale consists of ten values that the client is asked to rank in order of importance from 1 to 10. The Health Value Scale appears in Figure 6-3.

Interpretation of responses to the scale is straightforward. If health appears in the top four positions out of the ten positions possible, the client places a high value on health. If health appears in any other positions, the value placed on

Below you will find a list of ten values listed in alphabetical order. We would like you to arrange them in order of their importance to YOU, as guiding principles in YOUR life.

Study the list carefully and pick out the one value that is the most important for you. Write the number "1" in the space to the left of the most important value. Then pick out the value that is second-most important to you. Write the number "2" in the space to the left. Then continue in the same manner for the remaining values until you have included all ranks from 1 to 10. Each value will have a different rank.

We realize that some people find it difficult to distinguish the importance of some of these values. Do the best that you can, but please rank all 10 of them. The end result should truly show how YOU really feel.

_____ A COMFORTABLE LIFE (a prosperous life)

_____ AN EXCITING LIFE (a stimulating, active life)

_____ A SENSE OF ACCOMPLISHMENT (lasting contribution)

_____ FREEDOM (independence, free choice)

_____ HAPPINESS (contentedness)

_____ HEALTH (physical and mental well-being)

_____ INNER HARMONY (freedom from inner conflict)

_____ PLEASURE (an enjoyable, leisurely life)

_____ SELF-RESPECT (self-esteem)

_____ SOCIAL RECOGNITION (respect, admiration)

**FIGURE 6-3.** Health value scale. (*Adapted with permission from Rokeach, M. Value survey. Halpren Tests, Sunnyvale, Calif. Used with permission, from Wallston, B. S., Personal communication, 1980.*)

health is moderate (position 5, 6, 7) or low (position 8, 9, 10). In administering the scale, the nurse should encourage the client to rank the items in a way that most accurately reflects his or her value hierarchy. Care should be taken to avoid biasing the client and thus obtaining an inflated and inaccurate ranking of health as a personal value.

## CLARIFYING PERSONAL VALUES

The strategies suggested in this section are directed toward assisting clients in examining priorities, conflicts, or inconsistencies in personal value systems and congruency or lack of congruency between values and behavior. The strategies are based on the assumption that individuals set particular goals and wish to engage in behaviors that move them toward those goals. The purpose and procedure for each strategy will be described and appropriate materials for use with clients will be presented.

### Twenty Things I Love to Do[26]

*Purpose.* An important question for people of all ages to deal with is "Am I getting what I want out of life?" If living is to be rewarding, it should include activities that are prized highly and enjoyed. Clients may not know whether they are getting what they really want from life if they have not taken stock of their own needs and feelings. The purpose of this exercise is to help clients decide what activities bring them the most enjoyment.

*Procedure.* The client should be given the "Twenty Things I Love to Do" sheet presented in Figure 6-4 and encouraged to write down as many activities as possible that bring enjoyment or happiness. After the client has listed as many activities as possible, the nurse should ask the client to review the list and code all behaviors in the following way:

- A —Activities that I prefer to do alone
- P —Activities that I prefer to do with other people
- $ —Activities that cost more than $10 each time or require an initial major investment that I have not made yet
- PL—Activities that require advanced planning

In the *last time* column, the client should indicate how long it has been since engaging in each of the listed activities, and in the next column the client should rank from 1 to 5 (most enjoyable to less enjoyable) the five activities out of the list that are enjoyed most.

The content of the list can be reviewed with the client to assist in planning more frequent inclusion of enjoyable activities within his or her lifestyle. If possible, planning should center on the next few weeks or the next month, and encouragement should be given to the client to make concrete plans for engaging in the top-ranked activities in the near future. A projected time plan can be included in the "Plan Ahead" column. The client should achieve some degree of balance between things that he or she enjoys doing alone and activities that he or she enjoys doing with others. If the selected activities are expensive or require an initial outlay of money, the client may need to explore ways in which the necessary funds can be acquired or the cost of the activity decreased.

### The Real/Ideal Self

*Purpose.* The purpose of this strategy is to assist clients in comparing their value rankings on the Health Value Scale with what they picture as the ideal set of values for themselves.

*Procedure.* Before the client reviews the previous ranking of values, the personal ideal set of values should be completed on the scale shown in Figure 6-5. Most important value should be ranked "1" in the space to the left; the client continues

| Activities | A/P | $ | PL | Last Time | Rank Top Five (1–5) | Plan Ahead |
|---|---|---|---|---|---|---|
| 1 | | | | | | |
| 2 | | | | | | |
| 3 | | | | | | |
| 4 | | | | | | |
| 5 | | | | | | |
| 6 | | | | | | |
| 7 | | | | | | |
| 8 | | | | | | |
| 9 | | | | | | |
| 10 | | | | | | |
| 11 | | | | | | |
| 12 | | | | | | |
| 13 | | | | | | |
| 14 | | | | | | |
| 15 | | | | | | |
| 16 | | | | | | |
| 17 | | | | | | |
| 18 | | | | | | |
| 19 | | | | | | |
| 20 | | | | | | |

**FIGURE 6-4.** "Twenty things I love to do" sheet. (*Adapted from Simon S.B. Values clarification—a tool for counselors.* Personnel and Guidance Journal, *1973, 51, p. 616. With permission.*)

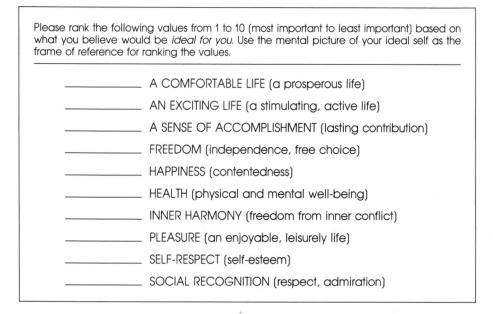

Please rank the following values from 1 to 10 (most important to least important) based on what you believe would be *ideal for you*. Use the mental picture of your ideal self as the frame of reference for ranking the values.

_____ A COMFORTABLE LIFE (a prosperous life)

_____ AN EXCITING LIFE (a stimulating, active life)

_____ A SENSE OF ACCOMPLISHMENT (lasting contribution)

_____ FREEDOM (independence, free choice)

_____ HAPPINESS (contentedness)

_____ HEALTH (physical and mental well-being)

_____ INNER HARMONY (freedom from inner conflict)

_____ PLEASURE (an enjoyable, leisurely life)

_____ SELF-RESPECT (self-esteem)

_____ SOCIAL RECOGNITION (respect, admiration)

**FIGURE 6-5.** My ideal set of values. (*Adapted from The Health Value Scale developed by Wallston, K.A., & Wallston, B.S., Health locus of control.* Health Education Monographs, *Spring 1978, 6.*)

ranking the remaining items until values are ranked from 1 to 10. The end result should be a picture of the client's ideal to which he or she can compare the rankings on the Health Value Scale during health assessment. If discrepancies are apparent between the real and ideal rankings, discussion can follow concerning how the client might move from the real toward the ideal.

**Values-Actions Review**
*Purpose.* The purpose of this strategy is to help the client determine how the values of most personal importance are expressed in activities of everyday living. Value-action discrepancies are major causes of frustration and conflict in life. Individuals identify goals that they are unable to reach because they do not engage in behaviors that consistently move them toward their desired goals. The consistency of personal values and actions is highly related to the level of satisfaction that a client experiences from a personal lifestyle.
*Procedure.* The client should use the form presented in Figure 6-6 and list the four most important personal values. Either real or ideal values may be used, or the same exercise can be completed with both if they differ considerably. Following each value, the client can identify those behaviors engaged in regularly that express important values. Upon completion of the Action-Values Review, additional behaviors that would assist the client in achieving personal goals can be discussed.

| Top Four Values | Actions I Take to Express These Values in Everyday Living |
| --- | --- |
| 1. | |
| 2. | |
| 3. | |
| 4. | |

**FIGURE 6-6.** Values-Actions review. This exercise uses responses from the Health Value Scale or the Value Survey—terminal or instrumental values.

The possibility of incorporating these new behaviors into personal lifestyle or daily activities can be explored.

### Pie of Life[27]

*Purpose.* This technique allows the client to inventory his or her own life in terms of how time is spent during typical work or leisure days. The Pie of Life can assist the client in identifying value/time inconsistencies. An analysis of how personal time is spent should show that values of highest priority are allocated the most time and effort. As an example, while the client may indicate that a high value is placed on health, review of a typical day may show that little time is devoted to protecting or enhancing personal health.

*Procedure.* The client is to indicate on the Pie of Life Form presented in Figure 6-7 how he or she spends a typical work day (in an occupation or, if a housewife, at home) and a typical leisure day. Each pie is divided into quarters that represent six-hour segments. The short lines around the circumference of the circle represent one-hour segments of time. In all, the pie totals 24 hours. The client may work with the categories listed below the circles or add additional categories to describe more appropriately how a typical day is spent.

Following completion of the two pies, the client should be directed to think about the following questions:

1. Are you satisfied with the relative sizes of your slices?
2. Ideally, how big would you want each slice to be?
3. Realistically, is there anything you can do to begin to change the size of some of your slices?

The nurse should stress to the client that there is no right way to section the pie. There is also no need to change if the client is happy with the way personal time is spent. If the client wishes to change, decisions about the direction of change must be made by the client. The nature of changes should be consistent with previously identified values and goals.

### Personal/Family Values

*Purpose.* The purpose of this exercise is to assist the client in determining what personal values are shared with family members. Shared values assist families in moving toward mutually desirable goals. If values of family members are very diverse, the exercise may have to be completed for each member.

*Procedure.* The client should work from a hierarchical list of personal values that has been completed. This may be the Value Survey (terminal or instrumental) or the Health Value Scale. The rank order number previously assigned each value should be placed within one of the segments of the two circles in Figure 6-8. The client should write in additional personal values not shared by his or her family or, conversely, values considered high-priority by the family but not of high-priority for the client. Review of the results will allow the client to determine

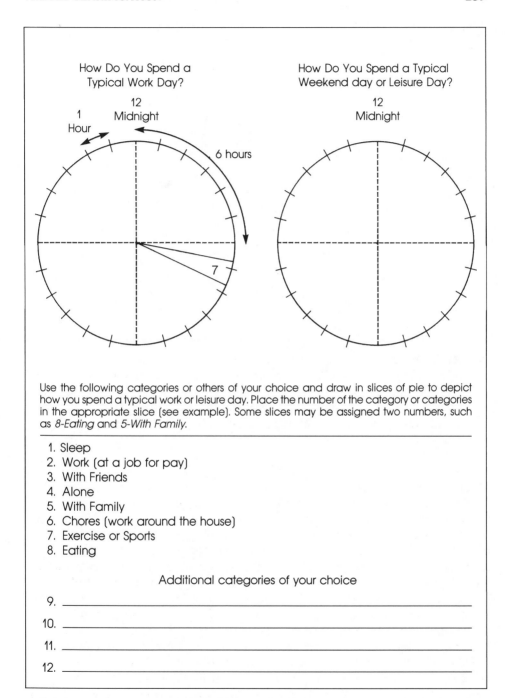

How Do You Spend a Typical Work Day?

How Do You Spend a Typical Weekend day or Leisure Day?

Use the following categories or others of your choice and draw in slices of pie to depict how you spend a typical work or leisure day. Place the number of the category or categories in the appropriate slice (see example). Some slices may be assigned two numbers, such as *8-Eating* and *5-With Family.*

1. Sleep
2. Work (at a job for pay)
3. With Friends
4. Alone
5. With Family
6. Chores (work around the house)
7. Exercise or Sports
8. Eating

Additional categories of your choice

9. _____

10. _____

11. _____

12. _____

**FIGURE 6-7.** The pie of life. (*Adapted from Simon, S.B., Howe, L.W.,Kirschenbaum, H.* Values clarification: A handbook of practical strategies for teachers and students. *New York: Hart, 1972. With permission.*)

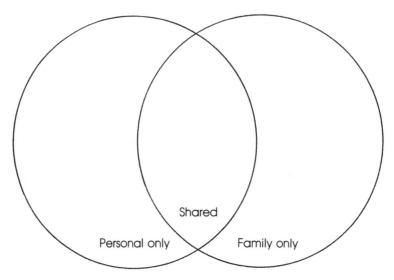

**FIGURE 6-8.** Personal-Family Values.

whether the highest-ranked personal values are shared with people who are close. This information can be used as a basis for discussion of family interactions, extent of agreement on important values, and ways that families can move together toward shared values and goals. A discussion of the mutuality of health as a value can provide insight into personal and family predisposition to engage in health behaviors.

**Alternatives/Consequences Search[28]**
***Purpose.*** The purpose of this strategy is to assist the client in considering alternatives to current lifestyle or ways of dealing with specific problems. Alternatives and the resultant consequences should be carefully considered before making a decision regarding a particular course of action to be pursued. The client is encouraged to identify challenge questions that set the stage for considering various action alternatives, for example, *How can I increase physical fitness? How can I make more friends?* and *How can I gain greater control over personal health status?* Instead of functioning primarily on the basis of habit, life should be lived in consideration of the full range of alternative actions available.
***Procedure.*** At the top of the form presented in Figure 6-9, the client should place a challenge question that represents the dilemma or problem that he or she wishes to address. As many alternative actions as possible that address the problem should be listed in the left-hand column of the form. The consequences of each alternative action should be enumerated. The extent to which the client is willing to try each alternative should be based on consideration of the consequences that are most appealing and the practicality of each action for that particular client.

### Blocks to Action[29]

*Purpose.* Acting on one's beliefs and values is a critical part of the valuing process. Blocks to Action is a strategy that should be used as a follow-up activity to the Alternatives/Consequences Search to assist clients in implementing the action alternatives selected. Barriers to action may be perceived or real, internal or external. Regardless of the source of the barrier, action may be inhibited if the barriers are not recognized and removed.

*Procedure.* On the Discovering Blocks to Action Form presented in Figure 6-10, clients should list the action alternatives that they are willing to try or consider as indicated in responses to the Alternatives/Consequences Search. In the second column, barriers to taking action should be listed. Each barrier should be coded in the third column as either within the client (*W*) or outside the client (*O*). In the right-hand column, steps that can be taken to remove or reduce barriers should be identified. Following completion of the written exercise, the extent to which perceived barriers actually exist can be discussed. The client is encouraged to look at personal strengths and potential for dealing with barriers that thwart purposeful health protecting and health-promoting activity.

### Value Support System

*Purpose.* The purpose of this strategy is to allow the client to identify individuals who support the values that are most important personally. This technique expands on the Personal/Family Values exercise presented earlier. Having people available for support is important in encouraging behaviors that move clients toward goals reflecting important personal values. If individuals who are close to the client do not share his or her values, this poses a threat to the personal value system and self-concept. The degree of threat depends on the personal strength of the client.

*Procedure.* The client can use the form presented in Figure 6-11, indicating at the top of the page a specific value that he or she wishes to consider. A different form can be used for each value. In the left-hand column, the client should list individual family members, friends, co-workers, and additional significant others. The client can indicate whether each person identified supports, is neutral to, or does not support the target personal value being considered. Important determinants of the effect of others on the client are emotional closeness and frequency of interaction. The client can include these factors in the analysis in the right-hand column. This exercise allows the client to look at the scope and strength of external support for important personal values.

### Review of Health-Related Behavior

*Purpose.* The purpose of this exercise is specifically to encourage the client to focus on health as a value and look at the impact of personal behaviors on health status. The client should be encouraged to look at health-promoting behaviors that were performed during the previous week, about which he or she felt proud or good. Health-damaging behaviors that were undesirable to the client should also be identified.

Challenge Question:

| Alternatives | Consequences | Place Check in Appropriate Column | | |
|---|---|---|---|---|
| | | I'LL TRY IT | I'LL CONSIDER IT | I WON'T TRY IT |
| 1. | 1. | | | |
| | 2. | | | |
| | 3. | | | |
| | 4. | | | |
| | 5. | | | |
| | 6. | | | |
| 2. | 1. | | | |
| | 2. | | | |
| | 3. | | | |
| | 4. | | | |
| | 5. | | | |
| | 6. | | | |

| | | | | |
|---|---|---|---|---|
| 3. | 1. | | | |
| | 2. | | | |
| | 3. | | | |
| | 4. | | | |
| | 5. | | | |
| | 6. | | | |
| 4. | 1. | | | |
| | 2. | | | |
| | 3. | | | |
| | 4. | | | |
| | 5. | | | |
| | 6. | | | |

**FIGURE 6-9.** Alternatives/Consequences Search Sheet. *(Adapted from Simon S.B.: Values clarification: A tool for counselors.* Personnel and Guidance Journal 51:*615, 1973. With permission.)*

| Alternatives I Will Try Or Consider | Blocks to Action | Source of Blocks W: Within O: Outside | Suggestions for Removing Blocks |
|---|---|---|---|
| 1. | | | |
| 2. | | | |
| 3. | | | |

**FIGURE 6-10.** Discovering blocks to action form.

| Alternatives I Will Try Or Consider | Blocks to Action | Source of Blocks W: Within O: Outside | Suggestions for Removing Blocks |
|---|---|---|---|
| 4. | | | |

**FIGURE 6-10** (continued).

*Procedure.* The client should be provided with a form similar to the one depicted in Figure 6-12. In the left-hand column, the client can list both health-promoting and health-damaging behaviors during the previous 7 days. Each health-promoting behavior should be considered in terms of when it could be repeated again. A specific time commitment should be made. For each health-damaging behavior, factors that encourage the behavior need to be explored and ways of discouraging the behavior identified. This exercise focuses the client on personal strengths in the area of health promotion and heightens awareness of behaviors detrimental to health.

## SUMMARY

The values-clarification strategies presented in this chapter are directed toward helping the client make important decisions about personal lifestyle. Each individual must ultimately choose those values that will serve as standards for personal actions and interactions with others. Some clients may have given little consideration to their own personal values and less attention to whether they hold conflicting values or whether their behavior is supportive of the values that they hold. Self-understanding is the first step toward taking action to reinforce and strengthen those behaviors that are consistent with established values.

Value:

| Individual | Support | Neutral | Do Not Support | Emotional Closeness VC: Very Close MC: Moderately Close D: Distant | Frequency of Interaction/Week |
|---|---|---|---|---|---|
| Family members | | | | | |
| Friends | | | | | |

| | | | | |
|---|---|---|---|---|
| Co-workers | | | | |
| Additional significant others | | | | |

**FIGURE 6-11.** Analysis of value support system.

What did you do this week that was health promoting or health damaging?

| Health Promoting | Can You Plan to Do It Again? | When? |
|---|---|---|
|  |  |  |
| Health Damaging | What Encouraged It? | What Could Discourage It? |
|  |  |  |

**FIGURE 6-12.**   Review of health-related behavior.

## REFERENCES

1. Rokeach, M. *The Nature of human values*. New York: Free Press, 1973, p. 5.
2. Rokeach, M., & Regan, J.F. The role of values in the counseling situation. *Personnel and Guidance Journal,* May 1980, 576–583.
3. Rokeach, 1973, *op. cit.,* p. 5.
4. *Ibid.,* p. 3.

5.  Conroy, W.J. Human values, smoking behavior and public health programs. In Rokeach, M.(Ed.), *Understanding human values: Individual and societal.* New York: Free Press, 1979, pp 199–209.

6.  Rescher, N. *Introduction to value theory.* Englewood Cliffs, N.J.: Prentice-Hall, 1969, pp. 111–115.

7.  Rokeach & Regan, 1980, *op. cit.*

8.  Raths, L.E., Harmin, M., & Simon, S.B. *Values and teaching: Working with values in the classroom.* Columbus, Ohio: Charles E. Merrill, 1966.

9.  Governali, J.F., Sechrist, W.C. Clarifying values in a health education setting: An experimental analysis. *Journal of School Health,* 1980, *50,* 151–154.

10.  Raths, Harmin, & Simon, *op. cit.,* p, 27.

11.  Casteel, J.D., & Stahl, R.J. *Value clarification in the classroom: A primer.* Pacific Palisades, Calif., Good Year, 1975.

12.  Glaser, B., & Kirschbaum, H. Using values clarification in a counseling setting. *Personnel and Guidance Journal,* May 1980, 569–575.

13.  Rokeach, 1973, *op. cit.,* pp. 357–361.

14.  Wallston, K.A., & Wallston, B.S. Health locus of control. *Health Education Monographs,* Spring 1978, *6.*

15.  Kavanagh, H.B. Some appraised instruments of values for counselors. *Personnel and Guidance Journal,* May 1980, 613–617.

16.  Allport, G.W., Vernon, P.E., & Lindzey, G. *Study of values,* (3rd ed.). Boston: Houghton Mifflin, 1960.

17.  *Ibid.*

18.  *Ibid..*

19.  Thomas, W.L. *The differential value profile.* Chicago: W. and J. Stone Foundation, 1963.

20.  Shostrom, E.L. *The personal orientation inventory.* San Diego, Calif.: Educational and Industrial Testing Service, 1963.

21.  Shostrom, E.L. *Actualizing therapy.* San Diego, Calif.: Edits, 1976.

22.  Morris, C.W. *Varieties of human value.* Chicago: University of Chicago Press, 1956.

23.  Buros, O.K.(Ed.). *The mental measurements yearbook* (8th ed.). Highland Park, N.J.: Gryphon Press, 1978.

24.  Rokeach, 1973, *op. cit.,* pp. 27–54.

25.  Kaplan, G.D., & Cowles, A. Health locus of control and health value in the prediction of smoking reduction. *Health Education Monographs,* Spring 1978, *6,* 129–137.

26.  Hawley, R.C., & Hawley, I.L. *Human values in the classroom: A handbook for teachers.* New York: Hart, 1975.

27.  Simon, S.B., Howe, L.W., & Kirschbaum, H. *Values Clarification: A handbook of practical strategies for teachers and students.* New York: Hart, 1972.

28.  *Ibid.* pp. 198–203, 207–208.

29.  *Ibid.*

# CHAPTER 7
# Health Education for Self-Care

Individuals spend the vast majority of their lives actively involved in caring for themselves. Self-care is a universal requirement for sustaining and enhancing life and health. The competence with which this task is accomplished determines the quality of life experienced and has a significant impact on longevity. Health education is the medium through which health professionals, such as nurses, physicians, and health educators, assist clients in achieving competence in self-care. Since the terms *self-care* and *health education* are encountered frequently in health-promotion literature, it is important to define both concepts early in this chapter.

- *Self-care* refers to activities that individuals personally initiate and perform on their own behalf in maintaining or enhancing life, health, and well-being.[1]
- *Health education* is a process that informs, motivates, and helps people to adopt and maintain healthful practices and lifestyles, advocates environmental changes as needed to facilitate this goal, and conducts professional training and research to the same end.[2]

Self-care is both an ongoing activity and a competence to be developed. Conceptually, the term includes much more than ability to carry out activities of daily living. While competence in such activities is part of self-care, care of self also includes actions directed toward minimizing threats to personal health, self-nurturance, self-improvement, and personal growth. The client serves as the primary resource within the health care system.[3] It has been estimated that informal self-care constitutes about 75 percent of all health care within the United States. In addition, at least 25 percent of the health problems seen by physicians could be taken care of by the individuals themselves without professional help.[4] While self-care within the medical model has been primarily defined as compliance with therapeutic regimens, self-care for health promotion requires that clients gain knowledge and competencies that can be used to maintain and enhance health in addition to the knowledge and skills required for self-care in illness.

**150**

## THE ROLE OF THE PROFESSIONAL NURSE

Professional nurses have a major responsibility for enhancing clients' capacity for self-care. Orem has developed a Self-Care Nursing Model that describes three systems within professional nursing practice: a compensatory system, a partially compensatory system, and an educative/developmental system.[5] In compensatory care, the nurse provides total care for the patient. Such care is most common in intensive-, acute-care settings within hospitals during severe illness. Partially compensatory care is implemented when the nurse and the patient share the responsibility for care. Care during rehabilitation from illness or in advanced chronic illness is partially compensatory. In contrast to the preceding two types of care, the educative/developmental nursing system gives the client primary responsibility for personal health, with the nurse functioning in a consultative capacity. It is this third nursing system that is most appropriate for health protection and health promotion.

Major areas of education for self-care that are important in maintaining or enhancing health include exercise and physical fitness, nutrition and weight control, stress management, maintenance of social support systems, and environmental control. All of these areas are addressed within the content of this book. Specific nursing functions to assist clients in developing competency in these self-care areas include enhancing self-care competencies, preventing loss of self-care competencies, overcoming self-care deficits, and enhancing clients' care capacities for others as well as care capacities of significant others for clients.[6]

Self-care is an appropriate area of health teaching for individuals of all ages. The public relies heavily on health care personnel as a source of such information. In a national sample of 659 adults, Freimuth and Marron[7] found that 71 percent of the population reported receiving information from health personnel, with the reliability of the information estimated to be 91 percent. Fifty-one percent of the population reported getting health information from public-service announcements, with an estimated 77-percent reliability. Forty-nine percent received information from family and friends, with a 50-percent estimate of reliability. Results of the study indicate that health personnel are the most frequent and most trusted sources of health information. The Health-Promotion Model presented in Chapter 4 makes it very clear that interactions with health professionals is an important interpersonal variable in facilitating self-care for health promotion.

Within the past five years, the public has indicated a marked increase in concern and motivation to take an active part in its own care. There are, of course, exceptions to this generalization; however, the trend is clearly evident in the proliferation of courses and materials to facilitate self-care. One of the earliest programs developed was *The Activated Patient: A Course Guide,* developed by Sehnert at Georgetown University.[8,9] The major thrust of this and similar programs is to assist clients in becoming knowledgeable partners in maintaining and promoting personal health.

Nurses have long recognized the right of clients of all ages to be both informed and active participants in care. Now as never before, nurses are faced with the exciting challenge of developing the educative/developmental component of nursing practice. Through health education and counseling, positive health practices can be encouraged and the overall impact of the health delivery system greatly improved as clients assume more responsibility for their own care.[10]

Many interesting examples of nurses actively involved in health education for self-care can be cited. Wherever nurses and clients interact, opportunities abound for educative/developmental intervention. As one example, Judy Igoe, a school nurse practitioner in Denver, Colorado, has developed programs for primary care of children of all ages within the school setting.[11] Use of games, such as "Winning at Wellness"[12] and Project Health P.A.C.T. (Participatory and Assertive Consumer Training),[13] prepare children and adolescents to engage in health-promoting behaviors and to assume a more active and responsible role in use of existing health care services.

Another nurse, Maureen Becker, of Minneapolis, Minnesota, working with a consortium of 110 physicians of various specialties in a large medical complex, is responsible for health education of clients. In addition, her responsibilities include the developing, marketing, and presenting of health education programs on self-care for prevention and health promotion within the community. Affiliation with a group of physicians provides access to clients for educative/developmental care, as well as third-party pay for such services.

## DOES EDUCATION FOR SELF-CARE WORK?

Health education is currently being challenged on many fronts in regard to its impact on health-related behavior and subsequently on the health status of individuals and groups. However, an increasing number of studies are providing evidence that health education can result in sustained behavioral change. The results of the Stanford Three Community Study are an outstanding example of the impact of health education on individual behavior. The study consisted of a two-year health education campaign directed at changing dietary behavior among the target populations to decrease the risk of cardiovascular disease. Mass media health education was carried out in two communities, with a third community serving as the control. In one of the experimental communities, mass media health education was supplemented by intensive personal counseling for high-risk individuals.

Analysis of the data on average daily consumption of cholesterol, saturated fat, and polyunsaturated fat revealed that the health education campaign had resulted in a 20- to 40-percent decrease in cholesterol and saturated fat consumption among both men and women. Intensively instructed men tended to outperform men exposed to mass media alone, while women responded equally well to mass media and counseling approaches. Mean changes in plasma cholesterol concentration for the various groups under study correlated with those that would have been predicted on the basis of self-reported changes in dietary behavior.

Personal counseling plus mass media resulted in more rapid changes, but repeated exposure to mass media tended to close the gap between the extent of behavior change in the two experimental communities. Improvements were maintained over the two years of the study, indicating the potential of health education for significantly changing health behaviors.[14] The critical aspect of health education in this study appeared to be the teaching of specific skills to promote the use of the information presented.

Rosenberg[15] reported that patients with congestive heart failure who attended a health education group had two-thirds less hospital readmission time in days and half the number of readmissions, compared to a control group without health education. The health education group also complied better with their medical regimen and achieved a lower intake of sodium in their diets than did the control group. Similar results were reported by Levine[16] for patients with hypertension. Individuals who received an educational program reported greater compliance with medical directions, greater weight loss, and more appointments kept than did a control group. In the experimental group, 66 percent had their blood pressure controlled, while only 44 percent showed control in the nonexperimental group. In a study of 88 hypertensive clients over a 5-month period, Given, Given, and Simoni[17] found a significant correlation between the level of knowledge and the extent of patient compliance with the therapeutic regimen.

At the Swedish Wellness Center in Englewood, Colorado, a 6-month pilot wellness program was conducted, with 100 hospital employees as participants. The wellness program included emphasis in the areas of nutrition, stress management, physical fitness, and environmental sensitivity. A battery of tests administered before the program and 6 months later showed that employees who completed all elements of the program experienced significant positive changes in all wellness areas.[18]

While many additional studies are needed to determine the parameters of effective health education and to identify factors affecting population responsiveness, research to date should encourage professional nurses to move ahead in the development and evaluation of health education programs for self-care.

## PUBLIC DEMAND FOR HEALTH EDUCATION

With the advent of modern medical technology, self-care fell into disrepute and was essentially ignored or relegated to "folk medicine" and "quackery."[19] Modern medicine brought with it an "exclusivity of health information" that incapacitated lay people in functioning as effective resources for self-care. People were defined as passive recipients of health care and expected to follow medical orders exactly and unquestioningly. While this philosophy may have worked for some acute diseases where little follow-through was necessary, the approach failed drastically when applied to chronic disease, illness prevention, and health promotion. In both illness prevention and health promotion, self-care is primary, with professional care in the form of education or guidance as supplementary.

The impact of this notion is only beginning to be felt within the United States, yet it has the potential for revolutionizing the American health care system.

Health professionals and the public are becoming increasingly aware that health education planned within the medical model is disease-specific, focusing on one problem at a time.[20] Rather than adhering to the medical model, health education should be directed by an educative/developmental model that is oriented toward assisting individuals and communities to achieve holistic changes toward higher levels of health. The educative/developmental model is by its very nature holistic, unlike the clinical/medical model.

The activated client must have the requisite values, attitudes, knowledge, and skills in order to care for him- or herself within the culture in a healthful way. Activated client's efforts to change personal health behaviors must be supported by attempts to change collective behavior, production patterns within industry, and national health policy. Altering collective behavior is discussed in Chapter 15.

The impact of public demand on federal legislation and programming for health is apparent in the passage of the National Consumer Health Information Act of 1976 and the establishment of the Bureau of Health Education, Center for Disease Control, and the Office of Health Information, Health Promotion, Physical Fitness, and Sports Medicine within the federal government.

Health education for the public was listed as one of the ten health priorities in the National Health Planning and Resources Development Act of 1974 (P.L. 93-641). In addition, HEW specified a set of health education initiatives as one of the goals of the Forward Plan for Health for Fiscal Years 1976–1980. The need to move from articulation to implementation of health education efforts is apparent from the fact that only 1 to 2 percent of the federal budget is currently spent on health education activities.[21] While education of the public for self-care has become an important part of federal policy, it has yet to become a highly viable and visible thrust for federal expenditures and programs.


## GOALS OF HEALTH EDUCATION

The goals of health education are holistic in nature and address behavior change at the individual, family, community, and national levels. Many health professionals have spoken to what those goals are. Vuori[22] identified the goals of health education as:

1. To influence directly an individual's health related behavior either by providing information for decision-making, by changing attitudes or by changing values
2. To change the 'value atmosphere' of society
3. To create a favorable attitude for the use of societal means (e.g., legislation, production, and price policies), in the form of political decision-making, to influence the health behavior of a population

Similar objectives have been offered by the Task Force on Health Promotion and Consumer Education, sponsored by the John E. Fogarty International Center for Advanced Study in the Health Sciences, National Institutes of Health and the American College of Preventive Medicine.[23] In the Task Force report, it is proposed that health education is a process that bridges the gap between health information and personal health practices. The ultimate goal of health education is the improvement of the nation's health and the reduction of preventable illness, disability, and death. Health education attempts to influence directly behavioral factors relevant to health. The specific objectives identified for health education within the report are as follows:

1. To improve the health of the people by (a) providing the necessary information to help prevent illness and disability insofar as possible and to maintain the highest possible level of well-being even when ill or disabled and (b) helping them to make the necessary modification in individual life style or behavior when necessary
2. To help restrain inflation in health care costs by relieving some of the preventable demand on health services
3. To involve the consumer/patient positively and constructively in his/her own health maintenance and in responsible effective use of the health care delivery system

Good health demands individual knowledge, motivation, responsibility, and participation in making choices related to health. Personal health behavior *can* be changed, but frequently this change must be made in the face of counterforces consisting of advertising, referent group norms, and the prevalent American lifestyle. It is obvious that a joint approach is needed in which personal commitment and competence for self-care are strengthened, and societal or environmental barriers to healthful behavior are weakened or eliminated.

Within the context of the above objectives, important activities for health education efforts are as follows:[24]

1. Inform people about health, illness, disability and ways in which they can improve and protect their own health
2. Inform individuals about relevant risk factors and ways in which they can decrease personal level of risk for specific diseases
3. Motivate people to want to change to more healthful practices
4. Help people learn the necessary skills to adopt and maintain healthful practices and life styles
5. Advocate change in the environment that facilitates healthful conditions and healthful behavior

The remaining parts of this chapter will be devoted to an examination of (a) factors that affect the response of individuals to health education, (b) the process of health education for self-care, and (c) potential outcomes of health education. A schema for health education directed toward health protection and health promotion is presented in Figures 7-1 and 7-2.

## FACTORS AFFECTING RESPONSE TO HEALTH EDUCATION

Individual responses to health education for self-care are multidimensional and thus extremely complex. The client brings to the learning situation a unique personality, established social interaction patterns, cultural norms and values, and environmental influences. Along with these factors, individual learning styles must be considered for effective health education.[25] The nurse providing education for self-care must also be aware of characteristic differences that exist between learning patterns of adults and children. Characteristics of the adult learner reported in the literature include:[26]

1. Previous experience that provides a rich resource to facilitate learning.
2. Self-direction rather than dependency in the learning process.
3. Problem-centered rather than subject-centered learning.
4. Interest in immediate rather than future application of knowledge.
5. High priority given to learning that facilitates mastery of current developmental tasks.

In contrast, health education experiences for children must be concrete, with emphasis on vivid visual, auditory, tactile, and emotional impact to facilitate learning. Limited experience restricts the extent to which children can call on past events to evoke meaningful feelings and images. Since teenagers represent an intermediate position on the age continuum, their level of maturity and ability to engage in problem solving and futuristic thinking must be carefully assessed. Selection of appropriate teaching strategies and self-care content must take into consideration the chronologic, intellectual, and emotional maturity of the client.

Individual perceptions identified in the Health-Promotion Model that affect readiness and motivation to learn self-care include:

- Importance of health
- Perception of health control
- Desire for competence in self-care
- Self-awareness
- Self-esteem
- Personal definition of health
- Perceived health status
- Perceived benefits of health-promoting behavior

Wallston, Maides, and Wallston[27] found that both the value placed on health and perceptions of control of health affected the extent to which young adults sought written information (pamphlets) on high blood pressure. Internal con-

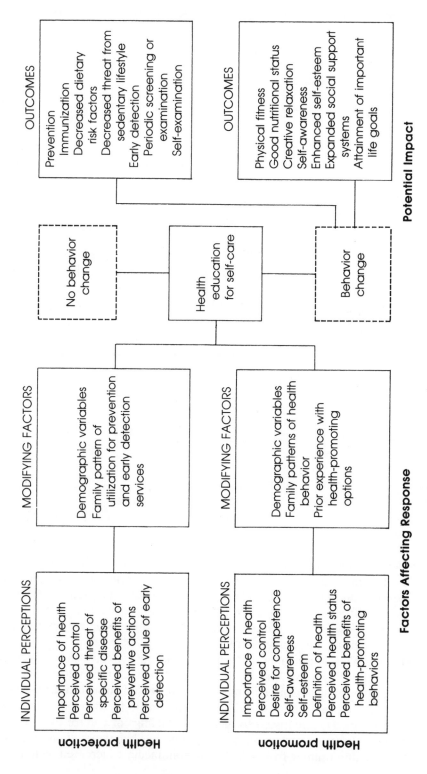

**FIGURE 7-1.** Client education for self-care.

157

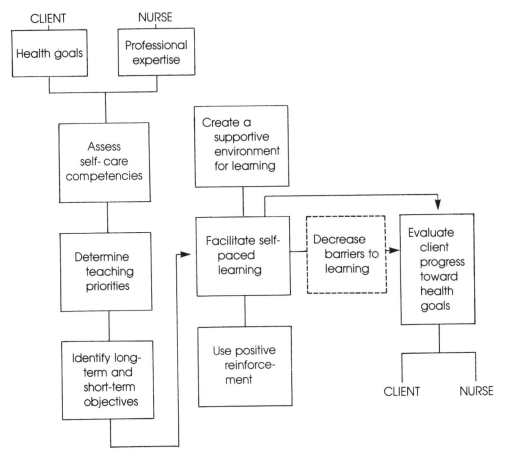

**FIGURE 7-2.** The health education process.

trol–high health value individuals chose more pamphlets (total) than did internal control–low health value, external control–high health value, or external control–low health value participants. These findings, which have been replicated, would indicate that people who value health and who perceive themselves to be in control of their own health status are more likely to be receptive, motivated, and active in acquiring information about self-care.

Clients who place little value on health and do not perceive themselves to be in control of their own lives present a special challenge to the nurse in health education and counseling. Values may have to be addressed through confrontation techniques described in Chapter 9 and/or attempts made to change perceptions of control of health. One approach to increasing feelings of control over health is to encourage clients to engage in health-promoting behaviors such as brisk walking or relaxation training from which almost immediate increased feelings of well-being are experienced. The rapid impact of such health behaviors can augment clients' perceptions of personal health control.

Each client's desire for competence in self-care must be taken into consideration. The fact cannot be ignored that some individuals do not want to be responsible for their own actions but instead wish to function within society in a highly dependent role. In many instances, the desire for competence has been frustrated and almost extinguished by a health care system that makes people feel infantile and helpless. It is critical that the nurse assess very early in interactions with clients the extent to which they desire to assume responsibility for their own care once they are given the requisite knowledge and skills to do so.

The level of self-awareness of clients is also important to determine very early in health education interactions. If clients are highly "attuned" to their bodily sensations, feelings, and responses, they will be better able to assess their need for additional knowledge, motivation, and skills to enhance self-care competencies. If little awareness is present, increasing self-awareness through self-exploration techniques (presented throughout the chapters of this book) may be necessary before the client can benefit fully from health education.

The self-esteem of the client is also a powerful determinant of response to health education. Does the client consider him- or herself capable of learning self-care skills? Does the client consider him- or herself worth taking care of? Does the client view him- or herself as a productive member of society? Does the client have high positive self-regard? Is self-preservation an important goal of the client?

The opposite of self-care is self-neglect. Self-neglect often results from low self-esteem. Valuing self is a prerequisite to serious and sustained efforts at self-care. Personal devaluation not only results in neglect but in disinterest and in overt health-damaging behaviors. The individual with high self-esteem is much more likely to be motivated toward healthful adaptation and self-actualization than is the individual with low self-esteem. Measures that allow for more systematic assessment of self-esteem than informal questioning and observation include the Coopersmith Self-Esteem Inventory and the Tennessee Self-Concept Scale.[28]

The nurse can help clients develop a positive image of what they are and what they can become. For example, the client interested in changing eating behaviors can be assisted in visualizing him- or herself as trim, attractive, and pleasant after weight loss rather than as deprived, bitter, and frustrated. Positive assets of the client should be stressed frequently during health education sessions.

Clients' personal definition of health will determine the content that they view as meaningful in health education. When health is defined as maintaining stability (norm) or avoiding overt illness, health-protecting behaviors such as immunization, self-examination for signs of cancer, and periodic multiphasic screening will be most important to the client. Defining health as self-actualization moves the client from reacting to the environment to acting on the environment. Health defined as self-actualization is the optimum use of personal, interpersonal, and environmental resources to sustain the continuing evolution of human potential. The emphasis of health education within this context is on health-promoting behaviors such as relaxation, exercise, or development of social support systems.

The client's definition of health may change during the health education process. As a result, an increased interest in health-promoting behaviors and health-protecting measures may emerge. The nurse must be sensitive to early signs of client change.

Perceived health status has also been shown to have an effect on response to health-promotion efforts. Sidney and Shephard[29] reported that those individuals who viewed themselves as very healthy indicated higher motivation to engage frequently and intensively in health-promoting behaviors than did individuals who viewed themselves as only moderately healthy. It appears that the experience of health is in itself a source of motivation, encouraging further health-promoting behaviors.

Clients develop expectations concerning the benefits of health protection and health promotion. These perceptions are based on previous life-experiences, contact with mass media, and interactions with health professionals. Expected outcomes range from belief in negligible effects to belief in major impact of health behaviors on the quality of life, morbidity, and mortality. Assessing the confidence of clients in the benefits of specific health behaviors will provide the nurse with information important in understanding individual responsiveness to health education interventions.

While individual perceptions that affect responses to self-care education have been considered, there are other modifying factors that must also be assessed in the health education process:

- Demographic factors, such as age, sex, ethnicity, education, and income
- Family patterns of health behavior
- Prior experience with health-protecting and health-promoting options

Demographic factors play an important role in the response of individual clients to health education. The importance of ethnicity cannot be too strongly stressed in planning for health education. Increasingly, health personnel provide care to people from a variety of ethnic backgrounds, including black, Hispanic, Asian, and others. An expanding volume of literature is available to assist health professionals in understanding cultures different from the middle-class, white American culture. Clark[30] and Martinez[31] provide excellent books on the Mexican-American culture, and Hill[32] on the black-American culture. Spector[33] also offers much helpful information on the impact of culture in health and illness. As an example of the need for understanding different cultural beliefs, since the Mexican-American family believes strongly in the effectiveness of *curanderismo* (folk medicine),[34] in working with individuals or families, emphasis must be placed on the beneficial aspects of *curanderismo* and an attempt made to incorporate these traditional cultural beliefs into health education for self-care.

A word of caution is in order concerning transcultural use of published health education materials. It is often supposed that simply translating materials into the language of another culture provides appropriate audio-visual teaching aids and pamphlets for client education. However, such is often not the case. The sense of modesty in some cultures may make pictures and illustrations of human anatomy offensive to clients. Materials prepared by people within the target culture or in consultation with them should be available to facilitate the effectiveness of nurses providing education for self-care to minority groups.

It is the responsibility of the nurse to become familiar with the cultural backgrounds of the people served. To do less is to avoid taking seriously the key aim of health education: changing the behavior and lifestyle of clients in the direction of a more positive and healthful one.

In studies of the impact of health education, education and income have also been shown to be important demographic factors. Ability to comprehend instruction varies with educational level, as does the background of knowledge and skills on which the client can draw in carrying out self-care. Income will affect the health priorities of families and the accessibility of services and materials to follow through with recommended behaviors. As long as access to health care is related to purchasing power, lower-income groups will experience limitations in their potential for acquiring the assistance needed to develop self-care skills.

The importance of family patterns of behavior in determining individual health practices has been stressed by White.[35] Family patterns that need to be considered for their impact on health education for self-care include:[36]

1. Communication
2. Reactions to stress
3. Eating
4. Activities
5. Rituals
6. Methods for identifying and accomplishing goals
7. Stages in family development (developmental tasks)
8. Formal and informal power and leadership
9. Socio-occupational orientation
10. Philosophy of life
11. Interpretation of health and health-related events

The family serves as the primary educational and support structure within the community. Most personal health practices are initially learned within the family by mandate, example, or informal instruction. Since self-care for many clients takes placed within a traditional or nontraditional family structure, the family or home setting is an ideal place for health education efforts.

Family members can actively support positive health practices, remain neutral, or thwart change. The degree of family support often determines the extent to which new behaviors that are health promoting will be adopted and sustained over a period of time. Family members can serve as important sources of motivation, reward, and reinforcement for specific health behaviors.

Prior experience with health-protecting and health-promoting activities can provide the client with self-care skills that are readily available for use or modification to meet new health care needs. In addition, past experiences in self-care can promote experiential, emotional, and physical readiness to learn. For instance, one client in the author's stress-management program learned relaxation skills readily because she had previously taken yoga classes and was familiar with yoga positions and stretching exercises. In providing health education for self-care, the nurse should capitalize on the existing knowledge and skills of clients. Assessing current and past experiences with health behaviors is an excellent way to accomplish this.

## THE PROCESS OF HEALTH EDUCATION FOR SELF-CARE

Health education consists of teaching and counseling activities in which information is imparted to clients and they are guided in applying what has been learned to everyday living. Meaningful health education provides learning experiences in which the traditional authoritarian relationship between health professionals and clients is replaced by an egalitarian relationship. The client is the controlling partner and as such must assume an assertive role in learning and subsequent behavior change.

The components of the health education process for self-care to be discussed in this chapter include: assessing self-care competencies, determining teaching priorities, identifying long-term and short-term objectives, facilitating self-paced learning, using positive reinforcement, decreasing barriers to learning, creating a supportive environment for learning, and evaluating client progress. Figure 7-2 presents an overview of health education as a collaborative process.

### Assessing Self-Care Competencies

Self-care competencies can be categorized into knowledge, motivation, skills, and orientation.[37] Knowledge can be assessed in a variety of ways: through informal discussion, health-knowledge checklists (Fig. 7-3), or structured tests of knowledge in specific content areas. The assessment approach that works best will have to be determined for each client, but, in general, informal discussion or a health-knowledge checklist is less threatening to the client than a structured test. Observation of actual behavior can also provide useful insights. However, frequently, the period available for client observation is too short to allow the nurse to draw reliable conclusions about the level of health knowledge that exists.

Motivation to engage in health education activities in order to develop greater expertise in self-care is critical to assess. Motivation for the client depends on a number of factors, such as importance of health, desire for competence, or mastery and self-esteem. The activated client shows evidence of motivation in aggressively seeking health information that will assist in self-care. The existence of apathy, disinterest, and inattention should alert the nurse to a lack of motivation on the part of the client. Reasons for lack of interest should be explored so that the nurse can knowledgeably intervene to increase motivation through appropriate use of reinforcement contingencies or behavioral contracts with the client. These approaches to motivation will be discussed further in Chapters 8 and 9.

---

In the list below, please check those behaviors that you are comfortable in performing for yourself without assistance from others.

_____ Counting my pulse at the wrist for 1 minute

_____ Counting my pulse at the neck for 1 minute

_____ Selecting comfortable and appropriate shoes for brisk walking or jogging

_____ Selecting appropriate clothing for walking or jogging activities

_____ Planning a progressive schedule of exercise to meet my personal needs

_____ Indicating the ideal weight range for my height

_____ Calculating my maximal heart rate during exercise

_____ Planning time for exercise that is convenient and possible

_____ Describing warm-up exercises that I could do before brisk walking or running

_____ Describing procedures for cooling down after vigorous exercise

_____ Exercising intensively at least four times a week for 30 minutes

_____ Integrating physical-fitness activities with my recreational interests

_____ Maintaining a record of my progress in physical fitness over a period of several months

_____ Eating appropriately before or after vigorous exercise

_____ Explaining how stress is released through physical exercise

_____ Describing how to avoid injuries during exercise

---

**FIGURE 7-3.** Health-knowledge check list for exercise and physical fitness.

Psychomotor skills of the client must also be assessed to determine the extent of fine and gross motor coordination available to carry out the physical aspects of self-care. Assisting the client in developing the behavioral skills to implement knowledge about health protection and health promotion is an essential step in health education. Initial assessment of skills allows the client to recognize his or her strengths and build upon them and to recognize areas in which further growth is possible.

What clients will learn about health also depends on their orientation to the world. Beliefs concerning the independence of man from nature, the importance of the future in contrast to the present or past, and the inevitability of death will determine predisposition to actively seek health-relevant information. Each of these beliefs either enhances or inhibits individual potential for self-care. Orientation is the most nebulous of the four competency areas to assess and is perhaps best addressed through informal discussion as the nurse becomes increasingly better acquainted with the client.

Through assessing the client's level of self-care competencies and motivation to learn at the beginning of the health education process, the nurse recognizes the centrality of the client in self-care. Failure to assess each client decreases the nurse's ability to individualize the content, approach, and materials used in health counseling.

### Determining Teaching Priorities

Deciding where to begin is often a dilemma for the nurse when the client needs information about a variety of different health behaviors. Futrell *et al.*[38] have suggested two criteria for determining where to start:

1. Start with the area most important to the client at the time.
2. Start with the area of knowledge that will contribute most to the maintenance or enhancement of health.

Clients have definite ideas about what they wish to know and what they consider important to them.

Often, interest does not lie in the area that poses the greatest threat to personal health. As an example, a client may smoke and also be particularly interested in beginning a personal exercise program. While smoking may constitute a more severe threat to health, inactivity is a risk factor also. It is obviously better to be a physically active smoker than an inactive smoker, since risks are synergistic. If the nurse assists the client to develop an exercise program, the client may also develop a heightened awareness of the negative impact of smoking on lung capacity and physical endurance. At that point, the client may exhibit readiness to discuss approaches to smoking cessation based on increased appreciation of its health-damaging effects.

Teaching priorities are not those of the nurse but those of the client. If the nurse starts where the client is, the client gains personal control over health education interactions, thus enhancing their meaningfulness.

### Identifying Short-term and Long-term Objectives

Goal setting is important in health education activities. In addition to goal iden-tification, long-term and short-term objectives should be identified. What are the specific knowledge, skills, motivations, and orientations that the client wishes to develop in order to achieve a desired health outcome? Goal setting should be cooperatively carried out by the client and nurse. The goals should be realistic, with each short-term goal fitting under a specific long-term goal so that learning proceeds in a logical sequence toward the desired health outcomes. An example of a goal-identification form is presented in Figure 7-4. Discussion of goals and their personal meaningfulness is essential to full participation of the client in the goal-setting process.

| Desired Health Outcome: Increased Physical Fitness | |
|---|---|
| Long-term goal: To take a brisk walk for 45 minutes four times each week. | GOALS ATTAINED |
| Related Short-term Goals:<br><br>1. To demonstrate how to check my pulse at the neck by counting beats for 1 minute.<br><br>2. To state submaximal heart rate that I should achieve during exercise.<br><br>3. To demonstrate two warm-up exercises for use before walking.<br><br>4. To describe how to cool down after brisk walking.<br><br>5. To construct a weekly schedule for brisk walking.<br><br>6. To demonstrate correct diaphragmatic breathing to be used during exercise.<br><br>7. To walk briskly for 10 minutes on two days during the first week.<br><br>8. To walk briskly for 15 minutes on three days during the second week.<br><br>9. To walk briskly for 25 minutes on four days during the third and fourth weeks.<br><br>10. To walk briskly for 35 minutes on four days during the fifth and sixth weeks.<br><br>11. To walk briskly for 45 minutes on four days during the seventh week. | |

**FIGURE 7-4.** Health education for self-care: goal-identification form.

Long-term goals or objectives guide large segments of learning. Each objective should address a single goal to be accomplished. Objectives may represent knowledge to be acquired, recalled, or remembered; values, beliefs, and attitudes to be developed; or complex overt behavioral responses to be learned. Short-term goals identify the specific content or activities that must be progressively mastered to achieve the long-term goal. Recall of information, return demonstration, or practice are some of the activities that may be appropriate as short-term objectives.

Use of the goal-identification form allows the client to identify long-term and short-term objectives, check off each objective as it is attained, and maintain awareness of the desired health outcome. Both the nurse and the client should retain a copy for continuing reference and update. If short-term objectives for health education are not clearly delineated during the decision-making phase, the client lacks a sense of direction and may not see how each step in the learning sequence can be accomplished during the action phase.

A word of caution for the nurse is in order concerning the overzealous client. Many individuals plan to achieve long-term goals in a single step. This is seldom possible. The client should be helped to understand that setting overly large sequential steps or trying to achieve the final goal immediately is highly likely to lead to frustration and discontinuation of desired behaviors. Good health habits take time to develop just as health-damaging habits do. Slowly increasing the time spent on a behavior or the frequency with which the behavior is practiced is likely to result in greater success in changing behavior in the long run than "all-or-none" approaches to behavior change.

### Facilitating Self-Paced Learning

The pace at which a client will learn depends on personal motivation, assertiveness, perseverance, skill, and learning style. The pace of learning may also vary with age, health status, and educational level. Self-pacing is important in order to allow the client to be self-directed and maintain control over the learning process. The pace at which the client meets each short-term objective will vary, and expectations of both the client and the health professional should be adjusted accordingly. The important factor is not how rapidly knowledge or skill is attained but the extent of mastery. The nurse should be attuned to small steps in client progress and use positive reinforcement frequently to enhance the client's feelings of success and sense of forward movement in developing competence in self-care.

The nurse must be realistic about teaching and learning and accept both good and bad days in clients of all ages. Sometimes the nurse and client will be elated with the results, sometimes discouraged.[39] When efforts are less rewarding than anticipated, the pace of learning should be reviewed carefully. It is possible that expanding the time frame for learning will result in increased success for the client. This is especially true for young children who have less experience to draw on in the learning process than do adults.

### Using Positive Reinforcement

Shaping behavior in sequential steps is an important concept from the psychology of learning that can be applied to health education. In shaping behavior, it is important for reinforcement to be immediate or contingent on desired behaviors or approximations of the desired behavior. In education for self-care, the client, the nurse, and the family of the client all play an important role in reinforcement. Praise should be liberally and meaningfully used to reward client behaviors that indicate progress toward stated goals or objectives. Cues should be used to facilitate successful responses and immediate feedback provided to correct errors in performance. When cues and error feedback are intermingled with positive reinforcement they are helpful, nonthreatening, and facilitate continued efforts of the client. Immediate and consistent reinforcement facilitates rapid learning and assists the client in deriving satisfaction from learning. Once learning has occurred, intermittent reinforcement of the desired behavior strengthens the behavior, making it more resistent to extinction.

Clients should be made aware of the importance of self-reward or self-reinforcement in the health education process. It is important that they learn to reward their own efforts and achievements since much of the time, contingent reinforcement for self-care cannot be supplied by others. As an example of self-reinforcement, the client may reward 15 minutes of jogging by a telephone visit with a favorite friend or by reading a magazine article or novel that is highly appealing. These reinforcements should be clearly identified by the client, and plans should be made for their use. A progress-and-reward sheet similar to the one depicted in Figure 7-5 can be helpful in formalizing the reward structure. The client should be discouraged from using foods as reinforcement, since this may encourage between-meal snacks that are undesirable. Obviously, rewarding 15 minutes of jogging with a chocolate sundae is self-defeating.

| Goal or Activity | | Successful Completion (check √) | Reward |
|---|---|---|---|
| Brisk walk today for 10 minutes | Day 1 | | A telephone conversation with Mary |
| | Day 2 | | 20 minutes set aside to read *Ladies Home Journal* |
| Brisk walk today for 15 minutes | Day 1 | | Allow an hour to relax on the patio |
| | Day 2 | | Buy myself a new novel |
| | Day 3 | | Go over to Joan's for coffee |
| Brisk walk today for 25 minutes | Day 1 | | Buy a new perfume |
| | Day 2 | | Spend time playing croquet with my family |
| | Day 3 | | Take time to enjoy my favorite TV program |
| | Day 4 | | Go to a movie with my husband |

**FIGURE 7-5.** Planning for self-reinforcement of health behaviors: progress-and-reward sheet.

It is important that the client also learn to use self-reinforcement that is internal as well as external. Self-praise, self-compliment, and feeling good about oneself are all forms of internal reinforcement. Learning to use internal self-reward in an appropriate manner permits the client to be less dependent on the availability of tangible objects to facilitate the learning process.

Family members need to learn to serve as sources of support for each other in developing health behaviors. For example, achievement of a specific goal may be rewarded by a family outing in the park or by the family spending time together in a favorite activity at home. This involves the family as a part of the reward network of the client. By providing mutual support, a sense of healthy interdependence rather than crippling dependence is created. Providing education for self-care in a family setting encourages mutual support. If home visits are not possible for the nurse, the family should be encouraged to come to the clinic with the client. It may be necessary to provide services during evening hours in order to make it possible for families to attend. Since the family serves as a primary reference group, their potential for reward and reinforcement of newly acquired health behaviors is much greater than that of the nurse.

### Identifying Barriers to Learning

Barriers to learning can result from various sources: personal values, beliefs, and attitudes; lack of motivation; poor self-concept; or inadequate cognitive or psychomotor skills. Whatever the source, if the client exhibits lack of progress, barriers within the individual as well as within the family, relevant social groups, and the environment should be explored. Barriers must often be identified and attenuated or eliminated before progress can continue.

Approaches to dealing with obstacles to healthy behavior should be an integral part of the health education plan. In this way, problems are addressed systematically, and progress in dealing with the barriers can be periodically assessed. The client may be unaware of what is inhibiting progress or reluctant to share such information with the nurse. An open climate of trust and empathy will facilitate communication between the client and the nurse concerning obstacles to learning.

### Creating an Optimum Environment for Learning

The environment in which health education for self-care is provided is vitally important to the success of educational efforts. Many clinic or health-center environments intimidate clients, thus making them reticent to participate openly in the learning process. If a clinic is used for health education, the rooms in which self-care is taught should be warm, comfortable, and informal. A desk should not be placed in the room; instead, there might be tables with chairs that can be rearranged or sofa and chairs in a conversational setting. Walls should be wallpapered or painted in pleasant colors, with pictures and textured materials used to create a supportive, nonthreatening climate. Visual aids in flip-chart form and on an easel at a comfortable height for the nurse to use while seated in a chair are ideal for teaching purposes.

Throughout health education, the nurse should avoid use of medical or nursing terminology that is unfamiliar to the client. If very young children are present during the teaching sessions, an area with attractive toys and books may need to be provided for their use. This will minimize distraction of the parents. If children are old enough to be included in the learning sessions, they definitely should be actively involved. Often, use of bright colors and interesting figures or designs on flip charts will amuse children and maintain their interest. Children can play an important role in reinforcing learning or in reminding parents to engage in recommended behaviors.

To the extent possible, actual materials available at home should be used in teaching clients. For instance, if a client is expected to use a booklet on low-cholesterol foods at home in preparing meals, the booklet to be used should be the basis for instruction. If the client is learning relaxation techniques, coaching audiotapes to be used at home should be demonstrated in the clinic, and questions should be answered regarding their use. Jogging or walking shoes and clothing to be worn for exercise should be used when learning appropriate pacing on a treadmill in the clinic setting. When health education in the home is not possible, the closer the clinic setting simulates the home setting, the more readily learning will be transferred and appropriately used. Well-illustrated materials should be liberally supplied to the client to take home in order to provide reinforcement of knowledge and skills gained during health education sessions.

Since minimal time for most health instruction is 15 to 30 minutes, the nurse must determine whether individual or small-group teaching methods are to be used. If time is at a premium and health education is provided to groups, the groups should be kept small to facilitate interaction and attention to the specific needs of group members. Groups can be formed on the basis of similar health-protection or health-promotion interests or by age, sex, or occupation. Over time, group members can develop a feeling of *esprit de corps* and can serve as sounding boards and support persons for each other in learning new behaviors. A combination of group and individual instruction may also be helpful. The author has found that relaxation techniques can be taught to a small group, but individualization of relaxation methods and use of biofeedback to assist clients in assessing their own progress is handled best in individual appointments. This combined approach allows for efficient use of professional time yet provides for individualization of educative/developmental care to maximize its effectiveness.

### Evaluating Client Progress

Evaluation is a process by which the nurse (teacher) and client (learner) in collaboration judge to what degree long-term and short-term goals have been attained. Three approaches to evaluation have been described by Green[40]: (1) evaluation of the health education process, (2) evaluation of impact (changes in knowledge, attitudes or behavior), and (3) evaluation of resultant morbidity and mortality. Green has proposed these approaches for evaluation research, but they are equally applicable to evaluation of client progress. While the nurse and client should periodically evaluate the health education process itself, major focus in evaluation should be placed on impact, that is, changes in attitudes, knowledge, or behaviors. Changes in morbidity can also be assessed for a large group of clients over a period of time by evaluating the impact of health education on the occurrence of chronic health problems within the group, compared to a group of cohorts without comparable health education.

All evaluation involves direct or indirect observation of behavior. Actual demonstration of the behaviors learned constitutes direct observation, while client report of participation in health behaviors represents indirect observation.[41] Both approaches are subject to measurement errors of which the nurse should be aware. The major source of error in direct measurement is inadequate sampling of the target behaviors during brief clinic or home visits. If the client is asked to demonstrate specific behaviors in the clinic, the artificiality of the setting may inhibit response. A source of error in indirect measurement is that clients may present a distorted picture of how they actually behave. That is, what they say they do may be different from what they actually do. The client may or may not be conscious of this distortion. Self-observation skills of clients may be inadequately developed, or clients may ascribe a "halo effect" to themselves, seeing performance of health behaviors as more frequent, more intensive, or more accurate than they actually are.

It is the position of the author that a combination of self-report and return demonstration should be used as a means of evaluating client progress. The primary purpose of evaluation is to provide an accurate picture for clients of where they stand in attaining their health goals. Several approaches to evaluation for this purpose will be presented for consideration.

*Checklists.* A checklist of objectives to be accomplished similar to the one presented in Figure 7-4 can be used for evaluation purposes. As each short-term and long-term goal is attained, it can be checked off on the list. In addition, specific knowledge or skills that the client has acquired can be checked off on a list comparable to the one presented in Figure 7-3. As each objective or behavior is checked off, the client is made aware of his or her own progress in developing positive health practices.

*Client Progress Notes.* Client progress notes can also be used to chart behavior change. Graphing changes in resting pulse, blood pressure, or electrical muscle activity can visually indicate progress in learning stress management or physical-fitness skills. Narrative notes about patient progress can also be used to provide more detailed information. Notes should be concise and brief and made by both the nurse and client on the progress forms.

*Laboratory Measurements.* Certain physiologic parameters available through laboratory tests can also be used to measure client progress. Serum cholesterol, triglycerides, blood glucose, lipoproteins, and serum albumin can be used as indicators of biologic change. Because of expense, the use of laboratory tests for this purpose should be carefully evaluated.

*Testing Devices.* Knowledge or performance tests can also be employed to assess client progress. This approach should be used with caution in the case of the client who becomes highly anxious in testing situations. The written test should be concise and provide for ease of response, and the nurse should be able to administer it in a half hour or less. The test should be quickly scored, and, if possible, feedback should be provided immediately to the client. An efficient and interesting approach to testing is through programmed learning. Programs can be written to evaluate the grasp of a particular concept, and immediate feedback and corrective information can be provided. Such an approach can decrease the stress of testing and provide reinforcement to the client.

*Verbal Questioning.* Progress can also be evaluated by questioning the client regarding his or her knowledge of a particular concept or behavior. This is a less formal approach than written testing, yet it allows for feedback from the client that assists both the nurse and the client in evaluating progress. Verbal questioning may be more comfortable for the client than written testing, and it should be done in a nonthreatening manner. Responses to questions can be evaluated and the client further questioned to clarify responses that are initially unclear.

*Direct Observation.* Direct observation of some health-protecting and health-promoting behaviors is possible. For instance, a client may be observed doing warm-up exercises to determine whether they are being done properly and with correct body alignment. The author asks clients that she has trained in relaxation to recline comfortably in a chair in the clinic setting; there they are left alone to achieve relaxation using the approach that they use at home. Following completion of the relaxation sequence, the author quietly enters the room to check pulse, blood pressure, and electrical muscle activity on monitors already comfortably placed on the patient.

*Dilemmas of Evaluation.* In an insightful article on the dilemmas of evaluating and measuring the outcomes of health education, Green[42] has identified potential problems in client evaluation. Conclusions drawn concerning client progress depend on the point in time following health education when observations are made. Curves showing possible trends in performance appear in Figure 7-6. The impact of health education could be interpreted in different ways, either as successful or unsuccessful, depending on the point in time when outcomes are measured. It is evident that client performance should be evaluated at several different points in time in order to draw accurate conclusions concerning the personal impact of health education.

What is desired, of course, is a sustained effect of the health education intervention that permanently changes lifestyle or behavior; that is the ultimate goal. However, clients experiencing decay of effect or backlash effect need to be evaluated carefully to determine why the new behavior patterns were not sustained. It is possible that a prolonged learning period or the development of stronger family or community support systems could have prevented recidivism and the return to earlier, less healthy patterns of behavior.

*Potential Outcomes of Health Education.* The content of health education for self-care will vary, depending on whether the primary emphasis is health protection or health promotion. Since the emphasis in health protection is on avoidance of disease, risk appraisal,[43-45] information about specific risk factors, ways of changing behavior or lifestyle to reduce risk, and methods for early detection of disease

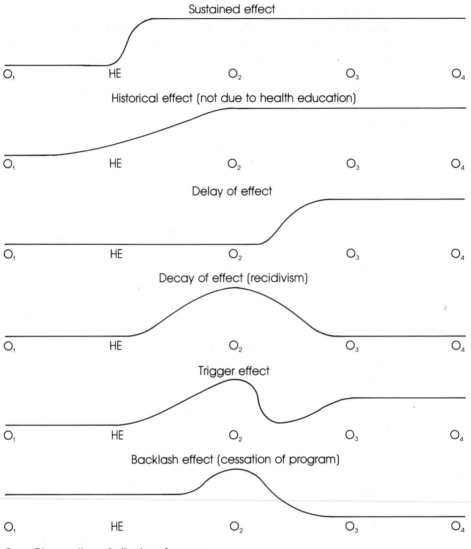

O = Observation of client performance
HE = Health Education

**FIGURE 7-6.** Performance trends following client education. *(From Green, L. W. Evaluation and measurement: Some dilemmas for health education. American Journal of Public Health, February 1977, 67, 155–161. With permission.)*

will be the focus.[46] As a result, specific outcomes to be expected include behaviors such as seeking immunization, changing diet to reduce nutritional risk factors, increasing physical activity to reduce the threat of a sedentary lifestyle, maintaining social support systems as buffers against disease, and use of screening and self-examination methods for early detection of disease.

The emphasis of client education for health promotion is on attaining higher levels of wellness, fulfillment, and life satisfaction. The content of such health education is not disease-specific but holistic in nature. Expected outcomes from education directed toward health promotion include physical fitness, good nutritional status, creative relaxation, self-awareness, enhanced self-esteem, expanded social support systems, and attainment of important life goals.

The close relationship between health-protection and health-promotion goals generally results in health education efforts directed toward both ends. Despite overlap of protective/promotive care in actual nursing practice, keeping in mind the conceptual distinction will result in more well-defined and effective health education activities.

## SUMMARY

Education for self-care assists the client in developing a health protection/promotion plan and in achieving modifications in lifestyle. The requisite knowledge and skills must be learned before desired changes in behavior can occur. Making decisions concerning what needs to be learned in light of desired health outcomes and long-term and short-term objectives provides the basis for planning individualized health education interventions. Assessment of self-care competencies that the client already has places emphasis on self-direction, self-responsibility, and control of learning experiences by the client. The nurse's primary role is that of a consultant. Educative/developmental care provided by the nurse should enable clients to achieve those health goals that they have set for themselves. The nurse in functioning as a valuable resource for instruction, motivation, and evaluation enhances the potential success of the client in learning.

## REFERENCES

1. Orem, D.E. *Nursing: Concepts of practice*. New York: McGraw-Hill, 1971.
2. Preventive Medicine U.S.A.: *Health promotion and consumer health education*. A Task Force Report sponsored by The John E. Fogarty International Center for Advanced Studies in the Health Sciences (NIH) and The American College of Preventive Medicine. New York: Prodist, 1976.
3. Levin, L. The layperson as the primary health care practitioner. *Public Health Reports,* May–June 1976, *91,* 206.
4. Levin, L.S., Katz, A.H., & Holst, E. *Self care: Lay initiatives in Health*. New York: Prodist, 1976, p. 13.
5. Orem, *op. cit.*

6.  Calley, J.M., Dirksen, M., Engalla, M., & Hennrich, M.L. The Orem Self-Care Nursing Model. In Riehl, J.P., & Roy, C. (Eds.), *Conceptual models for nursing practice.* New York: Appleton, 1980, pp. 302–314.
7.  Freimuth, V.S., & Marron, T. The public's use of health information. *Health Education,* July 1978, *9,* 18–20.
8.  Sehnert, K.W., & Nocerino, J.T. *The activated patient: A course guide.* Washington, D.C.: Center for Continuing Education, Georgetown University, 1974.
9.  Sehnert, K.W., & Eisenberg, H. *How to be your own doctor (sometimes).* New York: Grosset & Dunlap, 1975.
10. Arvidson, E., Connelly, M.J., McDaid, T., et al. A health education model for ambulatory care. *Journal of Nursing Administration,* March 1979, *9,* 16–21.
11. Igoe, J.B. Changing patterns in school health and school nursing. *Nursing Outlook,* August 1980, *28,* 486–492.
12. Schodde, G. *Winning at wellness game.* Seattle: University of Washington Hospital, 1978.
13. *Project Health P.A.C.T.* Denver: University of Colorado School Nurse Practitioner Program, University of Colorado Health Sciences Center, 1980.
14. Stein, M.P., Farguhar, J.W., Maccoby, N., & Russell, S.H. Results of a two-year health education campaign on dietary behavior: The Stanford Three Community Study. *Circulation,* November 1976, *54,* 826–832.
15. Rosenberg, S.G. Patient education leads to better care for heart patients. *HSMHA Health Report,* September 1971, *86,* 793.
16. Levine, D.M., Green, L.W., Deeds, S.G., et al.: Health education for hypertensive patients. *Journal of the American Medical Association,* April 20, 1979, *241,* 1700.
17. Given, C.W., Given, B.A., & Simoni, L.E. The association of knowledge and perception of medications with compliance and health states among hypertensive patients: A prospective study. *Research in Nursing and Health,* 1978, *1,* 76–89.
18. Adamson, G.J., Oswald, J.D., & Palmquist, L.E. Hospital's role expanded with wellness effort. *Hospitals,* October 1, 1979, *53,* 121–124.
19. Hentges, K. Health activation: Educating for self-care. *Health Education,* July–August 1978, *9,* 31–32.
20. Vuori, H. The medical model and the objectives of health education. *International Journal of Health Education,* 1980, *23,* 12–19.
21. Appelbaum, A.L. Who's going to pay the bill? (health promotion). *Hospitals,* October 1, 1979, *53,* 112–120.
22. Vuori, *op. cit.,* p. 18.
23. Preventive Medicine U.S.A. *Health Education,* op. cit., p. 21.
24. *Ibid.,* p. 3.
25. Mico, P.R., & Ross, H.S. *Health education and behavioral science.* Oakland, Calif.: Third Party Associates, 1975.
26. Knowles, M.S. *The modern practice of adult education.* New York: Association Press, 1970.
27. Wallston, K.A., Maides, S., & Wallston, B.S. Health-related information seeking as a function of health-related locus of control and health value. *Journal of Research in Personality,* 1976, *10,* 215–222.
28. Buros, O. *Mental measurements yearbook* (8th ed.). Highland Park, N.J.: Gryphon Press, 1978.
29. Sidney, K.H., & Shephard, R.J. Attitudes toward health and physical activity in the elderly. Effects of a physical training program. *Medicine and Science in Sports,* 1976, *8,* 246–252.
30. Clark, M. *Health in the Mexican American culture.* Berkeley, Calif.: University of California Press, 1970.
31. Martinez, R.A. *Hispanic culture and health care.* St. Louis: Mosby, 1978.
32. Hill, R. *The strengths of Black families.* New York: Emerson Hall, 1971.

33. Spector, R.E. *Cultural diversity in health and illness*. New York: Appleton, 1979.
34. Faick, V. Planning health education for a minority group: The Mexican Americans. *International Journal of Health Education, 1979, 22,* 113–121.
35. White, M. Inside family life: An arena for health education. *Nursing Forum* 1979, *18,* 245–252.
36. Kantor, D., & Lehr, W. *Inside the family*. San Francisco: Jossey-Bass, 1976.
37. Calley *et al., op cit.,* p. 311.
38. Futrell, M., Brovender, S., McKinnon-Mullett, E., & Brower, H.T. *Primary health care of the older adult*. North Scituate, Mass.: Duxbury Press, 1980.
39. Murray, R., & Zentner, J. Health teaching: A basic nursing intervention. In Murray, R., & Zentner, J. (Eds.), *Nursing concepts for health promotion*. Englewood Cliffs, N.J.: Prentice-Hall, 1975, p. 118.
40. Green, L.W. How to evaluate health promotion. *Hospitals*, October 1, 1979, *53,* 106–108.
41. Redman, B.K. *The process of patient teaching in nursing* (2nd ed.). St. Louis, Mo.: Mosby, 1972, p. 133.
42. Green, L.W. Evaluation and measurement: Some dilemmas for health education. *American Journal of Public Health*, February 1977, *67*:155–161.
43. Johns, R.E., Jr. Health hazard appraisal—a useful tool in health education? In *New concepts in health: A new horizon*. Proceedings of Twelfth Annual Meeting, Society of Prospective Medicine, San Diego, California, 1977, pp. 61–65.
44. Thorsen, R.D., Jacobs, D.R., Jr., Grimm, R.H., Jr., et al. Preventive cardiology in practice: A device for risk estimation and counseling in coronary disease. *Preventive Medicine*, 1979, *8,* 548–556.
45. Milsam, J.H. Health risk factor reduction and life style change. *Family and Community Health*, May 1980, *3,* 1–3.
46. Breslow, L., & Somers, A.R. Life-time health monitoring program. *New England Journal of Medicine*, 1977, *296,* 601–608.

# CHAPTER 8
# Developing a Health Protection/Promotion Plan

In the preceding three chapters, suggestions were made for conducting the health assessment, facilitating values clarification, and identifying the client's learning priorities. In this chapter, attention will be given to developing a holistic plan for health protection and health promotion that takes into consideration the client's values, attitudes, goals, competencies, and risk status for chronic illness. The health protection/promotion plan presented here provides a systematic course of action designed to assist the client in attaining desired health goals that are consistent with personal philosophy, ethnic heritage, life purpose, and human potential for growth.

Upon completion of assessment, the nurse has a great deal of information available regarding the beliefs, lifestyle, and health status of the individual client. Types of data obtained from assessment procedures described in previous chapters include:

- Health history
- Physical examination
- Physical-fitness evaluation
- Nutritional assessment
- Risk appraisal
- Life-stress review
- Lifestyle and health habits assessment
- Health beliefs review
- Values hierarchy
- Values/actions review (consistency between personal values and actions)
- Work and leisure (how time is spent)
- Extent of health knowledge
- Personal/family values (consistency between personal and family values)
- Family patterns of behavior
- Barriers to behavior change

Based on comprehensive assessment, the client's strengths, areas for improvement in self-care, and actual self-care deficits can be accurately identified in order to provide clear directions for health care planning. Just as a contractor would not begin construction of a house without a detailed blueprint from an architect, the professional nurse must have organized assessment data on which to base an effective health protection/promotion plan. By getting to know and understand the client prior to health care planning the following factors can be taken into consideration: individual perceptions that affect health and health-related behaviors, demographic characteristics including social and ethnic background, expectations of important referent groups, behavioral options available to the client, potential or actual barriers to self-care, environmental cues available to initiate health behaviors, and the existing support systems for health-enhancing behaviors. Increased self-awareness on the part of the client resulting from the assessment process provides a realistic rather than idealistic basis for the health protection/promotion plan.

To maximize positive outcomes from health planning, the client must be an active participant in the planning process. Relying on the client to make decisions concerning desirable health goals and approaches to their attainment affirms the client's ability to improve personal health status. The plan provides an opportunity for the client to express stabilizing and actualizing tendencies in concrete behaviors that result in increased wellness and more satisfying and productive living. Genuine dialogue between provider and client is also a prerequisite to sound health planning and effective implementation. In order to facilitate communication, it is important that the nurse accept clients as they are, encourage self-acceptance, and promote self-direction and independence. The role of the nurse is to *assist* clients with health planning rather than to *control* the process. The degree of responsibility that the client assumes for personal health status is an important factor in receptivity to planning and success in behavior change.

The health protection/promotion plan should be reasonable in terms of demands on the client, benefits accruing to the client, and the time frame allocated for accomplishment of desired goals. Health and health-related knowledge and skills already possessed by the client should be optimally used in the planning process. Capitalizing on positive health behaviors currently a part of personal lifestyle prevents overloading the client with a barrage of self-imposed or implied demands for major life changes.[1]

Effective change almost always proceeds gradually. The nurse should keep in mind that a few permanent changes that endure are more desirable than are many changes that are short-lived and from which the client rapidly regresses to less healthy or to health-damaging modes of behavior. The most productive approach often consists of involving the client in a single attempt at behavior change in an area of high personal priority before moving on to more comprehensive health planning described in this chapter. Once the interest of the client is captured and he or she is motivated to become more active in self-care, a holistic health plan can be developed.

Health planning is a dynamic process in which flexibility to meet the changing needs of clients and families is critical. The plan systematically lends direction but does not dictate goals that must be attained or behaviors that must be learned. It is possible at any point to revise the plan or return to a former step in order to create a more viable and positive growth experience for the client.[2] A viable health protection/promotion plan should assist the client in developing feelings of self-direction, purpose, and control within his or her own life, particularly in the area of health. Through implementation of the plan, the client learns both "to act on" and "to react to" the environment more effectively. Thus, the client experiences self-expression, positive change, and personal growth in self-selected directions. The ultimate goal of health planning and implementation is to make health protection and health promotion a way of living that the client enjoys and adopts as a permanent lifestyle. Only constructive patterns of behavior that persist over time will have major impact on health status.

## THE HEALTH-PLANNING PROCESS

The process for developing a health protection/promotion plan will be outlined below. Each step in the process will be discussed separately, and materials for actual use with clients will be presented. Tailoring the process and materials to meet the needs of specific individuals is the responsibility of each professional nurse providing educative/developmental care. The following nine steps actively involve both the client and the nurse in the health-planning process:

1. Review and summarize data from assessment.
2. Identify self-care strengths (competencies) of the client.
3. Identify personal health goals and related areas for improvement in self-care.
4. List possible behavior changes.
5. Prioritize behavior changes based on client's perception of desirability and difficulty.
6. Make a commitment to behavior change.
7. Identify effective reinforcements and/or rewards.
8. Determine barriers to behavior change.
9. Develop time plan for implementation.

Completion of the initial health protection/promotion plan moves the client from the decision-making phase to the action phase of health behavior. Specific approaches that can be used to initiate and sustain behavioral change will be discussed in Chapter 9.

### Summary of Assessment Data
During assessment, a wealth of information is collected about the client. From this data, there must be constructed a holistic picture of the client that summarizes the extensive data. The reduction of data to manageable proportions is an important step in developing the health protection/promotion plan. Through the summary process, the client can gain new insights concerning positive inner qualities and resources that may previously have been unrecognized. In addition, the client gains increased awareness of the range of behaviors that can be acquired or learned.

Summary statements in response to each of the 15 questions identified below can organize assessment data in concise and meaningful form. Both the nurse and the client should retain a copy of the assessment summary for continuing reference during the health planning process.

1. What are the client's most salient values?
2. To what extent are the values and actions of the client consistent?
3. Does the client have any existing health problems that need to be considered in developing a health protection/promotion plan?
4. To what extent does the client believe that he/she can personally control health status?
5. What is the level of physical fitness of the client?
6. What is the nutritional status of the client?
7. For what chronic illnesses is the client "at risk"?
8. What sources of stress does the client experience?
9. How does the client handle stress?
10. What positive health practices does the client already routinely engage in?
11. What are the patterns of health behavior within the client's family?
12. Who are the significant others that serve as a support system for the client?
13. What is the client's current level of health knowledge related to risk reduction or health promotion?
14. What does the client need to know in order to enhance self-care skills?
15. What potential or actual barriers to self-care exist?

Clients can be guided through the review and summary process by the nurse during clinic appointments or home visits. Collaborative efforts of the client and nurse during this stage of health planning promotes rapport and increases mutual understanding of client's health concerns and personal health status.

**Identifying Self-Care Strengths of the Client**
Every client brings unique personal strengths to the health-planning task. These assets should be identified early in interactions with clients, and acknowledged and reinforced by the nurse. Self-care strengths may be in any of the following areas: consistency between values and actions, physical fitness, weight management, ability to cope with stress, family patterns of health behavior, or extent of health knowledge. The nurse and client should achieve consensus on areas in which the client is already taking informed and responsible action in matters of self-care.

Each client who is seen by the nurse already has a system of self-care in place that includes conscious behaviors and unconscious habits. Self-care practices may be culturally or scientifically derived.[3] Folk medicine or common self-care practices passed down from one generation to another are always part of each individual's cultural and ethnic heritage. Information gleaned from health professionals, magazines, newspapers, and mass media supplement or modify culturally acquired self-care behaviors. The ability of the client to maintain or enhance his or her own health depends on the repertoire of knowledge, skills, motivation, and orientation that has been acquired during the course of living.[4] It is important to start at the client's level so that valuable time is not wasted in teaching what a client already knows or in trying to make minor changes in essentially desirable behaviors. Attention should be reserved for major changes that are needed, and the number of changes focused on at any one time should be limited.

For self-care directed toward health protection and promotion to be effective, it must be compatible with the environmental, cultural, and societal milieu of the client. The nurse must keep in mind that each client will carry out health-protecting/promoting behaviors in different ways that fit his or her individual lifestyle. Consider the following examples: foods that are rich sources of protein may vary from culture to culture; many different forms of exercise can be used to attain physical fitness; many different approaches are available for dealing with stress; and deep relaxation can be achieved in a variety of ways, from transcendental meditation to progressive muscle relaxation. Even though health behaviors already developed by the client may not be those personally preferred by the nurse providing care, they may achieve comparable beneficial results.

Through teaching, guidance, and support, the nurse nurtures and enhances existing competencies to meet self-care demands. The extent of self-care demands of any given client depends on chronologic age, developmental maturity, health status, and the sources of social support available. While clients will vary in their requirements for self-care and their competencies for self-management, it is important that the nurse emphasize to all clients their own importance as the "primary self-care agent." Constructive behavior on their own behalf remains a requirement during every stage of the life span.

The format for developing a health protection/promotion plan is presented in Figure 8-1. Placing self-care competencies early in the plan enhances self-awareness, self-esteem, and feelings of control on the part of the client. By pointing out to clients what they already do well for themselves, interest can be stimulated in developing further self-care assets.

### Identifying Personal Health Goals and Related Areas for Improvement in Self-Care

The next step in the planning process is to identify personal health goals and related areas in which the client could improve in self-care. Areas for improvement do not necessarily represent deficits in self-care or areas of self-neglect. While deficits may be present, some areas of improvement will represent opportunities for further growth and self-actualization. Systematically reviewing areas in which self-care could be improved, assists the client in making an informed choice concerning those areas that he or she will actually concentrate on in developing the initial health protection/promotion plan. The client may not be motivated to make all the changes in current lifestyle that are possible or even desirable. However, reviewing the possibilities for change provides freedom for the client to determine the direction in which he or she will proceed to improve current health status.

Designed for: _____

Home Address: _____

Home Telephone Number: _____

Occupation (if employed): _____

Work Telephone Number: _____

Birth Date: _____  Date of Initial Plan: _____

Current Health Problems (if any): _____

_____

Chronic Illness for Which at "Moderate or High Risk": _____

_____

List Major Risk Factors: _____

_____

_____

_____

_____

Physical Fitness Status:     Height _____  Weight _____

Percent Body Fat _____

Recovery Index _____

Current Dietary Patterns: Protein Intake (%) _____

Carbohydrate Intake (%) _____

Fat Intake (%) _____

Stress Status:              Life-Stress Score _____

Major Sources of Stress _____

_____

_____

Usual Signs of Distress _____

_____

STAI Scores:  State _____

Trait _____

**FIGURE 8-1.**  Format for health protection/promotion plan (continued on next page).

Perceptions of Control:

MHLC Scores: Internal _____

Chance _____

Powerful Others _____

Rank Order of "Health" in Health-Values Scale _____

Top-Ranked Five Priorities Health-Values Scale

_____

_____

_____

_____

### Self-Care Strengths of the Client

Self-Care Measures

Nutritional Practices

Physical or Recreational Activity

Sleep Patterns

Stress Management·

**FIGURE 8-1** (continued).

Self-Actualization


Sense of Purpose


Relationships with Others


Environmental Control


Use of Health Care System


Others

| **Personal Health Goals** | |
|---|---|
| GOALS | CLIENT PRIORITY<br>(1 = MOST IMPORTANT) |
|  |  |

**FIGURE 8-1**   (continued).

| Areas for Improvement in Self-Care | | | |
|---|---|---|---|
| Target Health Goal: | | | |
| HEALTH PROTECTION/ PROMOTION AREAS TO BE STRENGTHENED (MAY USE CATEGORIES UNDER SELF-CARE STRENGTHS OR ADD OTHER RELEVANT CATEGORIES) | CLIENT PRIORITY (1 = MOST IMPORTANT) | SPECIFIC BEHAVIOR CHANGES | CLIENT PRIORITY (1 = MOST DESIRABLE) |
|  |  |  |  |
| List below the top-priority areas for change as designated by client. | | | |
|  | | | |
| List below the two most desirable behavior changes in each area as designated by the client. | | | |
|  | | | |

**FIGURE 8-1**   (continued).

The nurse must avoid making clients feel guilty or inadequate in regard to current health care practices. The potential for increasing self-care competencies should be presented by the nurse as a challenging rather than threatening aspect of the health-planning process. The excitement of change and continuing growth should be clearly communicated by the nurse during health counseling sessions with clients.

On the health protection/promotion plan, areas for improvement in self-care should be listed. After the list has been made, the client must prioritize the areas in terms of personal importance. Letting the client determine priorities and supporting efforts to make changes in the areas selected is part of the educative/developmental role of the nurse.

Many clients will initially place high priority on areas of health protection where the threat of illness is tangible and easily understood. Decreasing risk for specific chronic health problems fits the medical orientation of the vast majority of Americans. Measures for risk reduction are often conceptualized by clients as being more concrete than measures for health promotion.[5] Mastery of health protection measures will frequently motivate clients to consider changes in specific areas of health promotion. It appears that once clients make changes to decrease specific threats to health, they gain new awareness of the many possibilities for further enhancing health and well-being.

### Listing Possible Behavior Changes

People evaluate their own behavior using internal subjective criteria or external standards established by others. Often, people are aware that "something is wrong" or that their current behavior is not as desirable as it might be, but they are unable to identify specific changes that can be made to improve health status. Clients may give emotional cues concerning the behavior that they wish to change. Examples of such cues include:

- "I don't like the way that I look!"
- "I'm so fat that I hate myself!"
- "I get mad at myself for being uptight!"

Emotions are legitimate feelings on the part of the client to which the nurse should be sensitive in order to recognize areas of behavioral concern. A constructive program of change can only begin after specific behavioral difficulties or dilemmas have been concretely identified.[6]

The two to three top-priority areas selected by the client for improvement need to be carefully examined to determine what behavior changes will result in desired outcomes. Without a clear view of the specific behavioral changes that may be accomplished in terms of enhancing self-care, the client will experience little motivation to modify personal lifestyle.

At this point, the client should be encouraged to look at each area of self-care in which improvement is desired and determine what behaviors currently practiced are supportive or nonsupportive of positive change. For instance, if the client values a slim, healthy figure and has the goal of losing weight, eating "junk" foods is inconsistent with both values and goal. The client should be assisted in examining major value/behavior inconsistencies that exist. Alternative actions that are both healthful and enjoyable need to be substituted for the inconsistent behaviors. It is unfortunate that what individuals have learned to prefer within the American lifestyle is often detrimental to health. While our bodies thrive on adequate intake of proteins, complex carbohydrates, and unsaturated fats, the American culture encourages consumption of simple carbohydrates and large amounts of saturated fats. Body needs and personal preferences developed as a result of social influences are frequently at odds with one another.

In identifying possible behavior changes, the client should be encouraged to concentrate on major changes that will have the greatest impact on health status. There should be no territory of behavior off-limits for exploration. The more open the client is in discussing health concerns with the nurse, the higher the probability of developing an exciting and challenging health promotion plan. Often, areas that are tempting to leave unexplored, such as marital relationships, human sexuality, or family cohesiveness, are the most crucial in which to make changes to increase potential for self-actualization.

*Prioritizing Behavior Changes.* Prioritizing possible behavior changes in terms of desirability to the client is a critical step in the development of a health protection/promotion plan. It is at this point that the client selects, from all the behavioral options available, those behaviors that are personally appealing, that he or she is willing to try. This brings the client full circle from assessing current health status and personal lifestyle, through considering areas of desired improvement and behavioral options, to actually identifying those behaviors to be learned in order to accomplish desired goals. At this point in the health-planning process, a cohesive plan of action begins to emerge.

The client's priorities for behavior change will reflect personal values; activity preferences; personal estimates of cognitive, affective, and psychomotor skills; subjective probabilities for success in learning; and ease with which target behaviors can be integrated into personal lifestyle. No one is in a better position than the client to know what changes are feasible given current health status, lifestyle, support systems, and environment. If the client is in control of new behaviors to be attempted and is confident of success in making the desired changes, he or she is well on the way toward integrating new health-protecting and health-promoting behaviors into current lifestyle.

### Making a Commitment to Behavior Change (Behavioral Contracts)
Through identification of new behaviors that the client is willing to try, a verbal commitment is made to change. However, the client may be more motivated to follow-through with selected actions if the personal commitment is formalized through a written contract. While contracts or written agreements between two or more parties have been used in business transactions for many years, use of a *behavioral contract* in helping relationships is relatively new. In a behavioral contract, the individual or client negotiates a realistic behavior change with another individual or with him- or herself. The contract contains specific information

about (1) the change to be made, (2) the way the change is to be accomplished, (3) the person who is to engage in the change, (4) the time frame in which the behavior is to be accomplished, and (5) the consequences of meeting or not meeting the terms of the agreement. Behavioral contracts used by the nurse are generally of two types: nurse–client contracts and self-contracts. Each type will be discussed separately, and illustrations of sample contracts will be provided.

*Nurse–Client Contract.* This type of contract can be defined as any working agreement, continuously renegotiable, among nurse, client, and family.[7] A contract provides direction for the helping relationships through identification of mutual objectives and responsibilities of each party to the contract. Although similar to a business contract, a nurse–client contract is generally less formal and seldom legally binding unless specific fee negotiations are included. Through mutual involvement of client and nurse in a meaningful contract, the signers recognize the responsibility of the client for his or her own health status and the caring, counseling, and supportive role of the nurse in preventive/promotive care. Contracts allow clients to participate actively in their own care by choosing goals that can be realistically accomplished.

An operational definition of the contracting process has been presented by Sloan and Schommer.[8] They identify components of the nurse–client contracting process as follows:

1. Mutual exploration of health problems, concerns, and goals between client and nurse (family and other health care providers may be included in discussion)
2. Establishment of mutually agreeable health goals
3. Mutual exploration of resources available to accomplish goals (terms of contract)
4. Development of a plan/steps/method to achieve goals
5. Negotiation of division of responsibilities that are mutually agreed upon in steps toward fulfilling goal(s)
6. Mutual agreement on time limit to accomplish goal(s)
7. Mutual evaluation of progress toward accomplishment of goal(s) in designated time frame
8. Modification, renegotiation, or termination of contract

Through nurse–client contracting, both parties to the contract are clear on who will be responsible for what. Generally, the client is responsible for carrying out certain behaviors, while the nurse is responsible for providing information, training, counseling, or specific reinforcement/rewards. The nurse as the health care professional involved in the contract bears the additional responsibility of providing helpful input and continuing feedback to the client concerning the adequacy of performance of activities identified in the contract. It is also critical that the nurse be consistent and conscientious in managing the reinforcement/reward contingencies of the contract. Failure in fulfilling this commitment will destroy the trust and confidence placed in the nurse by the client. A sample format for the nurse–client contract is presented in Figure 8-2.

### Nurse-Client Contract/Agreement

Statement of Health Goal: _____*Decreased feelings of stress and tension*_____

I _____*Jim Johnson*_____ promise to _____*use progressive relaxation*_____
         (client)

_____*techniques (four-muscle groups) upon arriving home from work each day*_____
                    (Client Responsibility)

for a period of _____*one week*_____ , whereupon,

_____*Nancy Turner*_____ will provide _____*a copy of*_____
         (nurse)

_____*Herbert Benson's book, Relaxation Response*_____
                    (Nurse Responsibility)

on _____*Saturday, March 7th*_____ to me.
                    (date)

If I do not fulfill the terms of this contract in total, I understand that the designated reward will be withheld.

Signed: _____*Jim Johnson*_____
                              (client)

_____*February 2, 1982*_____
                              (date)

_____*Kathy Turner*_____
                              (nurse)

_____*February 2, 1982*_____
                              (date)

**FIGURE 8-2.** Sample nurse–client contract.

Herje[9] has identified the following characteristics as important for nurse–client contracts:

1. Goals contracted for should be realistic.
2. Behavior related to achievement of goals should be measurable.

3. Goals should be stated in positive terms.
4. The contract should provide a definite time frame for accomplishment.
5. The contract should be written and signed by both nurse and client (a copy of the contract should be retained by each).
6. Behavior indicative of goal attainment must be rewardable.
7. The degree to which the goal is achieved must be able to be evaluated.

The nurse–client contract provides incentives for behavior change rather than relying on individual persistence and will-power. It is easier to follow through with a specific behavior if the client has made a definite commitment to another person to do so or will be rewarded upon achieving success. Goals included in the contract must be within the realm of accomplishment for the client, or experiences of failure and frustration will result in trying to meet contract terms.

Rewards selected should be immediate as often as possible and reinforcing to the client. Withholding reinforcement when the terms of the agreement have not been met is generally considered fair and acceptable by the client. However, penalties imposed by the nurse for failure to perform can create resentment and hostility on the part of the client and can threaten the integrity of the nurse–client relationship. For this reason, penalties or subtle forms of punishment, such as promoting guilt or shame, should never be used in implementing nurse–client contracts.

Since family members can support or inhibit clients from fulfilling the terms of the nurse–client contract, they should be included in goal-setting and contracting activities. Family members, because of their continuing contact with the client, can serve as important sources of encouragement, reinforcement, and reward. Family members, themselves may be a party to the contract, actively participating through fulfillment of specific responsibilities. As an example, a spouse may agree to accompany his or her mate during brisk walks or entertain children in order to provide a quiet time for client practice of relaxation. Entire families may be the clients in a contract and together identify health goals to be attained and plans for their accomplishment.

The extent to which the contract has worked must be evaluated. Did the client accomplish the goal(s) fully, partially, or not at all? What were the reasons for failure? How could the contract be reorganized so that the probability of successful completion is high? Does the contract need to be renegotiated? Should the contract be terminated? Careful analysis of the contracting process and evaluation of subsequent outcomes will permit the nurse and client to modify contracts as needed or to establish new contracts that successfully move clients toward desired health goals. Success in fulfilling the agreements in the contract enhances the client's self-esteem and problem-solving abilities. The client gains increased confidence and self-sufficiency in meeting future health needs.

As an example of nurses actively involved in the use of nurse–client contracts, one might cite Susan Steckel and her associates in Ann Arbor, Michigan. They have been highly successful in using contracting to increase the compliance of clients with their hypertensive regimens. Increasing health-protective practices, such as medication taking, adherence to low-sodium diets, and appointment keeping have been the major emphasis of their contracting activities with clients and families. The rate of successful management of hypertension among their clients is higher than in a comparable group not participating in the contracting process.[10] Nurse–client contracting as a means of eliciting participation and commitment of clients to health goals is also used by other nurses in a variety of community and ambulatory care settings.

*Self-Contract.* A self-contract is a commitment to oneself to perform specific behaviors for a previously identified reinforcement that is attractive and motivating.[11] Since the client is responsible for both the behavioral commitment and for conveying the reward, immediate reinforcement is possible. Numerous educational studies have emphasized the importance of reward contingencies for effective learning.

Self-contracting is an effective approach for enhancing the client's control over his or her own behavior, thus creating a sense of independence and autonomy. The client does not become overly dependent on the nurse for reinforcement but instead serves as the source of his or her own rewards for positive health behaviors.

Ultimately the client must learn to manage a personal reward system that is supportive of emerging positive health practices. The sooner the client can participate in self-contracting as an adjunct to nurse–client contracting, the more self-directive and self-confident the client will become. An example of a self-contract is presented in Figure 8-3.

A word of caution is in order regarding self-contracting. In many instances, the client with a low self-concept or little perceived control over health may not feel compelled to meet his or her own expectations and demands. The motto "to thine own self be true" is not taken seriously. Without the external expectations of significant others, there is little follow-through on specific activities to meet contract terms. When this occurs, the nurse should discuss with the client his or her personal feelings about independence in self-care. In addition, emphasizing the client's strengths and ability to accept responsibility in nurse–client contracts can enhance self-esteem and increase the probability of successful self-contracting in the future.

### Identifying Effective Reinforcements and Rewards

Identifying effective sources of reinforcement or reward for engaging in new health-protecting or health-promoting behaviors is an important step in planning for implementation of the health protection/promotion plan. The sources of reward may be the nurse, the client, or the client's family. The nurse and family can provide external rewards, while only the client can manipulate both external and internal reinforcement contingencies.

It is important to distinguish between external and internal reinforcement. External rewards generally refer to tangible objects or experiences that are reinforcing for the client. Objects that can be used for reinforcement include books, personal-care products, educational pamphlets, self-care materials, or passes to

---

**Self-Contract**

Personal Health Goal:                    *Change Dietary Habits*

I            *Doris Downs*            promise myself that I will    *follow*

    *the sample menus for a 1200 calorie diet for breakfast, lunch, and*

    *dinner*        for a period of                *one day*                ,

whereupon I will            *buy myself a new pair of earrings*

on         *Wednesday, June 8th*         .


Signed        *Doris Downs*

Date        *February 17, 1982*

---

**FIGURE 8-3.**  Sample self-contract.

exercise gyms or health spas. Cash value is not necessarily a good indication of reinforcement value. Experiential rewards may be 15 minutes with a nurse to talk about anything that the client wishes, an opportunity to meet with a physical-fitness consultant free-of-charge, or the opportunity to borrow a program of audio-cassettes from the nurse that address an area of health that is important to the client. Pleasurable family activities, such as trips, sports, or picnics, also can have strong reinforcement value. They should be used frequently to reward desired health behaviors, since increased family cohesiveness is often an additional benefit. Tailoring rewards to individual desires and preferences is important for their successful use in promoting positive health practices.

Praise or compliments from others are also forms of external reinforcement. The reinforcement value of any external reward depends on the client's perception of its desirability or utility and the probability with which the client believes that the target activity will be actually followed by the reward.[11,12] If the client highly values the reinforcement offered and believes that he or she is certain to obtain it if the appropriate behavior is completed, the probability of the client taking action is high. If the reward is of little value to the client, and he or she perceives the probability of obtaining it as low, little motivation will exist to engage in the target behavior.

Internal rewards are intangible, but they can be highly reinforcing to many individuals. Internal reinforcement can be defined as self-praise, increased self-satisfaction, or enhanced self-image or self-esteem as a result of completing a designated behavior. The important advantages of internal reinforcement include (1) the client's being in complete control of reward contingencies and (2) the fact that reinforcement can be administered immediately in any situation.

Reinforcements to be optimally effective in rewarding positive health behaviors cannot be left to accident or happenstance. Planning a reward system ahead of time insures that reinforcements will be available as they are needed and that they will be objects, experiences, or internal states that are highly valued by clients. In Figure 8-4, a sample reward-and-reinforcement list is presented. This form can be used by the client to list realistic sources of reinforcement to be used by the nurse, family, or self. An outline of a reward/reinforcement system is presented in Figure 8-5. The system provides a plan of action with reinforcement points carefully identified for shaping the specific behavior selected. Actual use of rewards for behavior and lifestyle change will be discussed in detail in Chapter 9.

### Determining Barriers to Change

All individuals experience barriers to making changes in behavior. While some obstacles cannot be anticipated, others can be planned for and overcome or their potential for impact considerably weakened before initiating the change process. If the client is aware of possible barriers and has formulated plans for dealing with them should they arise, successful behavior change is more likely to occur.

Barriers to effective health behavior can arise from inside clients themselves, from significant others, or from the environment. Internal barriers to change may be lack of motivation, fatigue, boredom, giving up, lack of appropriate skills, or disbelief that personal behavior can be successfully changed. Family members can impose considerable barriers if they encourage continuation of health-damaging behaviors or if they actively discourage attempts at behavior change. Attitudes of family members can be hostile, punitive, or apathetic toward new health practices, providing repeated negative reinforcement for the client. Barriers within the family may be overcome by developing contracts among family members that are mutually rewarding. For instance, a husband might contract with his wife in the following way:

*Wife will: brisk walk with husband for 30 minutes four days per week*
*(Monday, Tuesday, Thursday, Friday)*
*IF*
*Husband will: take her to the movies, leaving the children at home*
*with a babysitter, on Saturday evening.*

Children enjoy contracting too and are excellent in following through with the commitments they make. Contracting can be both fun and highly useful in supporting continued practice of positive health behaviors by clients and families.

Environmental barriers that may inhibit positive change include lack of space or appropriate setting in which to carry out the selected activity, dangers within the immediate environment, such as heavy traffic or high crime rate, and inclement weather or inappropriate climate (too hot or too cold). The client should be assisted

Developed by: _____
                                    (name)

External Rewards (list below and rank according to desirability, 1 = most
                          desirable)

Objects:

  Available



  Potentially Available



Experiences:

  Require Advanced Planning



  Do Not Require Advanced Planning



Internal Rewards (list below)

**FIGURE 8-4.** Reward-and-reinforcement list.

by the nurse in dealing with these environmental barriers or in locating a setting
for health activities where such conditions do not exist.

Barriers to new behaviors vary between clients. Recognizing potential blocks
or obstacles to positive health practices and dealing actively with them at the
beginning of behavior change can greatly reduce future difficulties.

Behavior: Learn to Use Progressive Relaxation as One Approach to Handling Stress

| Component of Behavior | Reward or Reinforcement |
|---|---|
| Attend first class session at 9 A.M. Saturday at the county health department | Watch the football game in the afternoon on TV |
| Use relaxation audiotape at home for 20 minutes of practice | |
| Sunday | Call John and visit for a while |
| Monday | Spend an hour at the driving range |
| Tuesday | Buy a new paperback novel |
| Wednesday | Praise myself for having practiced relaxation each day thus far |
| Thursday | Invite Harry and Jim over to play pool |
| Friday | Take my family to a movie |
| Attend second class session at 9 A.M. Saturday at the County Health Department | Take an orange juice break afterwards with Bret, a class member |
| Practice relaxation techniques for 20 minutes providing my own cues rather than using the tape | |
| Sunday | Go for a short drive and enjoy the scenery |
| Monday | Spend 30 minutes reading my new novel |
| Tuesday | Buy myself a new bottle of aftershave lotion |
| Wednesday | Praise myself for persistence and successful practice |
| Thursday | Allow myself to linger in a warm shower longer than usual |
| Friday | Go to stock car races with the family |
| Keep my weekly record of relaxation practice | The nurse will provide a copy of *Relaxation Response* by Herbert Benson |

**FIGURE 8-5.**   Reward/reinforcement plan.

### Developing a Time Plan for Implementation

Changes toward more positive health practices need to be made over a period of time in order to allow new behaviors to be learned well, integrated into one's lifestyle, and stabilized. Attempting to change or initiate a number of new behaviors all at once may result in confusion, discouragement, and abandonment of the health protection/promotion plan by the client. Whether the client is attempting to reduce risk for specific chronic diseases or to enhance personal health status, gradual rather than abrupt change is desirable. Just as health education for self-care must proceed at the pace of the learner rather than at that of the nurse, changes in behavior must be sequenced in reasonable steps appropriate for the client.

Developing a time plan for implementation allows appropriate knowledge and skills to be mastered before a new behavior is implemented. For example, it is difficult to warm up before brisk walking if the client has no idea of what appropriate warm-up exercises are. The time frame for developing a given behavior may be several weeks or several months. If the client is rewarded for accomplishing short-term goals, this provides encouragement for continuing pursuit of long-term objectives. A meaningful plan requires that deadlines be set for accomplishing specific goals. Adherence to deadlines should be encouraged, with changes made only when the time frame must be shortened or lengthened to make it more conducive to permanent behavior change.

Active involvement of the client in establishing a time frame for the development of new behaviors reinforces self-esteem, feelings of control, and self-responsibility in protecting and maintaining personal health. The client determines not only the areas in which changes will be made but also how time can be planned and managed to facilitate changes in behavior and lifestyle.

## REVISIONS OF THE HEALTH PROTECTION/PROMOTION PLAN

A schedule for periodic review of the health protection/promotion plan should be established. Revisions should be carried out during counseling sessions with both the client and the nurse contributing to the process. Impetus for changes in the plan may result from mastery of target behaviors, changes in client's values and priorities, or awareness of new options available to the client. Outdated plans fail to provide impetus or direction for change and thus become uninteresting and meaningless to the client.

Periodic revision and updating of the health plan provides a systematic approach for movement of the client toward higher levels of health. After experiencing success in behavior change, additional target behaviors to be learned and integrated into the client's lifestyle can be added. Level of physical fitness, dietary habits, ability to cope with stress, and social support systems can be remarkably changed over a period of time. Maintaining a viable and current health plan assists the client in managing personal behavior in order to achieve desired health goals.

## SUMMARY

The health protection/promotion plan presented in this chapter is intended to provide clients with a systematic approach to improving health practices and lifestyle. A sample plan is presented in Figure 8-6 to assist the reader in further understanding how the health protection/promotion plan can be used as the basis for individualized client care. Clients should be encouraged to keep and update their own health progress record or portfolio.

| | |
|---|---|
| Designed for: | *Jim Thorpe* |
| Home Address: | *486 N. Walden* |
| Home Telephone Number: | *(303) 875-3111* |
| Occupation (if employed): | *Chemical engineer* |
| Work Telephone Number: | *(303) 872-1334* |
| Birth Date: *8/3/41* | Date of Initial Plan: *4/2/80* |
| Current Health Problems (if any): | *Transient elevations in blood pressure* |
| Chronic Illness for Which at "Moderate or High Risk": | *Cardiovascular disease* |
| List Major Risk Factors: | *(1) Father died from heart attack at* |
| | *58 years of age, (2) 25% overweight,* |
| | *(3) 41–50% fat in diet, (4) sedentary* |
| | *occupation, (5) moderate to high stress,* |
| | *(6) periodic BP readings as high as 150/90.* |
| Physical Fitness Status: | Height *6'0"*    Weight *218 lbs.* |
| | Percent Body Fat *23%* |
| | Recovery Index *162* |
| Current Dietary Patterns: | Protein Intake (%) *13%* |
| | Carbohydrate Intake (%) *43%* |
| | Fat Intake (%) *44%* |

**FIGURE 8-6.** Sample health protection/promotion plan.

| | | | |
|---|---|---|---|
| Stress Status: | Life-Stress Score | | *154* |
| | Major Sources of Stress | | *Work* |
| | | | *Finances* |
| | Usual Signs of Distress | | *Difficulty sleeping;* |
| | | | *muscles tense and stiff* |
| | STAI Scores: | State | *40* |
| | | Trait | *38* |
| Perceptions of Control: | MHLC Scores: | Internal | *56* |
| | | Chance | *28* |
| | | Powerful Others | *38* |
| Rank Order "Health" in Health-Values Scale | | | *4* |
| Top Ranked Five Priorities Health-Values Scale | | | *Happiness* |
| | | | *Inner harmony* |
| | | | *A sense of accomplishment* |
| | | | *Health* |
| | | | *Self-respect* |

### Self-Care Strengths of the Client

Self-Care Measures

*Drinks 6–8 glasses of water/day*
*Does not smoke*
*Does not take laxatives*
*Knows what blood pressure and pulse readings should be*
*Uses soft toothbrush and dental floss regularly*

**FIGURE 8-6** (continued).

---

### Self-Care Strengths of the Client

Nutritional Practices

*Eats breakfast daily*
*Eats three meals/day*
*Adds little or no salt to food*

Physical or Recreational Activity

*Plays golf 1–2 times per week*
*Maintains good posture*
*Walks up stairs rather than riding elevator*

Sleep Patterns

*Gets 7 hours of sleep/night*
*Sleeps on a firm mattress*

Stress Management

*Can laugh at self*
*Understands the relationship between stress and illness*
*Enjoys spending time in unstructured activities*

Self-Actualization

*Maintains an enthusiastic and optimistic outlook on life*
*Is a member of two community-service groups*
*Is aware of personal strengths and weaknesses*
*Respects own accomplishments*

Sense of Purpose

*Believes that life has purpose*

Relationships with Others

*Is close to family and enjoys spending time with them in camping and*
  *recreational activities*
*Communicates easily with others*
*Perceives self as well-accepted by co-workers*

Environmental Control

*Does not permit smoking in house and car*
*Provides resources to meet personal needs*
*Maintains safe living area*

Use of Health Care System

*Reports unusual signs or symptoms to a physician*

---

**FIGURE 8-6** (continued).

| Personal Health Goals | |
| --- | --- |
| GOALS | CLIENT PRIORITY (1 = MOST IMPORTANT) |
| Decrease risk for hypertension | 1 |
| Learn to relax | 2 |
| Maintain desired weight | 3 |
| Achieve consistency between personal priorities and allocation of time | 4 |

| Areas for Improvement in Self-Care | | | |
| --- | --- | --- | --- |
| Target Health Goal: *Decrease risk for hypertension* | | | |
| Health Protection/ Promotion Areas to Be Strengthened (may use categories under self-care strengths or add other relevant categories) | Client Priority (1 = most important) | Specific Behavior Changes | Client Priority (1 = most desirable) |
| Increased physical activity | 1 | Brisk walk 4 times/week for 45 minutes | 1 |
| | | Begin jog-walk exercise | 4 |
| | | Swim at the "Y" 4 times/week | 2 |
| | | Play tennis at the "Y" 2 times/week | 3 |
| Monitor blood pressure | 2 | Have blood pressure checked at health department once a month | 2 |
| | | Have physician check blood pressure every 3 months | 3 |
| | | Buy blood pressure cuff and learn to take own pressure | 1 |

**FIGURE 8-6**   (continued).

| Areas for Improvement in Self-Care | | | |
|---|---|---|---|
| Target Health Goal: *Learn to relax* | | | |
| Health Protection/ Promotion Areas to Be Strengthened (may use categories under self-care strengths or add other relevant categories) | Client Priority (1 = most important) | Specific Behavior Changes | Client Priority (1 = most desirable) |
| *Understand my body's response to stress* | 3 | *Observe my own reactions in tense situations* | 2 |
|  |  | *Review my responses on "signs of distress"* | 1 |
|  |  | *Ask people close to me how I act when tense* | 3 |
| *Identify areas of stress in my life* | 2 | *Discuss my life-stress review with the nurse* | 1 |
|  |  | *Make a list of personally stressful situations as they occur* | 2 |
|  |  | *Talk to my wife about sources of stress in the home* | 3 |
|  |  | *Talk to my boss about sources of stress on the job* | 4 |
| *Learn specific relaxation skills* | 1 | *Read Relaxation Response by Herbert Benson* | 2 |
|  |  | *Attend series of classes on relaxation techniques* | 1 |
|  |  | *Attend classes in Yoga* | 3 |
|  |  | *Purchase a set of audiotapes on relaxation skills* | 4 |

**FIGURE 8-6**  (continued).

| Areas for Improvement in Self-Care | | | |
|---|---|---|---|
| **Target Health Goal:** *Maintain desired weight* | | | |
| Health Protection/ Promotion Areas to Be Strengthened (may use categories under self-care strengths or add other relevant categories) | Client Priority (1 = most important) | Specific Behavior Changes | Client Priority (1 = most desirable) |
| *Change eating habits* | *1* | *Decrease number and sodium content of between-meal snacks* | *1* |
| | | *Become familiar with basic food groups* | *3* |
| | | *Avoid eating anything after 7 P.M. at night except low-calorie snacks* | *2* |
| | | *Plan an 1800 calorie low-sodium diet to follow* | *4* |
| | | *Go on a crash diet* | *undesirable* |
| **Target Health Goal:** *Achieve consistency between personal priorities and allocation of time (family first priority)* | | | |
| Health Protection/ Promotion Areas to Be Strengthened (may use categories under self-care strengths or add other relevant categories) | Client Priority (1 = most important) | Specific Behavior Changes | Client Priority (1 = most desirable) |
| *Learn to use time at work more efficiently* | *3* | *Develop time-management plan* | *2* |
| | | *Arrive at work a half hour earlier* | *3* |
| | | *Learn to say "no" when asked to complete additional tasks outside my area of responsibility* | *1* |

**FIGURE 8-6** (continued).

| **Areas for Improvement in Self-Care** | | | |
| --- | --- | --- | --- |
| Target Health Goal: *Achieve consistency between personal priorities and allocation of time (family first priority)* | | | |
| Health Protection/ Promotion Areas to Be Strengthened (may use categories under self-care strengths or add other relevant categories) | Client Priority (1 = most important) | Specific Behavior Changes | Client Priority (1 = most desirable) |
| *Improve relationship with my wife* | *1* | *Arrange to take my wife out for lunch* | *1* |
| | | *Buy flowers or a special gift for my wife* | *3* |
| | | *Express appreciation to my wife for meal preparation* | *2* |
| *Improve relationships with my son and daughter* | *2* | *Set aside a specific time each week to go bike riding with my son and daughter* | *2* |
| | | *Arrange to take my son and daughter (wife, too) to a baseball game* | *3* |
| | | *Spend time one evening each week visiting with my son and daughter and listening to what they have to say* | *1* |
| | | *Take my son, daughter, and their friends roller skating* | *4* |
| List below the top-priority areas for change as designated by client. | | | |
| *Increase physical activity* *Learn specific relaxation skills* *Change eating habits* *Improve relationship with my wife* | | | |

**FIGURE 8-6**   (continued).

List below the two most desirable behavior changes in each area as designated by the client.

*Increase physical activity*
*Brisk walk 4 times/week for 45 minutes*
*Swim at the "Y" 4 times/week*

*Learn specific relaxation skills*
*Attend relaxation classes*
*Read* Relaxation Response *by Herbert Benson*

*Change eating habits*
*Decrease number and sodium content of between-meal snacks*
*Avoid eating after 7* P.M. *at night*

*Improve relationship with my wife*
*Arrange to take my wife to lunch*
*Express appreciation to my wife for preparing meals*

**FIGURE 8-6** (continued).

## REFERENCES

1. Litwack, L., Litwack, J.M., & Ballou, M.B. *Health counseling.* New York: Appleton, 1980.
2. Hames, C.C., & Joseph, D.H. *Basic concepts of helping: A wholistic approach.* New York: Appleton, 1980.
3. Caley, J.M., Dirksen, M., Engalla, M., & Hennrich, M.L. The Orem self-care nursing model. In Riehl, J.P., & Roy, C., (Eds.), *Conceptual models for nursing practice* (2nd. ed.) New York: Appleton, 1980, p. 304.
4. *Ibid.,* p. 311.
5. *Into the mainstream with health risk reduction.* Proceedings of the 15th Annual Meeting on Prospective Medicine and Health Hazard Appraisal, St. Petersburg, Florida, October 3–6, 1979. Available from Health and Education Resources, 9650 Rockville Pike, Bethesda, Maryland 20014.
6. Martin, R.A., & Poland, E.Y. *Learning to change: A self-management approach to adjustment.* New York: McGraw-Hill, 1980.
7. Sloan, M.R., & Schommer, B.T. The process of contracting in community nursing. In Spradley, B.W. (Ed.), *Contemporary community nursing.* Boston: Little, Brown, 1975, pp. 221–229.
8. *Ibid.,* pp. 224–225.
9. Herje, P.A. Hows and whys of patient contracting. *Nurse Educator,* January–February 1980, *5,* 30–34.
10. Swain, M.A., & Steckel, S.B. Influencing adherence among hypertensives. *Research in Nursing and Health,* March 1981, *4,* 213–222.
11. DeRisi, W.J., & Butz, G. *Writing behavioral contracts.* Champaign, Ill.: Research Press, 1975.
12. Ausubel, D.P. *Educational psychology: A cognitive view.* New York: Holt, Rinehart & Winston, 1968.
13. Fishbein, M., & Ajzen, I. *Belief, attitude, intention and behavior: An introduction to theory and research.* Reading, Mass.: Addison-Wesley, 1975.

# Part III
# STRATEGIES FOR PREVENTION AND HEALTH PROMOTION: THE ACTION PHASE

While the strategies in the preceding section have been focused on facilitating informed decision making by the client about health behaviors, this section will present specific actions that the client can take to protect and enhance personal health status. The strategies presented in each chapter can be used by the client in implementing the health protection/promotion plan. Since the dynamics of behavior change are important for both client and nurse to understand, attention will be given to various approaches for modifying lifestyle. Strategies for change will be presented and the roles of both nurse and client in the change process discussed. Approaches to exercise and physical fitness, nutrition and weight control, stress management, and building/strengthening social support systems will be presented. It is the intent of this section to provide the nurse with specific information and counseling strategies to be used in facilitating and supporting the client in efforts to attain better health, increased life satisfaction, personal growth, and fulfillment.

# CHAPTER 9
# Modification of Lifestyle

Every human being has the potential for becoming more competent, more purposeful, and more self-actualized by developing unique personal resources. Self-actualization is achieved primarily through progressive change, a natural part of the life process.[1] Lifton has described change as a formative process in human beings that consists of "creating, maintaining, breaking down and recreating viable form."[2] Because of man's creative and problem-solving abilities, change can be controlled and used to personal advantage. Self-directed change is also possible and can be defined as those behaviors that individuals deliberately undertake to achieve self-selected goals and desired outcomes. Acknowledgment of the potential of clients for self-modification recognizes their human dignity as individuals and their right to choose how they will live.[3]

Self-modification represents a set of skills that must be learned in order for the client to achieve control over his or her own behavior.[4] Change techniques involve the knowledgeable and productive use of self in self-monitoring (observation), self-instruction, self-reinforcement, and self-evaluation.[5] Self-modification has the following characteristics:[6]

*It applies the laws of learning.*
*It concentrates on specific actions, thoughts, or emotions.*
*It places heavy emphasis on positive reinforcement.*
*It occurs in real life situations.*
*It allows individuals to design and execute their own learning program.*

Self-control over one's own health status requires arranging the right set of internal and external conditions to support desired behaviors.

Behavior modification and lifestyle change represent the action phase of health behavior. A specific overt behavior is usually preceded by preparatory adjustments for action, such as learning, thinking, and deliberation.[7] These preparatory adjustments have been dealt with in the preceding chapters as the decision-making phase of health behavior. Nursing strategies during the action phase differ from those used to assist clients in making health-related decisions. During the action phase the nurse (1) assists the client in the identification and use of relevant cues to elicit desired behaviors, (2) sustains or increases level of readiness to engage in selected behaviors, (3) supports self-change approaches employed by clients, (4) reduces or eliminates potential or actual barriers to illness prevention and health promotion activities, and (5) assists clients in evaluating the impact of new behaviors on personal health status.

The action phase of health behavior is depicted in Figure 9-1. Level of readiness to act is largely a consequence of the decision-making phase. Cues of varying intensity (depending on level of readiness) are essential to activate behavior, while barriers can slow down or impede constructive health actions on the part of clients. Following initial action, the client may continue the new behavior without reservation, look for additional information to support the new behavior, or reconsider other action alternatives. Change is a two-phase process consisting of initiation and continuation of the target behavior. Research to date has dealt primarily with initiating behavior change. Interventions to facilitate long-term changes in behavior and integration of such behaviors as a permanent component of lifestyle need to be developed and empirically tested.

Factors that need to be considered in facilitating client change toward more positive health practices include the following:[8]

> *Reasons for change*
> *Available knowledge and skills to initiate and sustain change*
> *Ratio of payoffs for present behavior in relation to anticipated payoffs for change or new behaviors*
> *Extent of support for changed behavior within the social and physical environment*

The climate created for change is extremely important. Throughout the action phase, the client needs continuing awareness of personal resources that can make change possible. The client needs to benefit from others' perceptions of his or her strengths. Frequent recognition of clients' strengths and assets by the nurse, family, and significant others ("strength bombardment") will facilitate the client's ability to make changes personally deemed desirable.

The nurse as a helping person must have an accurate, empathetic understanding of the life situation of the client and provide support and warmth (positive regard) in order to facilitate change.[9] A client can best recognize and accept his or her strengths and potential for effective action if an interpersonal environment exists between the nurse and client that is characterized by caring, personal authenticity, and open communication.[10]

Nurses in all care settings attempt to affect client behavior in some way. Approaches generally used vary from direct information giving to planned programs of behavior change. As an example of client services focused on behavior modification, nurses at the Nursing Consultation Center, Pennsylvania State University, provide individual and family counseling as well as group programs to assist clients in evaluating and modifying lifestyle patterns that contribute to

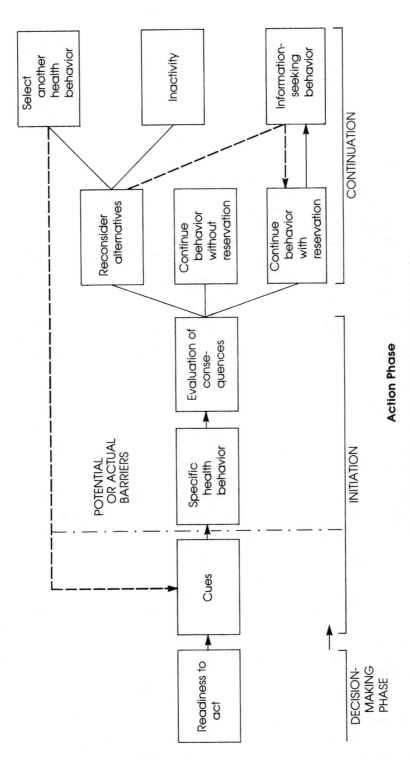

**Action Phase**

**FIGURE 9-1.** Action phase of health behavior.

209

health risks. In addition, the center also provides assistance to clients with chronic illness to enable them to develop a lifestyle that supports healthful and productive living. The services of the center are available to residents of the community as well as students, faculty, and staff of the university. The center represents a creative approach in providing innovative nursing services directly to the public.

Another example of services offered by a nurse to assist clients in changing their own lifestyles to achieve more healthful ones is the educative health counseling practice of Lynn Rew in Woodstock, Illinois. Rew is in collaborative practice with a group of physicians. She provides individual and family counseling for behavioral problems, marital dysfunction, midlife crises, and other health-related concerns, and she also consults with clients regarding personal behavior-modification programs. Areas of behavior modification on which Rew focuses in her practice are weight control, smoking cessation, stress management, divorce adjustment, sexual dysfunction, depression, and communication problems. The contribution of Rew to the care and well-being of clients within her practice setting is well recognized by the physicians with whom she works.

Nurses engaged in providing prevention and health-promotion services to clients must be skilled in facilitating self-directed change on the part of clients and families. In order to do this, nurses must understand the process of change and strategies for promoting the initiation and continuation of new health behaviors.

## STRATEGIES FOR CHANGE

Specific approaches to self-modification to be discussed in this chapter include (1) self-confrontation, (2) cognitive restructuring, (3) modeling, (4) operant conditioning, (5) counterconditioning, and (6) stimulus control. For an individual client, one particular technique may be chosen or several techniques may be combined in a more complex behavior-change program. It is critical that both nurse and client be mutually involved in decisions concerning behavior change approaches to be used.

### Self-Confrontation

At the core of every individual's value system is the self-concept. Self-concept represents beliefs about personal competence and worth. Personal values/beliefs and the values and beliefs of others provide standards of conduct by which the self-concept is evaluated. Threats to self-concept directly affect feelings of self-esteem. When a contradiction exists between values and self-concept or behaviors and self-concept, it can be resolved with the least effort by changing values that are less central or by changing behaviors to be consistent with self-concept.[11]

Self-confrontation as a counseling approach is based on the premise that change results from the arousal of an affective state of dissatisfaction within the client due to recognition of chronic inconsistencies in his or her values/beliefs/ behavior system or between the personal system and that of individuals whom the client admires and wishes to emulate. The extent to which dissatisfaction is aroused depends on the client's recognition of inconsistencies.[12] Once significant dissatisfaction is experienced, it is assumed that the person will *change* values, attitudes, and behaviors to make them more integrated with one another—and, more important, to make them more consistent with self-concept.[13]

$$\text{Self-confrontation} \rightarrow \text{Self-dissatisfaction} \rightarrow \text{Cognitive or}$$

(recognition of             behavioral

(inconsistencies)          change

Contradictions or inconsistencies that are of most concern to the client are the focus for intervention.

Self-confrontation has been shown to be effective in facilitating both values and behavior change. In reviewing a large number of studies in which self-confrontation techniques were used, value rankings changed in 21 of 22 studies, attitudes changed in 7 of 9 studies, and behavioral changes occurred in 6 out of 13 studies. Behavioral changes have been noted in some studies for as long as 13 to 90 weeks following a "single-dose" intervention.[14]

The Rokeach Value Survey presented in Chapter 6 is the instrument most frequently used in self-confrontation. However, the author suggests that "health" be added to the list of terminal values if the nurse intends to use the instrument for this purpose. The nurse may also wish to consider using the Health Values Scale discussed in Chapter 6 for self-confrontation counseling.

Administration of the Rokeach Value Survey or Health Values Scale provides the basis for discussing self-concept/values or values/values inconsistencies. Use of the Values-Actions Review presented in Chapter 6 can provide the information needed to explore self-concept/behavior or values/behavior conflicts.

Valuing *family security* but not *mature love* or *true friendship* represents a value/value conflict, while thinking of oneself as a robust and energetic person yet placing low value on *health* represents a self-concept/value inconsistency. The clients who consider themselves robust and healthy but find that they begin to breathe heavily and perspire when climbing stairs are experiencing a contradiction between self-conception and behavior. Recognition of this inconsistency may cause such clients to begin brisk walking or jogging to enhance physical fitness, thus meeting specific standards that are part of the self-concept.

Another approach to self-confrontation is to have the client examine personal value rankings compared to referent groups that the client admires or wishes to emulate.[15] For instance, the client might look at his or her value hierarchy in comparison to normative rankings of individuals who are in excellent health or who are avid health-promotion enthusiasts (joggers, bicyclists, or persons who meditate regularly). Seeing differences between personal values and those of important reference groups, the client may rethink his or her own values and reorganize the value hierarchy to approximate more closely that of the group that the client wishes to be like.[16]

While much of the clinical work that has been done with self-confrontation techniques has been in the area of racism and prejudice, the approach has excellent potential as a health protection/promotion intervention. It is highly possible that a fundamental shift in personal values may be required before there is acceptance of individual responsibility for health; that shift might be prerequisite to a significant health-related behavior change.

In an interesting study conducted by Conroy,[17] self-confrontation techniques were used as an approach to smoking cessation. He asked his experimental group to view two charts showing the instrumental value rankings of smokers and the instrumental value rankings for quitters (nonsmokers). The values of *self-discipline* and *broad-mindedness* were outlined in red. These values were selected because previous research had shown that smokers and quitters differed significantly on their ranking of these two values. Smokers ranked *broadmindedness* third and *self-discipline* eighth, whereas quitters ranked *broadmindedness* eighth and *self-discipline* first. The difference in rankings was discussed with the clients and they were asked to indicate their extent of admiration for people who had been able to quit smoking. They were then encouraged to compare their own value rankings with those of smokers and quitters.

After completion of the smoking clinic, values were again surveyed, the rank order of *self-discipline* in the experimental group had increased significantly while no significant changes had occurred in ranking of *broadmindedness* or other values. Increase in rankings of *self-discipline* were closely correlated with amount of dissatisfaction expressed by clients with their own preclinic value rankings. In reviewing the behavioral effects at the conclusion of the clinic period, the experimental group had reduced its smoking rate to 5 percent of its preclinic rate, whereas the control group still reported 28 percent of its preclinic rate.

A significant difference was apparent for a period of 2 months following termination of the experiment. This difference eventually became dissipated in a high rate of recidivism.[18] However, it is important to note that the self-confrontation treatment produced significantly greater short-term effects than a variety of other more typical smoking-clinic treatments. It is widely recognized that smoking represents an addictive behavior, like drinking, overeating, and misuse of drugs, that is highly resistant to change. Attempts to change addictive behaviors result in symptoms of withdrawal and psychologic difficulties because of the pervasive role that such behaviors play in lifestyle. Thus, successful use of self-confrontation in decreasing addictive behaviors portends even greater effectiveness for self-confrontation techniques in promoting positive health practices.

Several explanations have been proposed to explain the impact of self-confrontation as a counseling technique. One explanation is the value-mediation hypothesis, which states that since the individual functions holistically, a change in values will result in subsequent changes in behavior. A change in one part of the system results in a modification of the whole. Another explanation is that behavior change occurs directly from recognized inconsistencies between self-concept and behavior rather than indirectly through value change. The specific mechanisms whereby self-confrontation works still need to be identified.

Research to determine normative attitudes and values of individuals who routinely practice health-protecting and health-promoting behaviors would provide meaningful information on which to base nursing interventions. From this information, materials could be developed for use with clients to increase the incidence of protective/promotive behaviors and decrease the incidence of health-damaging behaviors. Conroy has suggested that in order for health professionals to change the American lifestyle significantly through individual and group interventions, the following steps must be taken:[19]

1. Educate the public as to its role and responsibility for health maintenance.
2. Identify through research the attitudes and values that support health-protection and health-promotion behaviors and sustain health-damaging behaviors.
3. Provide effective methods for altering not only attitudes and values but specific health-related behaviors.

The professional nurse is encouraged to use self-confrontation techniques in health counseling, carefully evaluating their impact on different client groups and with a variety of differing health values, attitudes, and behaviors. For further information on the clinical use of self-confrontation techniques, the reader is referred to additional sources.[20-22]

**Cognitive Restructuring**
Attention to clients' thinking, imagery, and attitudes toward self are relatively new areas for exploration in the change process. Cognitive restructuring as an intervention technique was developed by Ellis and Grieger to assist counselors in dealing with these phenomena. The approach is frequently referred to as rational-emotive therapy.[23] Not only a therapeutic technique, it also represents an interesting approach to increasing clients' beliefs in personal control of their environment. The basic assumption behind the approach is that the way that an individual labels or evaluates a specific situation determines his or her emotional reaction to the situation. Individuals as a result of experience develop generalized sets of beliefs about various situations or social interactions in their own lives, and these expectancies (self-generated) mediate or determine their emotional and behavioral reactions in any specific situation.[24] The critical factor in determining an individual's response is not the actual situation as much as what the person says to him- or herself (e.g., appraisals, attributions, and evaluations in the form of self-statements or self-generated images) before or during the target event.[25]

The self-statement is an important concept in cognitive restructuring. It can be defined as a covert verbalization that elicits emotional reactions. Since self-statements represent covert behavior, their impact is only indirectly observable through the client's self-reports and the overt actions for which the self-statements are assumed to be the mediating link between internal or external stimulus and behavioral response.

The process of self-statements and self-evaluation begins early in life. The child develops a self-directing and self-reacting verbal repertoire from observation of the self-administered praise and criticism of adults.[26] Self-administered praise can facilitate performance and feelings of esteem. Invariably self-criticism inhibits behavior. The nurse should be aware of the fact that what sometimes appears to be a skill deficit in self-care may be self-inhibition of the appropriate response. This inhibition is the result of inappropriate self-statements.

Maladaptive emotions are often mediated by irrational self-statements that the client generates in specific situations. If negative emotions are aroused because individuals unthinkingly accept certain illogical premises or irrational ideas, then there is good reason to believe that clients can be taught to think more logically and rationally and thereby create positive emotional states rather than negative ones that in return change behavior and life experiences in positive directions.

Velten[27] found that the reported moods of clients varied as a function of the self-referenced statements that they read. When individuals were given positive statements to read, such as "I feel great," and "My life is wonderful," positive moods prevailed. When individuals were given negative statements to read, such as "I have too many bad things in my life," or "I feel like my life is falling apart", negative moods were dominant. These data and those of other researchers support the ABC framework proposed by Ellis and Grieger[28] for explaining the impact of self-generated thoughts or ideas on responses to specific environmental events:

- A → Activating experience or event
- B → One's beliefs about A (rational or irrational)
- C → Emotional/behavioral consequences

While the *A* and *C* components are quite easy to identify, analyzing self-generated thoughts and emotions at the time of the event is more difficult. However, for effective cognitive restructuring to take place, self-generated thoughts (self-statements) must be accurately recalled and carefully analyzed.

Irrational self-statements are often brought about by overgeneralization from past unpleasant experiences ("I'll never lose weight"), self-blame ("I don't have any will-power"), and negative self-attributions ("I'm weak and no good"). Irrational self-statements result in decreased self-esteem, depression, and lack of success in attempts at behavior change.[29] Distortion of reality through overgeneralizations is a major source of irrational beliefs. Compare the following:

- Irrational belief (derived from         "I'll never be thin again!"
  overgeneralization)
- Rational belief                         "I have difficulty losing weight."

Ellis has suggested that irrational beliefs frequently can be identified by looking at the "shoulds" or "musts" in clients' lives or at their beliefs concerning powerlessness or lack of control. There are five common irrational beliefs:[30]

1. I must be loved by everyone. (Social rejection implies personal inadequacy.)
2. I should do everything that I do exceptionally well. (One must be thoroughly competent in all aspects of life).

3. I am powerless to determine whether I experience health and happiness or misery.
4. It is better to avoid life's difficulties rather than face them.
5. I cannot change myself or my surroundings.

To the extent that clients hold expectations that are inconsistent with reality (irrational self-statements), they are likely to experience failure in making the health-related changes in their lives that they wish to make. Self-statements constitute internal cues to behavior. If internal cues are irrational, desired behaviors will not occur. A number of studies have shown positive relationships between interpersonal anxiety, test anxiety, speech anxiety and the extent of irrational beliefs.[31-33] Further research is needed to determine the impact of irrational beliefs on health behaviors.

Goldfried and Sobocinski[34] have outlined the steps for applying the psychologic principles of cognitive restructuring to clinical intervention with clients. The goal of the intervention is to teach clients to think more rationally and thus gain greater control over their own lives and health. The specific steps of cognitive restructuring are the following:

1. *Help clients accept the fact that self-statements mediate emotional arousal.* Self-statements and emotional arousal to specific situations may occur automatically and without deliberate effort or conscious thought. Self-statements and associated emotions must be brought into conscious thought in order to deal constructively with their impact on health practices.
2. *Assist clients in recognizing the irrationality in certain beliefs.* Encourage the client to observe and challenge personal self-statements. The client should explore how he or she may be misinterpreting life events. The nurse should support the client in challenging irrational health-related beliefs, particularly those that are most troublesome. The client might ask the following questions:

   • What evidence supports my belief?
   • What parts of my beliefs are true? What parts are false?
   • Am I sticking close to reality (actual facts) in my self-statements, or am I overreacting and distorting events?

   The client should be encouraged by the nurse to offer arguments for the irrationality of self-defeating beliefs.
3. *Help clients understand that the inability to initiate or sustain desirable behaviors frequently results from irrational self-statements.* Negative emotional responses can be maintained by self-generated thoughts indefinitely and to the point where they automatically inhibit behavior without client awareness. Clients need to stop thinking irrationally in order to facilitate constructive behavior change.
4. *Help clients modify their irrational self-statements.* Have the client write down rational self-statements that represent responses to troublesome situations. Keep statements short so that they can be rehearsed in the target situation.

Rehearsal of rational self-statements decreases the incidence of irrational self-statements. The client can learn with practice to talk to him- or herself rationally and to give himself cues that support positive emotional states. Examples of rational self-statements are "calm down," "relax," "concentrate on the present," "this isn't so bad," "this situation is challenging," and "I'll conquer this one, given a little time."

Imagery can be used to assist the client in practicing rational self-statements.[35] Imaginary presentations of troublesome situations can be described to the client by the nurse and overt or covert rehearsal of rational self-statements carried out. The client should be encouraged to take at least 10 minutes each day for imagery and rehearsal of positive self-statements. Practice is essential to achieve cognitive restructuring. The ultimate goal for the client is to think about him- or herself and others more sensibly in the future. Through modifying internal thoughts and imagery, overt behavior can be changed.[36,37]

### Modeling

Another approach to assisting clients in changing toward more positive health practices is that of modeling. Modeling consists of observing the behavior of others who have successfully achieved the goal that the client has set for himself. Modeling is especially helpful when the client is aware of his or her specific goal but is uncertain about the exact behaviors that should be developed in order to move toward the goal.[38] In early life, children learn a great deal through modeling. This form of learning is continued into adulthood. Individuals acquire social skills and learn how to relate with others through observing the interactions of persons whom they respect and admire.

The nurse can serve as an important role model for health-protecting and health-promoting behaviors. Inherent in the nurse's professional role is the responsibility to provide a model of healthful living that is attractive to clients and consequently emulated by individuals to whom care is provided.

The following considerations are important in the effective use of modeling to facilitate behavior change:

- There must be models available with which the client can identify.
- The client must take an active role in the selection of appropriate models.
- The learner must have an opportunity actually to observe the desired behaviors and must attend to important aspects of the behavior.
- The client must have the requisite knowledge and skills to reproduce the behavior.
- The client must perceive incentives or rewards for imitating the target behaviors.
- The learner must have the opportunity for overt or covert rehearsal of the target behaviors.

By carefully choosing models that have achieved goals the client desires, opportunities can be provided to observe the model in events that contain the behaviors the client wishes to adopt. For example, how does an individual who is slim and trim eat? How much? Which foods? How long does eating take? What other behaviors does he or she engage in while eating? The client can acquire many useful ideas from models for modifying personal health behaviors.

Some clients may feel that it is undesirable to imitate others, that it results in artificial behaviors or that it is not genuine. However, the use of models does not imply that kind of imitation. Actually, the most economical kind of human learning is by imitation. By observing good models, complicated behavior sequences can often be repeated accurately on the first performance. This kind of imitation occurs throughout life and is a very natural process. Observing models gives ideas for behavior rather than a rigid sequence of actions that the client is expected to perform.[39] Observation of others also enriches the client's thinking regarding the range of behavioral options available.

It is important that the nurse and client mutually participate in the selection of appropriate models with whom the client can identify. This is particularly important when the cultural and ethnic backgrounds of the nurse and client differ. Models should be individuals who are frequently available during the initial learning stage and ones whom the client respects. The success of many self-help groups can be partially explained through modeling techniques that generate new ideas for behavior or coping strategies for specific problems. The fact that health professionals are generally held in very high esteem by clients places the nurse in an important position as a potential role model.

Actual observation of target behaviors is important to successful imitation. It is even more important that the client attend to key aspects of the behavior so as to benefit from the example. For instance, if verbal behavior rather than nonverbal behavior is the important point of observation, the client should be aware of this fact. If the nurse serves as the model, he or she can call attention to important aspects of behavior. If this is not the case, the client may have to be primed or assisted ahead of time to organize observations around the key points to be observed. Once attention has been directed to the critical aspects of a behavior sequence, learning from role models will be more efficient and effective.

It should be apparent to the nurse before model observation whether the client has the requisite knowledge and skills to reproduce the desired behavior. While it is optimum to develop the required skills prior to the modeling sequence, skills can be learned as part of the modeling process. The nurse as a model should not only demonstrate skills (e.g., warm-up exercises) that the client desires to learn, but also explain, provide needed information, and express personal feelings about the target behavior. This helps the client to think more holistically about and rehearse the behavioral sequence.

The client must perceive some incentive or reward for imitating the model's behavior. The incentive may be increased social effectiveness in relationships with others, improved eating patterns, or enhanced physical fitness. Verbal rewards by the nurse, such as praise and recognition, are often potent in promoting efforts to learn new behaviors. Self-praise and self-satisfaction are covert rewards that the client can administer for successfully performing modeled behaviors.

As a final note, opportunities for rehearsal of observed behaviors is critical to allow the client to internalize the verbal and nonverbal cues to behavior, such as limb position or muscle tension. Overt rehearsal is much more effective than covert rehearsal and should be encouraged immediately after observation whenever possible. Overt rehearsal allows the nurse to determine the efficacy of learning and provide feedback through suggestions for refining the client's performance of the target behaviors.

### Operant Conditioning

One of the most effective self-modification techniques available to clients is operant conditioning. It is based on the premise that all behaviors are determined by their consequences. If positive consequences result, the probability is high that the behavior will occur again. If negative consequences occur, the probability is low for the behavior's being repeated. A commonly repeated fallacy is that operant conditioning represents manipulation of the client by the nurse. This is not true: When self-modification is the focus of nursing intervention, the client controls the selection of behaviors to be changed and reinforcement contingencies to be used; that is, the client selects what he or she will change, how he or she will change, and the rewards that he or she will receive for change. Self-modification through operant conditioning gives the client the means of achieving personal health goals.

The client must be in complete control of the change process if new health behaviors are to be initiated and sustained. Positive reinforcement (reward) rather than negative reinforcement (removal of an aversive condition) or punishment (aversive experience) provide the motivation for behavior change. Behaviors that are to be reinforced must be clearly delineated in the health protection/promotion plan described in Chapter 8. The client must be aware of what marks the beginning and end of the target behavior and how the behavior that he or she wishes to reinforce is different from other related behaviors. A behavior such as "eats slowly" is too general and cannot be accurately observed. What is "slowly"? When does the specific behavior begin and end? "Pauses between bites during the meal and lays fork on plate" is a concrete behavior that can be clearly observed. Behaviors to be reinforced must be countable so that reinforcement can be appropriately used.

*Collecting Baseline Data.* If a client wishes to increase the incidence of a specific health-promoting behavior or decrease the incidence of a health-damaging behavior, it is important that an initial frequency count of the target behavior (baseline data) be obtained so that extent of progress toward the desired change can be accurately assessed. Counts of occurrence of the behavior may be made in total or in situation-specific or time-specific categories. The instrument or form on which behavior is to be recorded must be portable so that it is always available when the target behavior occurs. Total counts may be made on a small manual counter or calculator. Categorical counts are usually recorded with paper and pencil. A 3 × 5" index card is a convenient size for the client to carry.[40]

An example of a daily record of smoking behavior is presented in Figure 9-2. For many behaviors, times and situations are important because they rep-

| Behavior to Be Observed: | Smoking |
|---|---|
| Observation Categories: | Morning<br>Afternoon<br>Evening |

Method of Coding Behavior:

E = Smoking after or during eating and drinking
S = Smoking while nervous in a social situation
D = Smoking while driving the car
O = Smoking at other times

Smoking Record

Date: Tuesday, August 26

| Morning | Afternoon | Evening |
|---|---|---|
| E  E  D  O  S  S  S  E | O  S  S  D  S  E  E  E | E  O |

Date: Wednesday, August 27

| Morning | Afternoon | Evening |
|---|---|---|
| E  E  E  D  D  S  S  E  E | S  S  S  S  D  D  E  E  E  E | S  E  O |

**FIGURE 9-2.** Self-observation sheet. (*From* Self-Directed Behavior: Self-Modification for Personal Adjustment, *by D. L. Watson and R. G. Tharp. Copyright © 1972 by Wadsworth, Inc. Reprinted by permission of the publisher, Brooks/Cole Publishing Company, Monterey, California.*)

resent the configuration of cues in which the behavior occurs. The period of baseline data collection can end when (1) the client has a good estimation of how often the target behavior occurs, or when (2) the client is confident that he or she understands the patterns of occurrence of the target behavior.[41] Data from daily records can be compiled and graphed as illustrated in Figure 9-3.

Self-observation or monitoring can increase the client's awareness of the frequency of health-protecting, health-promoting, and health-damaging behaviors. Common reactions include "I didn't know that I smoked that much" or "I didn't realize that I smoke as much in the afternoon as I do in the morning." Self-observation before initiating a program to support behavior change provides a means of assessing client progress.[42]

It must be noted that while self-observation can be used to collect baseline data about the frequency with which health-related behaviors occur, studies of smoking cessation and other behavioral changes have failed to show sustained effects from self-observation or self-monitoring alone without use of other self-modification techniques.

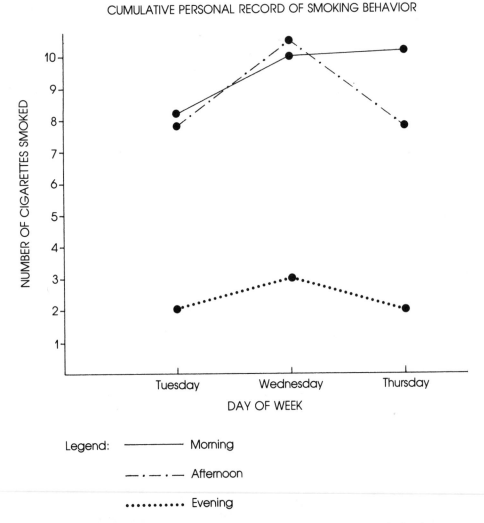

**FIGURE 9-3.** Sample cumulative graph of health-damaging behavior.

*Using Reinforcement Contingencies.* Appropriate use of reinforcement is extremely important in operant conditioning for self-directed behavior change. The reinforcements used in modifying health behaviors should be carefully selected, as described in Chapter 8. They should be important to the client, accessible for immediate use, and potent enough to motivate behavior.

Tangible or social reinforcers serve as effective sources of motivation. Activities as well as objects can be tangible reinforcers according to the Premack Principle.[43] This principle states that if Event A is more probable than Event B when the individual has both options available, Event A can function as a reinforcer if access to A is contingent on first performing B. For example, going to the movie (A) may be made contingent on brisk walking for 2 miles (B). When tangible and social reinforcers (praise, attention, approval) are paired they become synergistic, each enhancing the potency of the other.[44] A combination of both may be needed initially to facilitate the acquisition and practice of new health behaviors. As health practices become stabilized, less tangible sources of reinforcement are needed to sustain actions.

As soon as possible the client should be encouraged to use self-generated reinforcers such as complimentary thoughts or images. Covert self-reinforcement is the most versatile source of reward. The client has complete control over administration of self-praise and self-compliments. Once a new behavior is occurring regularly, the results of the behavior itself may provide adequate reinforcement. Losing weight, feeling more relaxed, or feeling more energetic all are consequences of health behaviors that have reinforcing properties.

The time frame for application of reinforcement is critical. Immediate reinforcement is highly desirable particularly in the early phases of self-change. Immediate reinforcement that is self-administered provides the client with moment-by-moment control over his or her own behavior. Initially, continuous reinforcement is also advisable. Continuous reinforcement promotes rapid learning of the desired behaviors. Intermittent reinforcement applied later stabilizes the behavior and makes it resistant to extinction. Over time, the nurse should decrease her active participation in the reinforcement system of the client. Fading can occur in a number of ways. The nurse may move from tangible reinforcers to social reinforcers or from continuous reinforcement to intermittent reinforcement and then to complete fading.[45] Reinforcement may also be increasingly delayed as a form of fading.

Using an organized approach for reinforcement of positive health behaviors generally promotes extinction of undesirable behaviors as a result of lack of reinforcement. Health-promoting and health-damaging behaviors are frequently incompatible. Increasing one automatically decreases the occurrence of the other. In fact, one of the reasons for infrequent occurrence of desired behaviors may be that an undesirable behavior competes with the desired behavior and interferes with its performance. Questions that the client can ask in order to identify a positive health behavior that is incompatible with a negative one include the following:[46]

> *Is there some directly opposite behavior that I would like to increase?*
> *What behaviors would make it impossible to perform the undesired behavior?*
> *If an incompatible positive behavior cannot be identified, is there a basically meaningless act that can be substituted for the undesirable behavior, e.g., folding hands in lap to prevent nail biting?*

This approach, which emphasizes substitution or replacement as opposed to denial, can maintain a positive climate for behavioral change even when health-dam-

aging behaviors that have become a habit for the client are being extinguished.
*Shaping Behavior.* Many behaviors are too complex to be acquired all at once.
Gradually shaping desired behaviors is an effective approach to making permanent
changes in lifestyle. Shaping occurs when closer and closer approximations of the
final behavior are rewarded. Reinforcement through the shaping process is contingent on increasingly higher levels of performance by the client. An example
of shaping is the following:

- Brisk walk for 15 minutes 2 days of first week
- Brisk walk for 20 minutes 3 days of second and third week
- Brisk walk for 30 minutes 3 days of fourth and fifth week
- Brisk walk for 45 minutes 4 days of sixth and seventh week
- Brisk walk for 60 minutes 4 days of eighth and ninth week

Each step toward the final behavior should be mastered before the next step is
attempted. The client can control the size of incremental steps to be rewarded
and the rate at which the desired behavior is acquired.

Problems that clients are likely to experience in the process of shaping behaviors include plateaus when progress seems impossible, cheating by reinforcing
inadequate levels of performance, and problems in persistence (sometimes referred to as willpower). These problems should be anticipated and dealt with
constructively, either through increased use of tangible reinforcers or through
potent social reinforcers during plateau periods when persistence is waning.

The nurse responsible for guiding the client in self-modification should be
skilled with shaping techniques. Two books have been written especially for
nurses on the subject: *Behavior Modification: A Significant Method in Nursing
Practice,* by LeBow,[47] and *Behavior Modification and the Nursing Process*, by
Berni and Fordyce.[48]

*Coverant Conditioning.* Efforts at conditioning within psychology have stretched
beyond operant conditioning of overt behavior to operant conditioning of covert
processes that precede behavior. Covert processes are self-generated thoughts or
images that are only indirectly observable through self-report of clients or observation of subsequent actions. A covert operant (coverant) is an idea that ini-
tiates behavior. It can serve as an internal cue for subsequent action. For example
the statement, "I'd really enjoy having a cigarette; it would make me feel relaxed
and calm," can be the first step to actual overt behavior (in this case, health-
damaging behavior). If occurrence of the thought or coverant can be decreased,
the behavior that generally follows will be less likely to occur. One approach to
conditioning coverants is the positive reinforcement of coverants that will result
in positive behaviors. One example is saying "stop" when the undesirable coverant occurs and substituting a desirable coverant, such as "If I don't smoke, my
breath will smell sweet and I will be more desirable to be around." Reinforcements
for coverants may be overt or covert. Overt reinforcement consists of using
objects, experiences, or interactions with others as rewards for appropriate cov-

erants, while covert reinforcement includes use of self-praise or self-encouragement.

Conditioning covert behaviors is an emerging area of exploration; more research needs to be conducted before the parameters for clinical use of coverant conditioning are clearly identified. For further information on this technique, a number of sources can be consulted.[49-52]

## Counterconditioning

Counterconditioning is a classical conditioning procedure that is frequently referred to as systematic desensitization. The aim of this approach to behavior change is to break an undesirable bond between a stimulus (conditioned stimulus) and a response (conditioned response). A conditioned response often represents an irrational or maladaptive response to one or more specific situations that has become automatic.

The goal of counterconditioning is to replace the undesirable stimulus–response bond with a more desirable one. For instance, anxiety may be replaced by relaxation in stressful situations, preventing the occurrence of the negative emotional response. Relaxation is actually incompatible with the previously conditioned response (anxiety). Stress management to be discussed in Chapter 12 is an excellent illustration of this clinical technique.

Counterconditioning can be carried out by use of imagery or in real-life situations. For example, when clients are being desensitized to stressful situations, they can be asked to imagine increasingly stressful events while they remain in a protected environment. Relaxation rather than tension represents the stimulus–response bond that the client is attempting to achieve. Once the client can relax during stressful imagery, relaxation techniques can be applied to stressful situations in real life. It is interesting to note that symptom substitution or displacement of anxiety seldom occur when counterconditioning is used to decrease the occurrence of negative emotions in specific situations.[53]

## Stimulus Control

By changing the antecedents of behavior, that is, the events that precede behavior, it is possible to decrease or eliminate undesired behavior and increase desired outcomes. The locus of attention in stimulus control is on the antecedents of behavior, rather than on its consequences as in operant conditioning. In order to use stimulus control effectively the client must have accurate information about when and where desirable behaviors could occur more frequently and/or under what conditions undesirable behaviors occur. The client must arrange for environmental cues to be encountered such as promote only desired behaviors. As indicated in the Health Belief Models and the proposed Health Promotion Model, cues are critical elements during the action phase.

During the decision-making phase, the client determines which health actions will be taken and achieves a certain level of readiness to act. This mobilized energy must be activated by an instigating event that can be either external or internal. The level of cue intensity needed to initiate behavior is directly related to the level of readiness of the client following the decision-making phase. People in a state of readiness to take a specific action appear to have a lowering of perception if not of sensory thresholds to specific stimulation relevant to their goal. Generally, the higher the level of readiness, the lower the intensity of the cue needed to activate appropriate behavior. Figure 9-4 illustrates this relationship. Cues that surpass optimum intensity usually inhibit behavior rather than facilitate it.[54]

Multiple cues potentiate each other. Internal cues can be coupled with external cues, for example, "feeling good after brisk walking" coupled with "the invitation from spouse to take a walk." Table 9-1 presents an overview of possible cues to taking health protecting/promoting actions.

Individuals define for themselves the cues that are relevant based on past knowledge and experience. For one client, a postcard reminding him or her of an exercise class may be an adequate prompting for attendance while for another client a personal call from the nurse and several reminders from spouse may be needed to initiate action. The nurse must be aware of effective cues for specific clients in order to prompt positive health behaviors with success. Dimensions of cues to be considered include relevance, strength (intensity), number, duration, and synergistic potential.

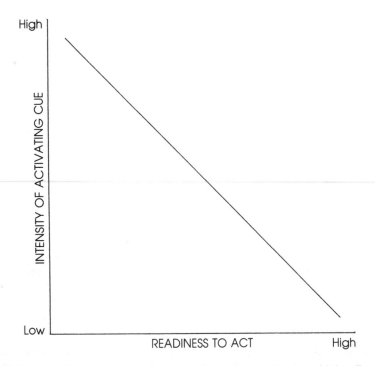

**FIGURE 9-4.** Relationship of readiness to take health actions and intensity of cues needed to activate behavior. *(From Rosenstock, I.M. Why people use health services. Milbank Memorial Fund Quarterly, July 1966. 44. 94–127. With permission.)*

---

**TABLE 9-1   POSSIBLE CUES FOR HEALTH-PROTECTING AND HEALTH-PROMOTING ACTIONS**

---

Internal Cues

Bodily states, e.g., feeling good, feeling energetic, recognizing aging, fatigue, cyclical discomfort

Affective states, e.g., enthusiasm, motivation for self-preservation, high level of self-esteem, happiness, concern

External Cues

Interactions with significant others, i.e., family, friends, colleagues, nurse, and physician

Impact of communication media, e.g., motivational messages from television, radio, newspapers, advertisements, and special mailings

Visual stimuli from the environment, e.g., passing a diabetic screening clinic, billboards, attendance at a health fair, passing a gym or exercise center, or viewing others participating in target activity

---

Some cues are successful in prompting a given behavior much of the time while others vary in effectiveness from one time to another or one situation to another. Cues may also be action specific. A configuration of cues that triggers relaxation may not be the cues that trigger exercise or appropriate eating behavior.

The nurse, family, environment, or client may serve as the source of behavioral cues. Since the extent to which the nurse can provide cues to action is limited, an important part of his or her role is to assist clients in (1) developing sensitivity to appropriate cues, (2) increasing chances for encountering appropriate cues, and (3) developing a system of internal cues that consistently trigger desired actions. It is important to remember that verbal and nonverbal cues, regardless of their source, must be consistent with each other. Any incongruity between cues can confuse and frustrate the client and inhibit action.

Antecedents of behavior need to be carefully analyzed in order to create a configuration of cues that will prompt specific health protecting/promoting behaviors. The client should describe the setting(s) in which the health-related behavior has occurred previously or could occur:

- *Physical setting*—Describe the setting(s) in which the behavior occurs. Describe when, where, and what is present.
- *Social setting*—Describe who is present when the behavior occurs and what they are doing.

• *Intrapersonal setting*—Describe what the client is thinking, feeling, or doing. What did the client say or think to him- or herself just before the behavior occurred?

Through controlling cues or antecedents, the incidence of target behaviors can be modified. The nurse can assist the client in learning how to change cue configurations to elicit desired behaviors. Specific approaches to stimulus control will be presented below.

**Cue Restriction or Elimination.** Situational cues for undesired behaviors can sometimes be eliminated. When such cues cannot be totally eliminated they can often be reduced. For instance, the cues to eating may be reduced to one room in the house, the kitchen/dining room. This is called stimulus narrowing or cue restriction. A setting can also be selected that is incompatible with an undesirable response (cue elimination). Examples include sitting in "no smoking" areas of restaurants or eating meals only with nonsmokers if cessation of smoking is the goal. Through stimulus narrowing or reduction, the target behavior comes under the influence of only a few cues. By localizing the cues that activate behavior, arrangements can be made for limited encounter with these cues. In successful cue elimination, extinction of the behavior should result.

**Cue Expansion.** In cue expansion, the number of stimuli that prompt desired behavior is increased. For instance, while personal preparation of food at home in one's own kitchen may prompt small servings of meats, fruit, and vegetables, the environment of a restaurant may prompt selection of rich entrees and desserts. An expanded configuration of cues can prompt health-promoting behavior in a variety of different settings. For instance, being given a menu at a restaurant can provide cues for looking at salad and vegetable options as opposed to less nutritious and higher caloric offerings. By expanding the range of cues that elicit specific responses, desirable behaviors can occur more frequently and with greater regularity. Gaining conscious control over behavior rather than responding automatically will assist the client in acting more rationally and more in line with personal health goals.

Controlling antecedents of behavior through the restriction, elimination, or expansion of cues can assist clients in creating internal and external cues supportive of positive health practices. Stimulus control is an important approach to successfully modifying behavior and lifestyle.

**Barriers to Change**

Interference with action can arise from external barriers within the environment, such as lack of facilities, materials, or social support, or from internal barriers, such as lack of knowledge, skills, or appropriate affective or motivational orientation on the part of the client. The professional nurse facilitates the action phase by assisting clients in minimizing or eliminating barriers to action. It is futile to encourage clients to take actions that are highly likely to be blocked or frustrated.

Internal barriers to self-modification toward more positive health practices can result from a variety of sources:

- Unclear short-term and long-term goals
- Insufficient skill to follow through with self-modification approach
- Perceptions of lack of control over environmental contingencies (cues, barriers) related to the target behavior
- Lack of motivation to pursue selected health actions

Barriers such as these often reflect insufficient planning or preparation for action during the decision-making phase.

Clients who find their course of action thwarted may reevaluate the decisions made regarding practice of specific health behaviors. They may seek more information to support change in behavior, discard the selected action in favor of another, rationalize the behavior as unnecessary, or deny the relevance of the related health goal.

The interaction of level of readiness and barriers to action is depicted in Table 9-2. Consequences for the client and appropriate nursing actions are also presented. Conflict, action, or inactivity can result from differing levels of readiness and blocks to action. When clients evidence a high level of readiness to engage in health-protecting/promoting behaviors and barriers are low, only a low-intensity cue is needed to activate behavior. A high-intensity cue under these conditions may actually be aversive. When readiness is high and barriers to action are also formidable, barriers need to be reduced or eliminated. When both readiness and

TABLE 9-2   INTERRELATIONSHIPS BETWEEN LEVEL OF READINESS TO TAKE HEALTH ACTIONS, BARRIERS, CONSEQUENCES FOR CLIENTS, AND NURSING INTERVENTIONS

| Level of Readiness | Barriers to Action | Consequences for Client | Nursing Interventions |
|---|---|---|---|
| High | Low | Action | Support and encouragement; provide low-intensity cue |
| High | High | Conflict | Assist client in lowering barriers to action |
| Low | Low | Conflict | Provide high-intensity cue |
| Low | High | No action | Assist client in lowering barriers to action and then provide high-intensity cue |

barriers are low, readiness to act should be increased in order to initiate action. When readiness is low and barriers high, both factors should be addressed in order to allow constructive behaviors to occur.

Significant others can serve as barriers to health actions. When family members or other persons or groups disagree or are neutral or apathetic toward health behaviors, the extent of inhibition created for the client depends on the following factors:

• The relevance of disagreeing persons or groups
• Attractiveness to the client of disagreeing persons or groups
• Extent of disagreement of relevant persons or groups
• Number of persons relevant to the client who are in disagreement with behavior.

As the nurse listens to the client's account of efforts at implementation of health practices, he or she may well be able to provide insights concerning blocks to desired behavior. By analysis of the environment in which the behavior is to occur and preparation of the client with the appropriate knowledge and skills to deal constructively with potential or actual barriers to implementation, the nurse can facilitate accomplishment of personal health goals meaningful to the client.

### Maintaining Behavior Change
Changes in behavior that are transient accomplish little in enhancing client health status. Not only must behavior be sustained in the environment in which it is learned, but the behavior must be generalized to other situations. Factors that affect continuation of positive health behaviors include:

• Number of personal beliefs and attitudes that support the target behavior
• Extent of affective and cognitive commitment to target behavior
• Ease of incorporating behavior into lifestyle
• Extent to which behavior is intermittently reinforced or rewarded
• Degree of future orientation of the client
• Amount of activity involved in making the decision to take action
• Personal attractiveness of incompatible actions
• Centrality of health as a value
• Extent to which decision to take action has been communicated to others

At this point in time much more is known about interventions to initiate change in health behaviors than about effective methods for maintaining positive health practices as an integral part of personal lifestyle. Maintaining change, however, is important if long-term effects are to be anticipated from the nursing care provided. The continuation phase is indeterminate in length, extending from beginning stabilization of the new behavior throughout the client's life span. Three approaches for maintaining new behaviors will be discussed briefly below.

*Publicizing Commitment.* Commitment to a specific course of action to improve health should be communicated to as many people as possible. Making commitment to change behavior a matter of public knowledge will provide support or subtle pressures from others to maintain behavior after it is stabilized. By informing others of the intention to adopt more positive health practices, significant individuals can provide cues or reinforcements for the desired behaviors. In fact, individuals who also believe that they should take similar actions may join the client in a collegial endeavor that provides continuing support and camaraderie.

*Recording Progress.* Clients can be encouraged to keep a graph that depicts their progress over time in developing and continuing positive health practices. The frequency, intensity, or duration of the behavior may be graphed depending on which parameter best depicts the client's accomplishments. A sample of a progress chart for brisk walking is presented in Figure 9-5.

*Intermittent Reinforcement.* Intermittent reinforcement has been shown to be more effective than continuous reinforcement in sustaining behaviors. Intermittent reinforcement is carried out by requiring greater frequency, intensity, or duration of the target behavior before reward is given, as compared to continuous reinforcement. The amount of reinforcement may be varied, and the latency of reinforcement may be varied as well. These reward contingencies can be manipulated by the client, family, or nurse.

Intermittent reinforcement maintains the novelty of rewards and the interest of clients while avoiding saturation and decreased effectiveness of reinforcement contingencies. Without certainty of reward but with some probability of attaining it, positive behaviors have been shown to persist over long periods of time.

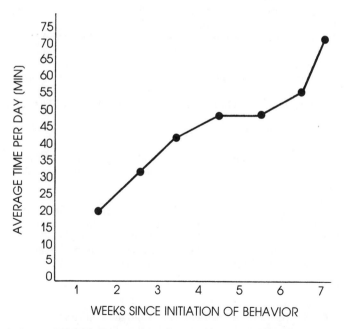

**FIGURE 9-5.** Progress chart for brisk walking.

## SUMMARY

Within this chapter an attempt has been made to familiarize the reader with selected strategies for behavior change that can be used with clients to assist them in self-modification toward healthier states. The nurse is encouraged to consult suggested sources for more in-depth information on each technique. The usefulness of each strategy for individual clients will depend on their personality, social and physical environment, and usual patterns of learning. The nurse in assisting clients to modify personal health behaviors not only promotes desired changes but provides the client with skills for continuing self-change and self-actualization.

## REFERENCES

1. Schwitzgebel, R.K., & Kolb, D.A. *Changing human behavior: Principles of planned intervention.* New York: McGraw-Hill, 1974.
2. Lifton, R.J. *The life of the self.* New York: Simon & Schuster, 1976.
3. Kanfer, F.H. The many faces of self-control, or behavior modification changes its focus. In Stuart, R.B., (Ed.), *Behavioral self-management: Strategies, techniques and outcomes.* New York: Brunner/Mazel, 1977, p. 5.
4. Kanfer, F.H., & Karoly, P. Self control: A behavioristic excursion into the lion's den. *Behavior Therapy,* 1972, *3*, 398–416.
5. Kazdin, A.E. *Behavior modification in applied settings* (2nd ed.). Homewood, Ill.: The Dorsey Press, 1980.
6. Watson, D.L., & Tharp, R.G. *Self-directed behavior: Self-modification for personal adjustment.* Monterey, Calif.: Brooks/Cole, 1972.
7. Shibutani, T. A cybernetic approach to motivation. In Buckley, W. (Ed.), *Modern systems research for the behavioral scientist.* Chicago: Aldine, 1968.
8. Kanfer & Karoly, *op. cit.,* p. 5.
9. Sauber, S.R. *Preventive educational intervention for mental health.* Cambridge, Mass.: Ballinger, 1973, p. 74.
10. Otto, H. *Group methods to actualize human potential.* Beverly Hills, Calif.: Holistic Press, 1970.
11. Rokeach, M. *The nature of human values.* New York: Free Press, 1973.
12. *Ibid.*
13. Lockwood, A.L. Notes on research associated with values clarification and value therapy. *The Personnel and Guidance Journal,* May 1980, pp. 606–608.
14. *Ibid.,* p. 608.
15. *Ibid.,* p. 608.
16. Rokeach, M., & McLellan, D.D. Feedback of information about the values and attitudes of self and others as determinants of long-term cognitive and behavioral change. *Journal of Applied Social Psychology,* 1972, *2,* 236–251.
17. Conroy, W.J. Human values, smoking behavior, and public health programs. In Rokeach, M. (Ed.), *Understanding human values: Individual and societal.* New York: Free Press, 1979.
18. *Ibid.,* p. 200.
19. *Ibid.,* pp. 202–207.
20. Rokeach, M., & Cochrane, R. Self-confrontation and confrontation with another as determinants of long-term value change. *Journal of Applied Social Psychology,* 1972, *2,* 283–292.

21. Greenstein, T. Behavior change through value self-confrontation: A field experiment. *Journal of Personality and Social Psychology,* 1976, *34,*254–262.

22. Grube, J., Greenstein, T.N., Rankir, W.L., & Kearney, K. Behavior change following self-confrontation: A test of the value-mediation hypothesis. *Journal of Personality and Social Psychology,* 1977, *35,*212–216.

23. Ellis, A., & Grieger, R. *Handbook of rational-emotive therapy.* New York: Springer, 1977.

24. Goldfried, M.R. The use of relaxation and cognitive relabeling as coping skills. In Stuart, R.B. (Ed.), *Behavioral self management: Strategies, techniques and outcomes.* New York: Brunner/Mazel, 1977, pp. 82–116.

25. Meichenbaum, D.H., & Turk, D. The cognitive, behavioral management of anxiety, anger and pain. In Davidson, P. (Ed.), *Behavioral management of anxiety, depression and pain.* New York: Brunner/Mazel, 1976.

26. Kazdin, *op. cit.,* p. 259.

27. Velten, E., Jr. A laboratory task for induction of mood states. *Behavior Research and Therapy,* 1968, *6,*473–482.

28. Ellis & Grieger, *op. cit.,* pp. 8–9.

29. Martin, R.A., & Poland, E.Y. *Learning to change: A self-management approach to adjustment.* New York: McGraw-Hill, 1980, pp. 159–160.

30. Ellis, A. *Reason and emotion in psychotherapy.* New York: Lyle Stuart, 1962.

31. Meichenbaum, D.H., Gilmore, J.B., & Fedoravicious, A. Group insight versus group desensitization in treating speech anxiety. *Journal of Consulting and Clinical Psychology,* 1971, *36,*410–421.

32. Trexler, L.D., & Karst, T.O. Rational-emotive therapy: Placebo and no treatment effects on public speaking anxiety. *Journal of Abnormal Psychology,* 1972, *79,*60–67.

33. Osarchuk, M. *A comparison of a cognitive, a behavioral therapy and a cognitive plus behavioral therapy treatment of test anxiety in college students.* Unpublished doctoral dissertation, Adelphi University, 1974.

34. Goldfried, M.R., & Sobocinski, D. The effect of irrational beliefs on emotional arousal. *Journal of Consulting and Clinical Psychology,* 1975, *43,*504–510.

35. Goldfried, M.R., *op. cit.,* pp. 97–99.

36. Redd, W.H., & Sleator, W. *Take charge: A personal guide to behavior modification.* New York: Random House, 1976.

37. Blittner, M., Goldberg, J., & Merbaum, M. Cognitive self-control factors in the reduction of smoking behavior. *Behavior Therapy,* 1978, *9,*553–561.

38. Watson & Tharp, *op. cit.,* p. 134.

39. *Ibid.,* pp. 74–75.

40. *Ibid.,* p. 84.

41. *Ibid.,* p. 97.

42. *Ibid.,* p. 108.

43. Martin & Poland, *op. cit.,* p. 21.

44. Deibert, A.N., & Harmon, A.J. *New tools for changing behavior.* Champaign, Ill., Research Press, 1978, pp. 18–25.

45. Berni, R., & Fordyce, W.E. *Behavior modification and the nursing process.* St. Louis: Mosby, 1977, p. 68.

46. Watson & Tharp, *op. cit.,* p. 137.

47. LeBow, M.D. *Behavior modification: A significant method in nursing practice.* Englewood Cliffs, N.J.: Prentice-Hall, 1973.

48. Berni & Fordyce, *op. cit.*

49. Daniels, L.K. An extention of thought-stopping in the treatment of obsessional thinking. *Behavior Therapy,* 1976, *7,*131.

50. Wolpe J., & Lazarus, A.A. *Behavior therapy techniques.* New York: Pergamon, 1966.

51. Girdano, D.A., & Everly, G.S. *Controlling stress and tension: A holistic approach.* Englewood Cliffs, N.J.: Prentice-Hall, 1979, pp. 153–154.

52. Hays, V., & Waddell, K.J. A self-reinforcing procedure for thought stopping. *Behavior Therapy*, 1976, *7,*559.
53. Agras, W.S. *Behavior modification: Principles and clinical applications.* Boston: Little, Brown, 1972.
54. Edgell, S.E., & Castellan, N.J. Configural effect in multiple cue probability learning. *Journal of Experimental Psychology*, 1973, *100,*310–314.

# CHAPTER 10
# Exercise and Physical Fitness

Today, the average American is older physically than his or her chronologic age because of long-term neglect of bodily needs. Most urban dwellers are underactive but overstimulated, leading to lack of energy, low productivity, and limited enjoyment of daily life. These individuals have been labeled "physically disadvantaged" by Cantu.[1] While the physically impaired are often considered to be persons with chronic health problems such as cardiac disorders or stroke, individuals who are overweight, elderly, and sedentary should also be included in this category. Modern lifestyle fosters unfitness. While some individuals are genetically endowed with stronger physical constitutions than others, most Americans cheat themselves out of months, years, or even decades of good health by inappropriate physical-activity habits.[2] Years of inactivity are a major causative or contributing factor for many chronic health problems.

Physical fitness is critical for dynamic, fulfilling, and productive living. It is an important expression of both the stabilizing and actualizing tendencies in human beings. No health protection/promotion plan is complete without an individualized exercise or activity program that takes into consideration the present level of fitness of the client and existing health problems.

Unfortunately, the lifestyle of the majority of Americans is a sedentary one. While growing up, most individuals have focused on the competitive aspects of sports in school athletic programs and have not developed a commitment to physical exercise as an important lifetime activity.[3] Fortunately, over the past few years, regular exercise has been increasingly recognized by many Americans as contributing to personal health. The President's Committee on Physical Fitness and recent research findings concerning the health benefits of physical exercise have contributed to this movement.

## BENEFITS OF EXERCISE

Many studies have indicated that frequent strenuous exercise associated with a continuous and significant elevation of pulse for 20 to 30 minutes helps protect individuals against the threat of heart attacks, improves physical well-being, and

**233**

increases feelings of vitality. Paffenbarger,[4] in a study of Harvard alumni, found that individuals who exercised only casually ran a 64 percent greater risk of heart attack than fellow alumni who exercised vigorously and frequently (expending more than 2000 calories/week in vigorous exercise). Evidence also suggests that there is a relationship between regular exercise and longevity, productivity, and improved psychologic states (e.g., decreased depression, increased self-esteem).[5-7] Sidney and Shephard[8] found that adults who participated vigorously in a physical-training program showed decreased anxiety and improvement in body image. The major positive effects of systematic endurance exercise are summarized in Table 10-1.

Decline in physical fitness often occurs with age. However, this process can be markedly slowed by a systematic physical-activity program. The basic components of fitness include the following:[9]

> *Cardiorespiratory endurance—capability of heart, blood vessels, and lungs to function at optimum efficiency in delivering nutrients and oxygen to tissues and removing wastes*
> *Muscular strength—capacity of muscles to exert maximal force against a resistance*
> *Muscular endurance—capacity of muscles to exert force repeatedly over a period of time*
> *Flexibility—ability to use muscles and joints through maximum range of motion*
> *Motor skill performance—ability of nerves to receive messages that result in smooth, coordinated muscle movement*

A physically fit person generally has a lower heart rate and more rapid recovery (return to resting rate) for any given exercise work load than does a person who is unfit. Maximal oxygen uptake (aerobic capacity) is an important measure of fitness. During treadmill stress test or bicycle ergometer test, use of special equipment that analyzes oxygen and carbon dioxide content of expired air allows determination of maximal or submaximal oxygen uptake.[10] Maximal uptake can be used for young adults, while submaximal uptake (50 and 75 percent of the age-computed maximal rate) is a safer procedure for older or sedentary individuals. Maximal oxygen uptake is expressed in milliliters of oxygen consumed per kilogram of body weight in a minute. Figure 10-1 depicts maximum oxygen uptake values for selected activity groups.

A well-planned physical-activity program can increase aerobic capacity by 20 to 30 percent, improve cardiorespiratory endurance, enhance muscle strength, and improve flexibility. A significant change in level of physical fitness can be achieved. The rest of this chapter will be devoted to discussion of various types of exercise and fitness programs. The reader is referred back to Chapter 5 for information concerning physical-fitness evaluation.

## TABLE 10-1   POSITIVE INFLUENCES OF CHRONIC ENDURANCE PHYSICAL EXERCISE

Blood Vessels and Chemistry
    Increase blood oxygen content
    Increase blood cell mass and blood volume
    Increase fibrinolytic capability
    Increase efficiency of peripheral blood distribution and return
    Increase blood supply to muscles and more efficient exchange of oxygen and carbon
       dioxide
    Reduce serum triglycerides and cholesterol levels
    Reduce platelet cohesion or stickiness
    Reduce systolic and diastolic blood pressure, especially when elevated
    Reduce glucose intolerance

Heart
    Increase strength of cardiac contraction (myocardial efficiency)
    Increase blood supply (collateral) to heart
    Increase size of coronary arteries
    Increase size of heart muscle
    Increase blood volume (stroke volume) per heart beat
    Increase heart rate recovery after exercise
    Reduce heart rate at rest
    Reduce heart rate with exertion
    Reduce vulnerability to cardiac arrythmias

Lungs
    Increase blood supply
    Increase diffusion of $O_2$ and $CO_2$
    Increase functional capacity during exercise
    Reduce nonfunctional volume of lung

Endocrine (Glandular) and Metabolic Function
    Increase tolerance to stress
    Increase glucose tolerance
    Increase thyroid function
    Increase growth hormone production
    Increase lean muscle mass
    Increase enzymatic function in muscle cells
    Increase functional capacity during exercise (muscle oxygen uptake capacity)
    Reduce body fat content
    Reduce chronic catecholamine production
    Reduce neurohumeral overreaction

Neural and Psychic
    Reduce strain and nervous tension resulting from psychologic stress
    Reduce tendency for depression
    Euphoria or "*joie de vivre*" experienced by many

Reprinted from Cantu, R.C. *Toward fitness: Guided exercise for those with health problems.* New York: Human Sciences Press, 1980. With permission.

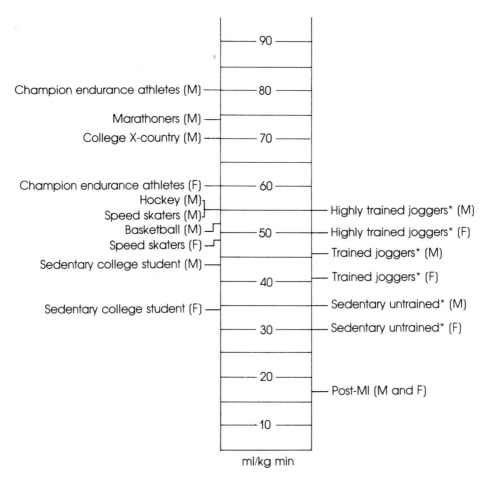

**FIGURE 10-1.** Maximal oxygen uptake values for selected activity groups. F: female; M: male. An asterisk indicates that values are for middle-aged adults. (*Reprinted from Getchell, B.* Physical fitness: A way of life *(2nd ed.).* New York: Wiley, 1979. With permission.)

## THE ROLE OF THE NURSE

Nurses are generally familiar with the importance of exercise such as passive or active range of motion for the bed-ridden patient or ambulation during hospitalization to prevent the undesirable and hazardous effects of immobility. The nurse's role in preventing deterioration of fitness for the patient is a well-defined one. In contrast, the concept of promoting physical fitness for purposes of health protection and promotion in the well adult has been largely ignored in nursing curricula. As a result, most nurses know little about this aspect of health promotion even though it is one of the most important factors in preventing disability and increasing health and wellness.[11]

The nurse should be able to evaluate physical fitness of clients and incorporate knowledge of physiology, chemistry, and anatomy (e.g., Krebs cycle, cell physiology, cardiovascular dynamics) into practical approaches to exercise. The nurse should not only instruct, support, and evaluate clients during physical-fitness activities but should serve as a role model of the physically fit adult. Personal experience with exercise and fitness activities increases the enthusiasm of the nurse for such programs and promotes understanding and empathy for clients during the early experiences of muscle soreness, fatigue, and slow progress.

Many nurses are actively involved in providing exercise and weight-control programs for adults in the community and children in school settings. Wellness programs in many hospitals are coordinated by nurses and place major emphasis on group physical-training programs.

## PRE-EXERCISE CONSIDERATIONS

All individuals who have a family or personal history of cardiovascular disorders, present previous signs or symptoms of cardiovascular disease, or are over 35 years of age should obtain a complete physical examination before beginning an exercise program. The physical examination should include a family history, blood lipid profile, resting blood pressure, resting 12-lead electrocardiogram, and exercise 12-lead electrocardiogram.[12] A treadmill stress test or bicycle ergometer test is also recommended. If the client's personal physician is not familiar with these physical fitness tests or does not have the proper equipment to administer them, the client should request the name of a physician qualified to conduct such an evaluation.

The aerobic capacity of the client as well as heart rate and rhythm patterns during testing are important considerations in structuring an appropriate exercise program. The nurse should work closely with the client and his or her physician in implementing a physical-activity program. This facilitates early detection of problems that the client may encounter and periodic reevaluation of the program.

## PROPER BREATHING

Learning to breathe is the first thing that newborn infants do, but many children, adolescents, and adults develop inefficient and improper breathing patterns. When breathing is inappropriate or inadequate, all parts of the body, including muscles and brain, are affected by a shortage of oxygen. Proper breathing is not just a matter of the inhalation and exhalation of air; it includes the expansion of all parts of the lungs as well as correct posture to make this expansion possible. The proper movement of the diaphragm is critical for effective breathing. It should lower (contract) during inhalation and curve up into the thorax (relax) during exhalation. This type of breathing, referred to as diaphragmatic or abdominal breathing, is important throughout each day, but it is particularly important during exercise, when cells of the heart and muscles need increased oxygen.

Because of limited space, the physiology of breathing will not be discussed here. Instead, several breathing exercises will be described that the nurse can teach clients in order to promote maximum expansion of lungs and increased benefits from exercise.

### Nickolaus Breathing Technique[13]

This exercise increases the client's awareness of breathing patterns, helps gain control of breathing, increases lung capacity, and relaxes the total body in preparation for exercise. It can be incorporated as part of the warm-up routine.

The client should be instructed to lie on the floor (rug or mat is preferred, but a blanket may be used), with knees bent to keep lower back against the floor and knees and feet 6 to 8 inches apart. The body should be aligned as illustrated in Figure 10-2, with feet on the floor, toes turned slightly inward so that the arches are lifted. Chin should be toward chest, with mouth slightly open. The client should imagine lying in bed, relaxed, letting everything go, just before drifting off to sleep. The hands should be placed on the stomach, with middle fingers meeting at the navel so that the client can feel the up-and-down movement of abdominal muscles. The client should inhale slowly through the nose to the count of 4, letting the diaphragm descend and abdomen rise. The breath should flow upward into the chest, expanding the upper part of the torso. The air should then be allowed to flow out through the nose and mouth, gently contracting muscles of the chest then those of the abdomen. With abdominal contraction, the lower part of the back should make solid contact with the floor. This exercise should be repeated six times.

It is important to maintain an even flow in breathing with inhalation and exhalation performed in a steady and continuous fashion. The only tension that should be felt during exhalation is in the abdomen.

### Diaphragmatic Breathing (Sitting Position)[14]

If the client prefers, diaphragmatic breathing can be performed while sitting in a straight-backed chair. The client should assume a comfortable position, with feet resting flat on the floor and hands placed one over the other at the navel as illustrated in Figure 10-3. Eyes should remain open. The client should imagine a

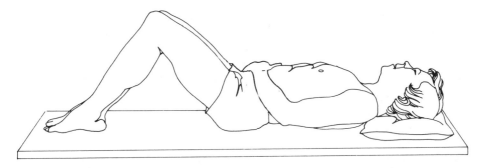

**FIGURE 10-2.** Body position and alignment for Nickolaus breathing technique.

giant balloon in the abdomen below the hands that he or she is attempting to fill with air. The hands will raise as the imaginary balloon is filled. The client should continue inhalation through the nose until the balloon is "filled to the top." Total length of inhalation should be 5 to 7 seconds. The client should inhale through the nose since this allows the air to be warmed and moistened and the removal of impurities. Air inhaled through the mouth may be too cold for comfortable deep breathing.

The breath should be held momentarily while the phrase "I feel calm" is repeated slowly. The air can then be exhaled to "empty the balloon." During exhalation the raised abdomen and chest recede. This breathing exercise should be repeated four to five times in succession at least eight or ten times per day. If lightheadedness occurs, decrease length of inhalation or number of repetitions.

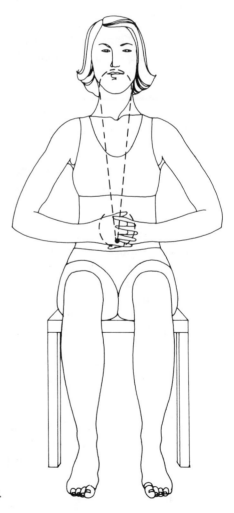

**FIGURE 10-3.**
Sitting position for diaphragmatic breathing.

**Complete Breathing[15]**
This technique is taken from yoga and is a combination of coordinated postural movements and breathing. The starting position for complete breathing is illustrated in Figure 10-4a. Knees should be together, with hips resting on heels and frontal part of head resting on the floor. This position is assumed after complete exhalation. The body should be raised as in Figure 10-4b when air is inhaled; abdomen should move out, and the hollow in the back should be prominent. The client should raise arms above his or her head while holding his or her breath for 1 to 2 seconds (Fig. 10-4c). During exhalation, the starting position is slowly assumed again (Fig. 10-4d) in preparation for the next sequence. This exercise should be practiced six to eight times in succession three to four times per day; it can be modified for the elderly or disabled as illustrated in Figure 10-5.

**Summary**
Correct breathing is essential for good cardiopulmonary function. As with any skill, practice is important in mastering appropriate breathing techniques. Use of appropriate diaphragmatic breathing will greatly enhance vitality and facilitate endurance during active exercise.

**CHARACTERISTICS OF GOOD EXERCISE**

A program of exercise that promotes physical fitness should have the following characteristics from the client's perspective:[16]

• It should be enjoyable
• It should be vigorous enough to make use of a minimum of 400 calories
• It should sustain the heart rate at 70 to 85 percent of maximum potential for 20 to 30 minutes (approximately 120 to 150 beats)
• It should produce rhythmical movements, with muscles alternatively contracting and relaxing
• It should be repeated for 30 to 60 minutes, 4 to 5 days per week
• It should be systematically integrated into the client's lifestyle

Recreational activities that achieve target heart rate and thus develop cardiopulmonary and muscular endurance include running, swimming, cross-country skiing, cycling, rowing, handball, basketball (if played vigorously), and squash.[17] Brisk walking can also be used since it is continuous, rhythmical movement. However, walking takes a longer period of time than the above recreational activities to achieve target heart rate. Table 10-2 presents target heart rate and heart-rate range by age. Sports not recommended as beneficial in conditioning include golf, bowling, baseball, softball, and volleyball.

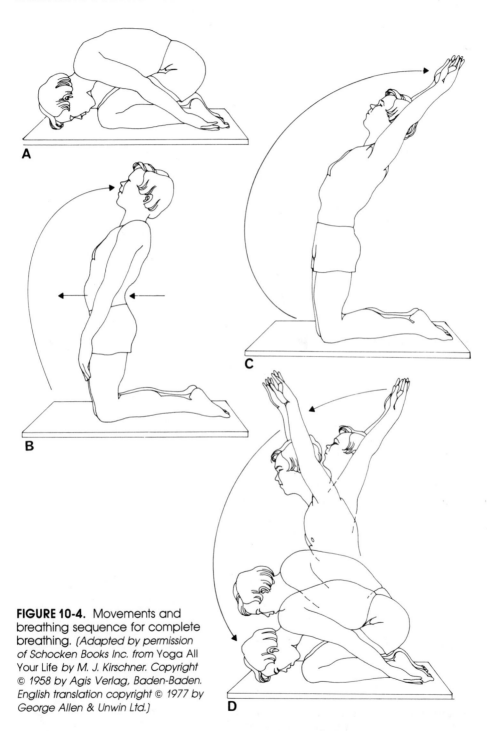

**FIGURE 10-4.** Movements and breathing sequence for complete breathing. *(Adapted by permission of Schocken Books Inc. from* Yoga All Your Life *by M. J. Kirschner. Copyright © 1958 by Agis Verlag, Baden-Baden. English translation copyright © 1977 by George Allen & Unwin Ltd.)*

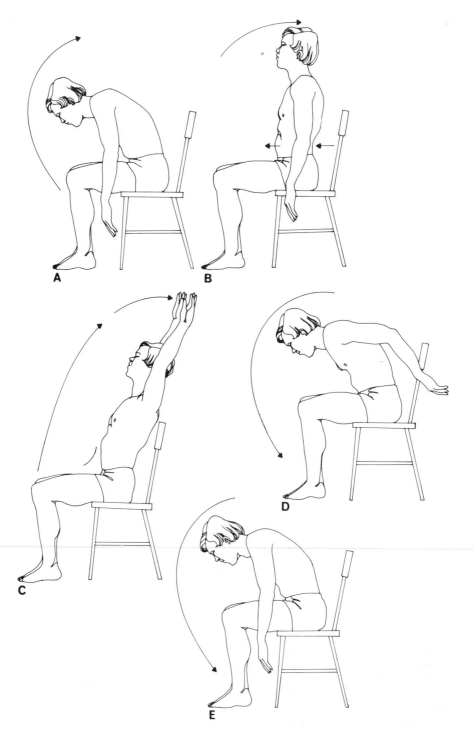

**FIGURE 10-5.** Modified complete breathing technique for the elderly or disabled. *(Adapted by permission of Schocken Books Inc. from* Yoga All Your Life *by M. J. Kirschner. Copyright © 1958 by Agis Verlag, Baden-Baden. English translation copyright © 1977 by George Allen & Unwin Ltd.)*

---

**TABLE 10-2   TARGET HEART RATE AND HEART-RATE RANGE BY AGE GROUP**

Maximum heart rate is the greatest number of beats per minute that your heart is capable of. During exercise, your heart rate should be approximately 70 to 85 percent of this maximum.

| Age | Your Maximum Heart Rate (beats/min) | Your Target Heart Rate (75% of the maximum in beats/min) | Your Target Heart-Rate Range (between 70 and 85% of the maximum in beats/min) |
|---|---|---|---|
| 20 | 200 | 150 | 140 to 170 |
| 25 | 195 | 146 | 137 to 166 |
| 30 | 190 | 142 | 133 to 162 |
| 35 | 185 | 139 | 130 to 157 |
| 40 | 180 | 135 | 126 to 153 |
| 45 | 175 | 131 | 123 to 149 |
| 50 | 170 | 127 | 119 to 145 |
| 55 | 165 | 124 | 116 to 140 |
| 60 | 160 | 120 | 112 to 136 |
| 65 | 155 | 116 | 109 to 132 |
| 70 | 150 | 112 | 105 to 123 |

Reprinted from Kuntzleman, C.T. *The Complete Book of Walking.* New York: Simon & Shuster, 1979, p. 96. With permission.

## WARMING UP FOR EXERCISE

A warm-up period before extended exercise is important in order to increase blood flow to heart and skeletal muscles, enhance oxygenation of tissues, and loosen (decrease tension) and strengthen muscles. The warm-up period need take no longer than 10 to 15 minutes and should be immediately followed by endurance exercise. Some exercise specialists differentiate between warm-up and stretching exercises and believe that there is less likelihood of injury from stretching exercises if they are carried out after the endurance regimen but prior to cool down. The following is a suggested warm-up sequence of exercises:

1. Walk briskly for 1 minute
2. Jog for 45 seconds
3. Walk briskly for 30 seconds
4. Arm circles
5. Jumping jacks
6. Lateral bend
7. Head rotation
8. Side leg raises
9. Single leg raise and knee hug
10. Push-ups (floor or wall)

Each of the warm-up exercises except jogging and walking will be described below. Jogging and walking will be dealt with at length later in this chapter under Endurance Exercises. The reader is referred to the references at the end of the chapter for other activities that can be used in warm-up routines.

### Arm Circles

This warm-up exercise increases the flexibility of muscles in the arm and shoulder region. The client should stand with feet shoulder-width apart and arms at sides. Arms should make large sweeping circles, with elbows straight, swinging arms from the shoulders.[18] The inward cross-body and outward cross-body arm circles and forward (swimming crawl motion) and backward (backward swimming crawl) arm circles are illustrated in Figure 10-6. Ten repetitions of each type of arm circles are recommended.

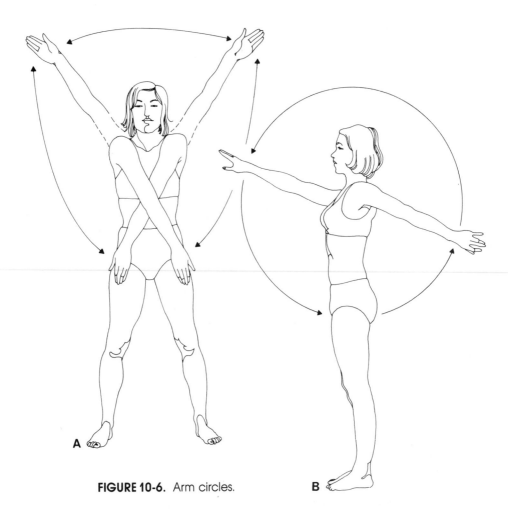

**FIGURE 10-6.** Arm circles.

**Jumping Jacks**

This exercise is frequently used as part of the warm-up routine. It stretches and loosens major muscle groups within the arms and legs. The client should start with feet together and hands at sides. When jumping to the position with feet apart, arms should be kept straight and swung up over head. Ten to twenty jumping jacks should be repeated at a comfortable tempo. Figure 10-7 illustrates the jumping-jack exercise.

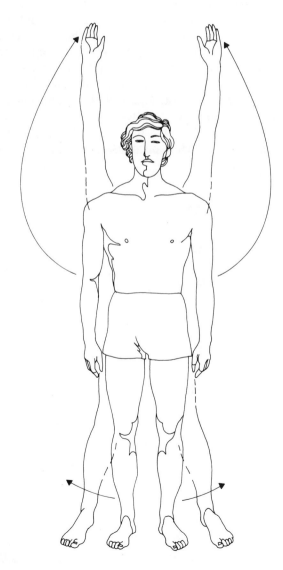

**FIGURE 10-7.** Jumping jacks.

**Lateral Bend**

This warm-up exercise is intended to loosen and stretch the lateral muscles of the trunk and back. Feet should be about shoulder-width apart, arms at sides. By bending laterally, the client should reach down the right leg with the right hand until he or she feels a pulling sensation in the back. At this point, the client should straighten to upright position and repeat the same stretching movement on the left side. Ten repetitions are recommended. The lateral bend is illustrated in Figure 10-8.

**Head Rotation**

The client should assume a sitting position, with arms comfortably resting at sides. While the client breathes in, the chin should be dropped forward to the chest. The client should roll the head to the left, then to the back, stretching the chin toward the ceiling. As the head is rolled to the right and forward again, the client should exhale. This is an excellent exercise for increasing the flexibility of neck muscles and is particularly recommended for individuals who spend a great deal of time at desk work. Figure 10-9 illustrates head rotation. Repetitions should be increased from five to fifteen, as tolerated. The client should be informed that initially some dizziness may occur; therefore, this exercise should never be performed in a standing position.

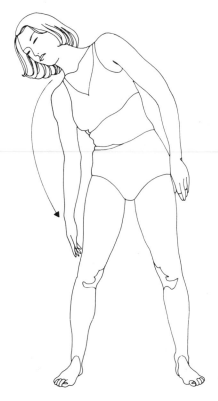

**FIGURE 10-8.** The lateral bend.

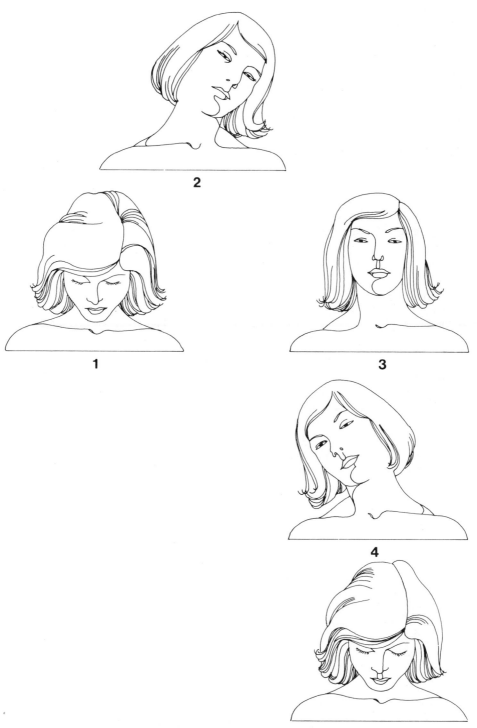

**FIGURE 10-9.** Head rotation.

**Side Leg Raises**
This exercise stretches and strengthens the lateral hip muscles and is a good conditioning exercise. The client should lie on his or her right side in extended position, with head resting on right hand as shown in Figure 10-10. The client raises the left leg as high as possible above the horizontal position and then returns to starting position. After completing repetitions for one side, the client repeats the exercise on the other side. Fifteen to 25 repetitions are recommended.

**Single Leg Raise and Knee Hug**
This exercise is intended to strengthen low back and abdominal muscles while increasing the flexibility of hip and knee joints. The client assumes a reclining position as illustrated in Figure 10-11 and raises extended left leg about 12 inches off the floor, slowly bending the knee and moving it toward the chest. The client then places both hands around the knee and pulls it gently toward his/her chest as far as possible. The leg is then slowly extended to the starting position. This exercise is repeated three to five times with each leg.

**Wall Push-ups**
This exercise is intended to strengthen arm, shoulder, and upper back muscles while stretching chest and posterior thigh muscles. The client should stand erect facing the wall with feet about 6 inches apart, arms extended, and palms of hands against the wall. The client slowly bends the arms and lowers body toward the wall, until cheek almost touches the wall. The body is then slowly pushed away from the wall, extending arms and returning to original position. This exercise should be repeated five to ten times as illustrated in Figure 10-12. Traditional floor push-ups can also be used if the level of fitness of the client permits more exertion than required by wall push-ups.

The client who is just beginning a physical exercise program will need to select three or four warm-up exercises initially, completing 5 to 10 repetitions of

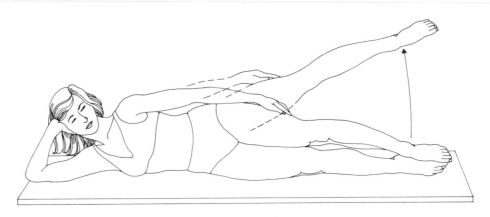

**FIGURE 10-10.** Side leg raises.

each. As endurance exercise is continued, repetitions can be increased, different warm-up exercises can be selected for variety, or others can be added to extend the time spent in warm-up. Cool weather usually requires a longer warm-up period than does warm weather.

## STRETCHING EXERCISES

Loss of joint and muscle flexibility occurs more frequently with aging than does loss of strength and endurance. Flexibility is defined as the extent to which the client is able to move joints and muscles through full range of motion. Since walking and running do little for flexibility, stretching exercises are extremely important in the maintenance of physical fitness.

Stretching exercises put more strain on muscle than do warm-up exercises. Excessive stretching, just like excessive jogging, can produce injuries. After the body is warmed up or after the endurance phase of exercise, stretching can be carried out with much less discomfort and concern for injury. Stretching exercises should be done slowly, and positions should be held for a few seconds. As the client becomes more flexible, stretching positions can be held for longer periods of time.[19] Because of limited space, only a few stretching exercises will be presented. The reader is referred to the references at the end of the chapter for more detailed information on stretching routines.

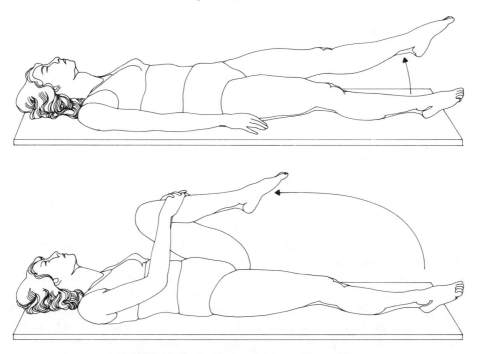

**FIGURE 10-11.** Single leg raise and knee hug.

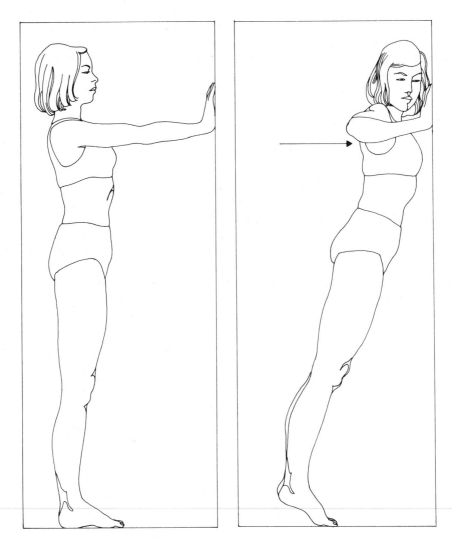

**FIGURE 10-12.** Wall push-ups.

**Back Stretch**
The back is extremely vulnerable to injury and many Americans suffer from chronic back problems. This exercise stretches the back and neck muscles and promotes greater strength and flexibility. The client should stand erect with feet shoulder-width apart and bend forward at the waist, letting arms, shoulders, and neck relax. The client should go to the point where a slight stretch is felt in the back of the legs. If the client cannot reach the floor, the hands can be placed on the legs to provide support. When straightening back up, the knees should be slightly bent to avoid pressure in the lower back. Figure 10-13 illustrates the back-

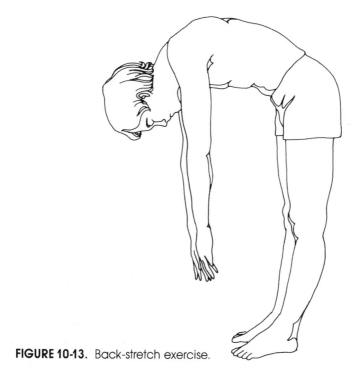

**FIGURE 10-13.** Back-stretch exercise.

stretch exercise. Five to seven repetitions are recommended initially. If the client is elderly or disabled, back-stretch exercise can also be done sitting in a chair. Knees are placed apart, feet flat on the floor, with the body gently lowered between the knees. The fingers and palms of the hands should touch the floor. This exercise is particularly effective in dealing with postural strain following typing, driving, sewing, or other forms of sedentary work.[20]

**Leg Overs**
The purpose of this exercise is to stretch the rotator muscles of the lower back and pelvic region. The client should lie on back with legs extended and arms extended at shoulder level with the palms up. The leg should be kept straight as it is raised to the vertical position (toes pointed). The opposite leg should remain on the floor in extended position. The vertically extended leg should reach across the body to the opposite hand and then be returned to the vertical position as shown in Figure 10-14. The exercise should be repeated with each leg for four to ten repetitions.

**Hamstring Stretcher**
This exercise can be done in three different positions as illustrated in Figure 10-15.

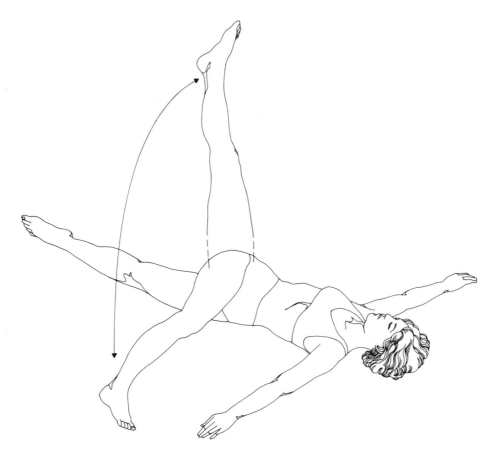

**FIGURE 10-14.** Leg overs.

In the standing position (Fig. 10-15a), one leg is raised and the heel of the foot rests on a table or chair. The client should lean toward the raised foot until stretching is felt in the thigh. This position should be held for several seconds with care being taken not to overstretch.

In the sitting position (Fig. 10-15b), knees should be extended with legs spread apart at a 45-degree angle. The client should bend forward at the waist, grasping one ankle with both hands and trying to touch the head to the knee until stretching is felt in the back of the leg. This position should be held for 5 to 7 seconds.

In the lying-down position (Figure 10-15c), the client is on his or her back on the floor or bed. Arms are raised perpendicular at right angles to the body. Each leg should be kept straight but swung up gently toward the fingers. Five to ten repetitions with each leg are recommended.[21] The lying-down position may be easier for elderly individuals to use. The purpose of the exercise is to stretch the lower-back muscles and hamstring muscles, which shorten considerably with age or in women from wearing high-heeled shoes.

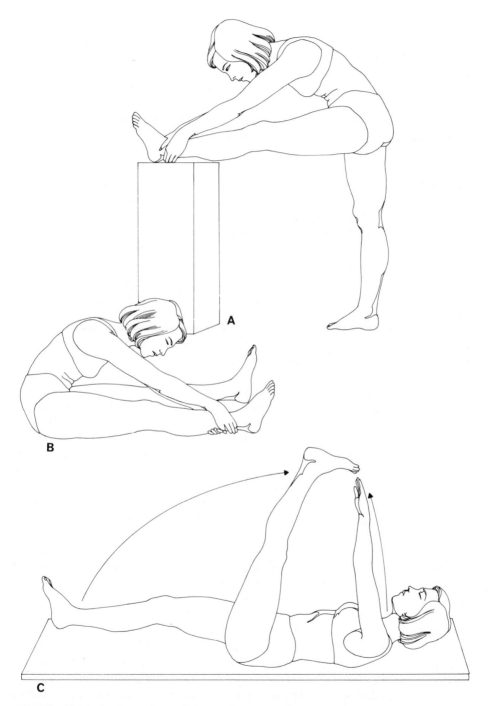

**FIGURE 10-15.** Hamstring-stretching exercises. **a.** Standing hamstring stretcher. **b.** sitting hamstring stretcher **c.** Lying-down hamstring stretcher.

### Trunk Rotator

This exercise is performed to stretch the muscles of the lower back, buttocks, and waist. The client should begin by standing with feet shoulder-width apart and hands with fingers interlaced behind head. First the client should lean to the right and continue moving in a clockwise direction, down and up to the left and back to the original position, in a circular motion. The circular motion should be repeated in a counter-clockwise direction.[22] Six to eight repetitions in each direction are recommended. The body motion for the trunk rotator is depicted in Figure 10-16.

### Cat's Arch

This exercise is intended to stretch the muscles of the lower back, waist, and stomach. The client should begin by getting down on hands and knees, keeping elbows straight and knees bent at a 90-degree angle. The stomach should be pushed toward floor and the back bent downward. This will cause extension of the back muscles. Then the client should arch his or her back like an angry cat. In attempting to do this, the client should pull in the stomach muscles as much as possible and push the lower back towards the ceiling. This exercise is excellent for increasing the flexibility of the lower back, particularly after sitting behind a desk for long periods of time.[23] Figure 10-17 depicts the two different positions to be assumed during this stretching exercise. Six repetitions are recommended initially, increasing to 15 to 20 as tolerated.

### Stretching Exercises for Feet and Ankles

The feet and ankles are extremely important in most endurance activities and thus should be given careful attention in stretching and flexibility exercises. Lying in the position shown in Figure 10-18, with the knee flexed, the foot can be circled clockwise until the toe is pointed away and then flexed back to its starting position. This exercise should be repeated only five times with each foot since cramping may occasionally occur. If cramping does occur, the foot should be relaxed until cramping subsides, and then the exercise can be continued.

Foot flexion is also illustrated in Figure 10-18. In this exercise, the foot is arched by extending the metatarsal but keeping the toes flexed. The toes are then pointed and flexed again, and then the entire foot is flexed. This exercise should also be repeated five times with each foot. These exercises can be carried out while sitting in a chair with the leg slightly raised if the physical condition of the client makes this position more feasible.

### Summary

Stretching exercises strengthen muscles, ligaments, and tendons and develop flexibility in the body's muscles and joints. This increases physical readiness to engage in endurance exercise as well as greater ease and comfort in carrying out the activities of daily living. The number and type of stretching exercises appropriate for each individual must be determined through mutual discussion and planning between the nurse and the client.

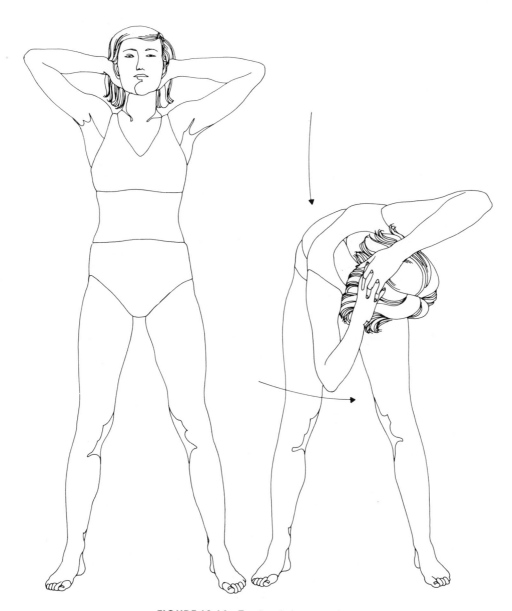

**FIGURE 10-16.** Trunk-rotator exercise.

## ENDURANCE EXERCISES

A systematic program of endurance exercise can result in cardiopulmonary and muscular conditioning. Endurance exercises should be integrated into the personal lifestyle since continued practice is essential for long-term health-protection and

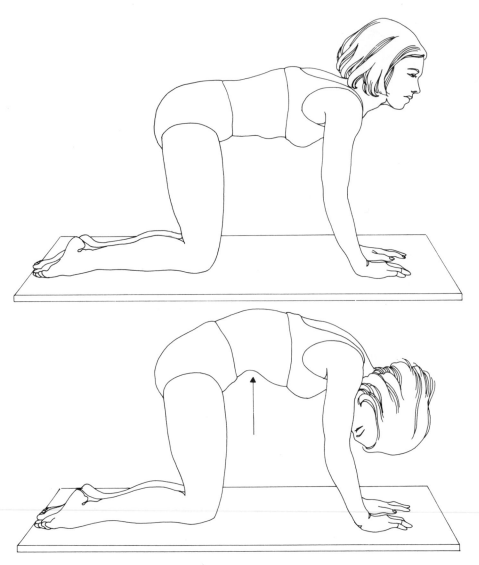

**FIGURE 10-17.** The cat's arch.

health-promotion benefits. Maintaining physical fitness is a lifelong process that can be enjoyable, rewarding, and challenging to the client. Endurance exercises to be discussed in this chapter include walk-jog, jogging, and walking. These are the least expensive and usually the most convenient endurance exercises for clients to perform.

Critical aspects of self-care important for all individuals engaged in a physical fitness program include the following:

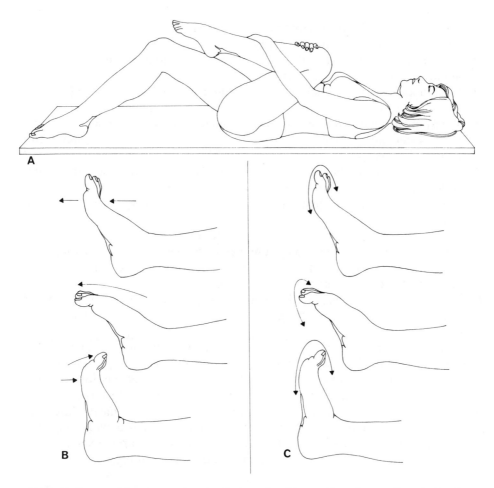

**FIGURE 10-18.** Stretching exercises for feet and ankles. **a.** Exercise position. **b.** Foot flexion. **c.** Foot/ankle circles.

1. The feet should be well cared for since they are subjected to increased stress and friction during endurance exercise.
2. A good pair of running shoes should be worn for all endurance exercises. Characteristics of good shoes include:[24]
   - Cushioned soles
   - Ample toe room
   - Heel elevation from $\frac{1}{2}$ to $\frac{3}{4}$ inches above sole
   - Good support
   - Oxford type
   - Leather, allowing feet to breathe
   - Sole that flexes at the ball of foot but not at the midpoint.

3. Clean, snug-fitting socks should be worn during exercise to prevent the development of pressure points and blisters.

4. Endurance exercises should not be carried out during the hottest or most humid hours of the day in warm weather.

5. Endurance exercise should not be carried out immediately following a meal. The client should wait $1\frac{1}{2}$ to $2\frac{1}{2}$ hours after eating a full meal.

6. Workout should be preceded by drinking an increased amount of clear liquids (e.g., water, juice). Water loss from the body is markedly increased during endurance exercise.

7. From $1\frac{1}{2}$ to $2\frac{1}{2}$ hours before exercise, ingestion of small to moderate amounts of high-carbohydrate foods can increase glucose reserves.

8. Maintenance of an adequate intake of salt and potassium prevents muscle cramps.

9. Excessive stretching during warm-ups should be avoided.

10. Shin splints can be prevented by running or walking on soft or semisoft rather than hard surfaces. The surface should also be relatively flat rather than hilly to prevent excessive fatigue.

11. If injury to achilles tendon (inflammation, partial rupture, or complete rupture) occurs, ice should be applied immediately, and activity should be reduced.

The nurse is responsible for assisting the client in developing specific competencies related to efficient and effective use of endurance exercise for physical conditioning. Borgman[25] has identified competency-based objectives for a teaching plan on exercise as an aspect of health maintenance. These objectives are presented in Table 10-3. Review of the competencies required indicates the complexity of physical-endurance activities. The client must be able to plan adequately for exercise, prepare for exercise, monitor physical status during exercise, take appropriate actions if problems arise, and appraise personal progress.

**Walk-Jog**
This endurance exercise is appropriate for clients of all ages. Interspersing walking and jogging provides variation and distributes periods of physical stress over a span of time. Following warm-up exercises, the client should begin a period of jogging that lengthens throughout the conditioning program. In the beginning, jogging for 30 seconds followed by walking for an equal amount of time allows the client to adjust to increased physical activity. The client should jog erect, with the spine extended to maximize comfort. As the amount of time spent in jogging increases, the client will develop greater concentration on the smoothness and rhythm of body movement. Increased awareness of breathing, muscular contractions, relaxation, sensations of lightness, and enjoyment will characterize the activity.

The client should be able to take his or her radial or carotid pulse for 15 seconds and multiply by 4 during both jogging and walking segments of the walk-jog. The heart rate should be within the target heart rate range during jogging (see Table 10-2), dropping somewhat during walking segments. If heart rate is not

---

**TABLE 10-3   COMPETENCY-BASED OBJECTIVES FOR A TEACHING PLAN ON EXERCISE**

---

The consumer of health should be able to:

Express personal concept of health.

Examine personal views in regard to health and physical fitness.

Relate his or her general health and illness history.

Relate his or her specific (if available) health–illness information (e.g., blood pressure, weight, diet, smoking habits, electrocardiogram results, specific blood chemistry results such as cholesterol and triglyceride levels, personality characteristics, etc.).

Express personal likes and dislikes of physical activity.

Recognize that exercise is a part of but not the sole factor of health maintenance.

Locate exercise resources in the community.

Plan a time schedule when exercises could be included without altering the client's lifestyle.

Conjointly plan an exercise program with his or her doctor and nurse/teacher.

Recognize aerobic exercises that either are or are not appropriate for the client.

Describe suitable clothing to wear during exercising.

Explain the importance of a warm-up period.

Describe the symptoms of angina and muscle strain that would indicate cessation of activity.

Demonstrate how to monitor a pulse before, during, and after exercise.

Compare vital signs and physical changes during and after exercise to resting vital signs.

Demonstrate emergency actions (CPR) that may be necessary during group exercising activities.

Question exercise fads and nonprofessional literature on exercise.

Compare his or her progress over a period of time.

Plan for medical and nursing/teaching follow-up.

Value his or her progress and perseverence in habit formation and health maintenance.

Choose by virtue of his or her individual right to terminate the program.

---

Adapted from Borgman, M.F. Exercise and health maintenance. *Journal of Nursing Education,* January 1979, *16,* 6–10. With permission.

initially at target level, it will increase as the jogging periods are lengthened. If heart rate is above this level during jogging, changing to brisk walking and shortening the next jogging segment is suggested. A plan for developing a walk-jog program is presented in Table 10-4. The client should continue at each level until he or she has mastered that walk-jog combination and then move on to the next. If problems are encountered in moving to the next step, such as excessive fatigue, marked breathlessness, or faintness, the client should return to the previous level for a period of 3 to 5 days before attempting the next level of conditioning the second time.

The client should be cautioned to proceed judiciously. If he or she is over 50 years of age and has been following a sedentary lifestyle, it is wise to have the client brisk walk on a progressive schedule for 10 to 12 weeks before beginning the walk-jog routines.

### Jogging

Through jogging, the client reaches target heart rate (70 to 85 percent maximum) more rapidly than in a walk-jog routine. However, continuous jogging is more physically demanding than walk-jog and should never be attempted as the initial endurance exercise. It is recommended that the client complete the previously described walk-jog routine before attempting continuous jogging.

#### TABLE 10-4   PROGRESSIVE WALK-JOG PROGRAM

| Level | Jog | Walk | Repeats |
|-------|-----|------|---------|
| 1 | 30 sec | 30 sec | 4 sets (work up to 12 sets for 3 consecutive days) |
| 2 | 1 min | 30 sec | 6 sets (work up to 12 sets for 3 consecutive days) |
| 3 | $1\frac{1}{2}$ min | 30 sec | 6 sets (work up to 12 sets for 2 consecutive days) |
| 4 | 2 min | 30 sec | 6 sets (work up to 10 sets for 2 consecutive days) |
| 5 | 4 min | 1 min | 4 sets (work up to 6 sets for 2 consecutive days) |
| 6 | 8 min | 2 min | 2 sets (work up to 4 sets on 2 consecutive days) |
| 7 | 12 min | 2 min | 2 sets |
| 8 | 15 min | 3 min | 2 sets |
| 9 | 20 min | 3 min | 2 sets |

Jogging or running are the forms of endurance exercise that result in the highest caloric expenditure per minute. Females expend 9.1 kcal/min$^{-1}$ at 81.9 percent VO$_2$ maximum, as compared to males who expend 15.5 kcal/min$^{-1}$ at 81.1 percent VO$_2$ maximum. Weight makes a difference in the amount of calories burned, particularly for jogging, although similar patterns are found for walk-jog and walking.[26] The higher the weight, the more calories that are burned.

Following completion of the walk-jog routine, continuous jogging should be carried out initially for a period of time no longer than 20 minutes. The client should carefully evaluate his or her tolerance of continuous endurance activity by checking his or her pulse every 5 minutes during jogging and by noting any unusual physical symptoms. After 10 to 14 days of jogging continuously for 20 minutes, the client can increase jogging time to 30 minutes. If this is tolerated well for a period of 2 weeks, the jogging period can be increased to 35 or 40 minutes. This is an adequate length of time to allow heart rate to rise and to sustain target heart rate at conditioning level for 30 minutes.

Many individuals who jog continuously have reported altered psychologic states, such as euphoria, heightened inner awareness, or increased feelings of control during jogging. Many report decreased attention to environmental surroundings or that jogging results in a "natural high."[27] Because of increased internal focus and decreased attention to surroundings during jogging, the client should take precautions to minimize chances of injury. The client should never jog at night when unseen obstacles may cause serious trauma or jog in an area of heavy traffic.

Discussion of jogging as an endurance exercise in this chapter has been brief. For additional information, the reader is referred to the references at the end of the chapter and to several excellent books.[28-30]

### Walking

This endurance exercise is safe for people of all ages. It can be tailored to individual differences and a wide range of fitness levels. Since fewer calories are expended in walking when compared to jogging, the client must walk briskly twice as long to achieve comparable levels of conditioning. Kuntzleman[31] has stated that an adult male burns the number of calories equivalent to one pound of fat (approximately 3500 calories) in 12 hours of brisk walking. The number of calories expended depends on walking rate (mph) and body weight. For comparable amounts of walking, individuals who weigh more expend greater energy than do individuals who weigh less. Brisk walking is extremely important during periods of attempted weight loss as it prevents the loss of lean body tissue.

The positive outcomes from a systematic walking program are many and varied. Walking can result in the following:

- Decreased percentage body fat
- Improved circulation
- Increased muscle tone in legs
- Decreased problems of constipation

- Improved mental state, with decreased depression and anxiety
- Improved recovery index following exercise
- Lowered blood pressure
- Improved physical fitness
- Decreased risk of coronary heart disease

Walking at 70 to 85 percent of maximum heart rate for at least 20 minutes three times per week will improve physical fitness. Walking at 70 to 85 percent of maximum heart rate for 30 minutes or longer four times per week can decrease the risk of coronary heart disease. If at the rate of walking selected by the client, pulse does not reach target level, rate of walking or length of walk must be increased to achieve a training effect. The barometer for how much walking the client can tolerate early in the walking program is the level of fatigue, breathlessness, or uncomfortable symptoms experienced. If after walking, the client seems excessively tired for more than an hour, the walk may be too strenuous. The client can walk more slowly or for a shorter period of time until tolerance is increased for more sustained efforts.

Regarding the psychologic effects of walking, a study of a group of men over 50 years of age indicated that after several weeks of walking for 15 minutes per day, neuromuscular tension was decreased more effectively than it was from using standard dosages of tranquilizers over the same period of time.[32] Walking can promote feelings of serenity and relaxation. Consequently, it is an important adjunct to other stress-management techniques that the client may choose to use.

In order to maximize the benefits from a walking program, a number of suggestions can be made to the client:

- Walk naturally.
- Wear good shoes with adequate support.
- Let arms hang loosely at sides.
- Hands, hips, knees, and ankles should be relaxed.
- Feet should strike the ground at the heel.
- Push off with toes when walking.
- Use heel-to-toe rolling motion.
- Breathe naturally.
- Walk for fitness and for fun.

Several ways that the client can make walking more enjoyable include inviting someone to walk along and visit, varying the route taken for the walk, and "getting into the walk" (appreciating the pleasurable body sensations of smooth, coordinated movement).

Other endurance exercises that are beyond the scope of this book include swimming, running, bicycling, and rope skipping. The reader is referred to references at the end of this chapter for further information on these activities.

## Summary

In summary, all clients engaged in endurance exercise should have well-developed self-monitoring skills. The client participating in endurance exercises should not only understand how and when to check his or her own pulse but should also know what symptoms to look for as an indication of a possible problem. The nurse should counsel the client concerning the following symptoms and emphasize the need for the client to seek medical attention if they occur:[33]

- Chest or arm pain
- Marked increase in shortness of breath
- Irregular heart beat
- Light-headedness, fainting
- Nausea and vomiting with exercise
- Unexplained weight changes
- Muscle or joint problems
- Prolonged fatigue
- Muscle weakness
- Unexplained changes in exercise tolerance

## COOLING DOWN

Following warm-up, stretching exercises, and endurance exercise, cooling down is important. This phase of the workout provides a 5- to 10-minute recovery period following strenuous activity to allow circulation to gradually return to normal, preventing pooling of blood in muscles and possible fainting. Cooling down is important since in endurance exercise, blood pressure, body temperature, heart rate, and lactic acid within the muscles are all increased. Cooling down appropriately promotes elimination of waste products from the muscles, maintains blood flow to and from the muscles, and allows body temperature and heart rate to decrease slowly. Inappropriate cooling down can make the client feel sore and nauseated. At the end of the cooling-down period, the heart rate of the client should be below 100.

Several exercises can be used during the cooling-down period. Five will be presented in this chapter for the client to consider. Exercises selected for cooling down should not allow a rapid drop in heart rate; there should be a gradual change over a period of time (usually 5 to 10 minutes).

### Walking and Deep Breathing

An excellent exercise for cooling down is to continue walking briskly for 5 minutes, breathing deeply. Diaphragmatic breathing fully aerates the lungs and facilitates continuing oxygenation of blood following endurance exercise. As the client walks, he or she can also shake head and arms in a relaxed manner (shakedown). The shakedown further loosens tight muscles.[34]

**Straight Arm and Leg Stretch**
This exercise strengthens abdominal muscles while stretching the muscles of the arms. The client should lie flat on the floor with legs together and arms at the sides. The buttocks and abdomen are tensed so that the back is flat against the floor. The client should slowly move arms and legs outward along the floor as far as possible, hold for 5 seconds, and return to a starting position. Five to ten repetitions of this exercise are recommended. The two positions to be assumed during the exercise are shown in Figure 10-19.

**Achilles Stretcher**
This exercise is helpful in stretching the heel cord on the lower part of the calf muscle (achilles tendon). The client should face the wall, an arm's distance away, with knees straight, toes slightly inward, and heels flat on floor. With hands resting on the wall, the client should lean his or her body forward by bending elbows slowly. It is important that legs and body be kept straight and heels be on the floor. Five to ten repetitions of this exercise are recommended. See Figure 10-20 for illustration of this exercise.

**Half Knee Bend**
This exercise is helpful in toning the hips, thighs, and buttocks, as well as in allowing gradual cooling down following endurance exercise. The client should assume a starting position with hands on hips and feet separated about shoulder

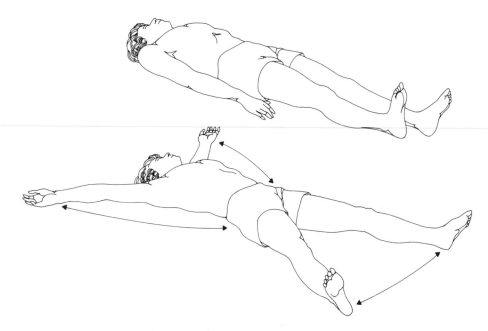

**FIGURE 10-19.** Straight arm and leg stretch.

width. As the exercise begins, the arms should be swung forward up to shoulder height and the knees bent about half-way, with heels kept on the floor. From this position, the client should return to the starting position. Figure 10-21 depicts the action sequence. Six to eight repetitions are recommended initially, with frequency gradually increased to twelve to fifteen. The client can also progress to full knee bends as personal tolerance allows.[35]

### Bent-Knee Half-Curl[36]
This exercise strengthens abdominal muscles and maintains activity during cooling down. The client should assume a lying-down position, with knees bent at a 45- to 90-degree angle and feet flat on the floor. Hands should be interlaced behind head. Tucking chin into chest, the client should curl forward until shoulders are

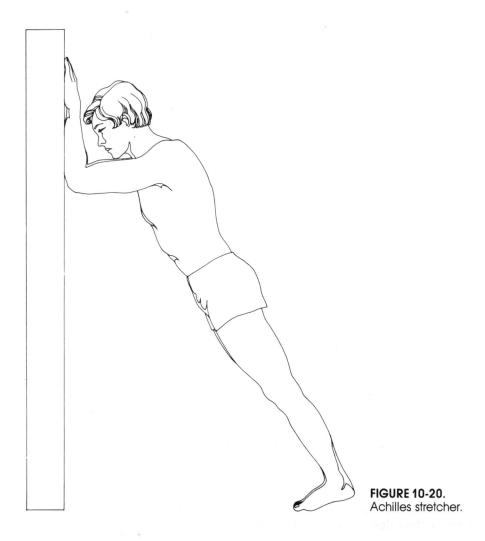

**FIGURE 10-20.**
Achilles stretcher.

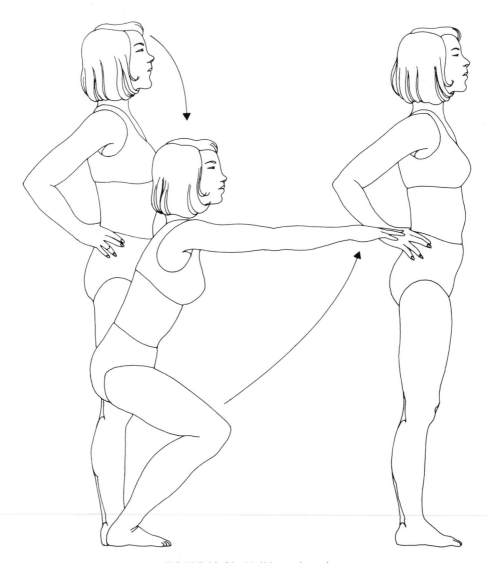

**FIGURE 10-21.** Half knee bend.

about 10 to 14 inches off the floor. This position should be held for 2 to 4 seconds. The client should slowly return to the starting position. Three to four repetitions are recommended initially, with frequency increased to six to eight as conditioning progresses. The sequence to be followed in completing this exercise is depicted in Figure 10-22.

**Conclusion**
Any of the activities described in the section on Stretching Exercises can also be used for cooling down. The client should vary his or her routine to maintain

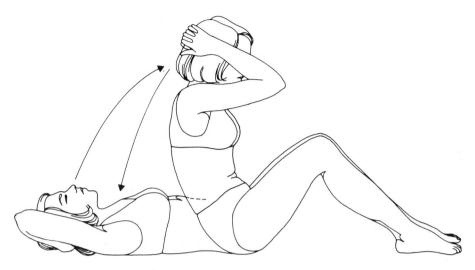

**FIGURE 10-22.** Bent-knee half-curl.

personal interest and also to determine those exercises that are most effective for him or her in allowing a slow decrease in heart rate.

## CONTINUATION OF EXERCISE PROGRAM

To maintain physical fitness, it is critical that clients continue their exercise program as an integral part of their personal lifestyle. Drop-out rates as small as 11 percent and as large as 70 percent have been reported for physical-activity programs within the first 6 weeks. What can the nurse do to promote consistent practice of behaviors directed toward improving and maintaining physical fitness? Some suggestions for assisting the client in maintaining behavioral consistency include the following:

- Setting both short-term and long-term goals
- Recording progress
- Making a time commitment
- Choosing the best time of the day and establishing a pattern (habit of regular physical activity).
- Selecting a specific place in which to exercise.
- Dressing the part in clothing appropriate for exercise.
- Thinking the part by concentrating on bodily movements during exercise; this provides important biopsychologic feedback, an important part of endurance exercise
- Varying warm-up and cool-down exercises
- Walking or running with others

- Picking an interesting and pleasing route for endurance exercise and periodically varying the route
- Alternating "hard" and "easy" days. On some days, exercise may be more intensive than on others. If exercise has been particularly strenuous one day, a less intense exercise session may be planned for the next day

Eischens[37] has suggested four approaches for assisting clients to persevere with exercise and conditioning activities. These include intent, regularity, limits capacity, and concentration. The major intent of exercise should be clear to the client, and he or she should recognize what endurance exercise means personally. Is the goal to improve personal health, to reap psychologic benefits, to lose weight, or to decrease the risk of coronary disease? Once personal health goals to be attained through physical activity have been identified, setting short-term as well as long-term goals sustains motivation.

Regularity in endurance exercise is also important to optimize positive health effects. As mentioned above, the client may alternate between "hard" and "easy" days. This alternation is considered by some exercise physiologists to lead to more rapid increases in strength then does repetitive strenuous exercise. Options for easy days can be (1) warm-up, stretching, and walking for 20 minutes, or (2) warm-up, stretching, and walk-jog for 15 minutes. Several days of complete rest are not recommended since this interferes with the conditioning process and breaks up the pattern established by the client. For conditioning, 4 days per week are recommended as a minimum, with 7 days preferred.

Each client will discover his or her physical and psychologic limits capacity for endurance exercise; these are subject to change throughout the conditioning process. Exercise should be a stimulating but manageable challenge for the client; it should not result in excessive stress or discomfort.

Discovering personal capacities through exercise or physical activity is an important expression of the actualizing tendency. Increased awareness of breathing, muscle movement, relationship to terrain, body temperature, and skin sensations through concentration can be an exciting experience for the client. A different part of endurance exercise can be focused on each time. At one time the focus may be on breathing, at another on sensations and positions of legs and feet, still another on skin sensations. Concentration or fully experiencing endurance exercise can provide short-term benefits that are highly reinforcing to the client.

In addition to the above, depicting progress in physical fitness on a graph can provide motivation for continuation of exercise and conditioning activities on the part of the client. Awareness of progress in itself can make exercise rewarding; there may be no need for tangible or social reinforcement. A graph of cardiovascular status in terms of resting heart rate that can be used to chart progress is depicted in Figure 10-23. Other parameters of fitness may also be charted in a personal-growth notebook kept by the client, with assistance from the nurse. Recognizing tangible progress toward desired health goals supports continuation of exercise and physical-fitness activities.

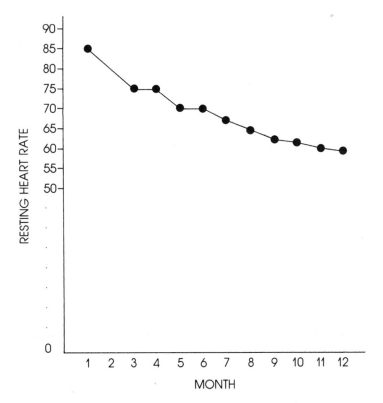

**FIGURE 10-23.** Cardiovascular status.

## EXERCISE FOR INDIVIDUALS WITH SPECIAL PROBLEMS

Diabetics, postcoronary patients, the obese, and individuals with chronic illnesses that limit mobility need special assistance in structuring exercise programs. While these clients present health problems to be taken into consideration in structuring an exercise program, few such individuals are restricted from engaging in some form of systematic physical activity. Almost always, they can improve their health by doing so. Close supervision by a physician and/or nurse is essential for these individuals during the time that an exercise program is being planned and stabilized. The program of physical activity must also be reevaluated periodically to insure that it is within the capabilities of the client.

### Diabetics
David Costill, director of the Human Performance Laboratory, Ball State University, has observed that a diabetic who exercises for 30 minutes or more daily may show as much as a 30 to 40 percent decreased need for insulin.[38] Glucose uptake is increased 7 to 20 times during exercise. When exercise stops, blood flow

to muscles decreases, but uptake of glucose remains three to four times that of resting level for an hour.[39] During exercise, insulin levels decrease, while muscle intake of glucose increases. This appears to indicate that during exercise, muscles can take glucose from the blood stream without requiring insulin. This effect is primarily responsible for the reduced insulin requirements and improved glucose tolerance in exercising diabetics. Exercise not only burns calories but lowers blood glucose without insulin. The insulin-dependent diabetic runs a risk of hypoglycemia if he or she does not decrease intake of insulin or increase intake of carbohydrates before strenuous exercise.[40]

Exercise for the diabetic is likely to retard vascular complications and is mandatory for optimum control of the disease. The cardiovascular system of the diabetic can be conditioned to the same extent as that of the nondiabetic. While there are no major limitations on exercise, special precautions that should be kept in mind, including the following:

- Care of feet: good shoes and wrinkle-free socks are a must for the diabetic, to prevent trauma to lower extremities.
- Ingestion of a controlled amount of carbohydrates before exercise prevents hypoglycemia.
- The physician will most likely have to adjust (decrease) the insulin dosage to accommodate exercise.
- Steps in the conditioning program may be more gradual to accommodate any existing cardiovascular impairment.
- Becoming overly fatigued should be avoided.

Current approaches to the treatment of diabetes recognize the critical role of systematic exercise in therapy, health protection, and health promotion.

**Postcoronary Patients**

The recovery of many coronary patients has been facilitated through regular systematic exercise. Before beginning an exercise program, the patient should be carefully evaluated by the physician to determine the potential effects of exercise on cardiac status. A step test, bicycle ergometer test, or exercise stress test may be used for this purpose. Through these diagnostic procedures, the physician may be able to detect ischemia not evident during rest (depressed ST segment of EKG), heart rate during activity, and arrhythmias or conduction defects.

Vigorous exercise should be avoided during the first 6 months after myocardial infarction. Under a physician's supervision, walking can begin during this time, but it is usually limited to short distances. By the twelfth week of walking, the patient may be able to begin a slowly graduated jogging program. Cantu[41] describes post-heart attack conditioning programs for individuals under 45 years of age and 45 years of age or older at the time of the attack. The reader is referred to this excellent source for detailed description of such programs. Kuntzleman[42] describes a walking program for cardiacs;[42] this source can provide helpful information for the nurse working with clients following myocardial infarction.

The only contraindications for beginning a postcardiac patient on an exercise regimen are the following:[43]

*Heart muscle damaged to extent of aneurysm or weakness in heart muscle wall*
*Acute heart failure*
*Myocarditis*
*Grossly irregular heart beats (multifocal ectopic arrhythmias)*
*Progressive or sudden onset of severe chest pain with exertion*
*Some types of congenital or valvular heart disease*
*Recent pulmonary embolism or thrombophlebitis*
*Complete heart block*

In summary, the importance of systematic exercise to the postcoronary client cannot be overemphasized. The client will reap both physical and psychologic benefits that are critical to full recovery. The exercise program for such a client must be carefully monitored by the physician and the nurse and cooperatively planned and modified as needed to meet individual needs.

### The Obese

The individual who is markedly overweight presents special needs that must be considered in structuring an exercise program. A stress electrocardiogram or step test is essential before beginning systematic exercise. Increased body weight results in greater stress on the heart, muscles, and joints than in a person of normal weight. Body size may also decrease mobility and flexibility. While description of a complete physical-activity program for the obese is beyond the scope of this book, a number of suggestions for modifying exercises for overweight individuals will be provided:

- Correct breathing should be stressed as critical to maximize ventilatory efficiency during exercise.
- Warm-up exercises should be selected that can be done in a standing position or in a chair, since obese individuals may have difficulty with floor exercises.
- Incremental steps in exercise program should be more gradual than for normal-weight individuals.
- Weight loss should be the primary goal of endurance exercise.
- Jogging is not recommended for the obese individual.
- Swimming is an excellent endurance exercise for the obese person since water provides buoyancy and weight support.

The obese individual can gain major health benefits from a well-planned exercise program. The intent of exercise must be clearly identified by the obese client in order to provide continuing motivation toward physical fitness over an extended period of time. Short-term and long-term goals should be realistic and reinforcement carefully planned to facilitate persistence in exercise and physical activity.

### Chronic Illness (Limited Mobility)

The chronically ill client with limited mobility or decreased tolerance for exercise should be encouraged to develop a physical activity program to meet his or her special needs. Clients with multiple sclerosis, Parkinson's disease, arthritis, amputation, paralysis, and chronic obstructive pulmonary disease all fit into this category. While the pathology may differ, the need for exercise in spite of physical limitations is characteristic of all clients with disabling health problems.

The nurse, in caring for clients with a physical disability, should promote the use of active exercise to the extent possible. Passive range of motion can supplement active exercise as needed. Active exercise of unaffected body parts maintains muscle tone, coordination, and flexibility, while passive range of motion facilitates joint mobility and prevents muscle atrophy. Guidelines for structuring exercise programs for the chronically ill include the following:

- Begin physical activity program gradually, since clients tire easily.
- Teach clients relaxation skills to reduce muscle tension or anxiety during exercise.
- Avoid excessive force against joint or muscle resistance during exercise.
- Provide feedback as needed to facilitate the correct sequence of movements.
- Maintain good posture and body alignment during exercise.
- Provide positive reinforcement to encourage persistence despite difficulties and slow pace of progress.

**TABLE 10-5  SUMMARY OF SUGGESTED PHYSICAL ACTIVITIES**

| Warm-Up | Stretching | Endurance | Cool-Down |
|---------|-----------|-----------|-----------|
| Walk briskly (1 min) | Back stretch | Walk-jog | Walking and deep breathing |
| Jog (45 sec) | Leg overs | Jog | Straight arm and leg stretch |
| Walk briskly (30 sec) | Hamstring stretcher | Walking | |
| Arm circles | Trunk rotator | Swimming* | Achilles stretcher |
| Jumping jacks | Cat's arch | Running* | Half knee bend |
| Lateral bend | Stretching exercises for feet and ankles | Bicycling* | Bent-knee half-curl |
| Head rotation | | Rope skipping* | |
| Side leg raises | | | |
| Single leg raise and knee hug | | | |
| Wall push-ups | | | |

*Not discussed in text

Maintaining optimum fitness in the chronically ill is an important part of illness prevention and health promotion. While detailed discussion of special exercise techniques is beyond the scope of this book, the reader is referred to additional sources for assistance.[44–48]

## SUMMARY

The purpose of this chapter has been to provide an overview of the conditioning process for physical fitness. The nurse as a key health professional will assume responsibility in many instances for assisting clients in structuring and implementing individual exercise programs. The skill with which the nurse is able to accomplish this will determine her or his professional and personal contributions to the client's optimum health and wellness.

In conclusion, Table 10-5 provides a summary of suggested warm-up, stretching, endurance, and cool-down exercises. This list can be further expanded by the individual nurse to include physical activities described by other authors.

## REFERENCES

1. Cantu, R.C. *Toward fitness: Guided exercise for those with health problems*. New York: Human Sciences Press, 1980, p. 12.
2. *Ibid.*, p. 14.
3. Fielding, J.E. Successes of prevention. *Milbank Memorial Fund Quarterly/Health and Society*. 1978, 56,274–302.
4. Paffenbarger, R.S., Wing, A.L., & Hyde, R.T. Physical activity as an index of heart attack risk in college alumni. Paper presented at the Annual Meeting of the American Heart Association, Miami Beach, Florida, November 19, 1977.
5. Greist, J.H., Klein, M.H., Eischens, R.R., & Faris, J.W. Running as a treatment for non-psychotic depression. *Behavioral Medicine*, 1978, 6,19–24.
6. Greist, J.H., Klein, M.H., Eischens, R.R., et al. Running as a treatment for depression. *Compr Psychiatry*, 1979, 1,41–54.
7. Morgan, W.P. Influence of acute physical activity on state anxiety. *NCPEAM Proceedings*, 1973, 113–121.
8. Sidney, K.H., & Shephard, R.J. Attitudes toward health and physical activity in the elderly. Effects of a training program. *Medicine and Science in Sports*, 1976, 8, 246–252.
9. Getchell, B. *Physical fitness: A way of life* (2nd ed.). New York: Wiley, 1979, pp. 10–13.
10. *Ibid.*, pp. 22–29.
11. Borgman, M.I. Exercise and health maintenance: A teaching program with competence based objectives. *Journal of Nursing Education*, January 1977, 16,6–10.
12. Cantu, R.C., *op. cit.*, pp. 154–155.
13. Isaacs, B., & Kobler, J. *What it takes to feel good: The Nickolaus technique*. New York: Viking Press, 1978, pp. 47–49.
14. Everly, G.S., Jr., & Girdano, D.A. *The stress mess solution*. Bowie, Md.: Brady, 1980, pp. 121–122.
15. Kirschner, M.J. *Yoga all your life*. New York: Schocken Books, 1977.

16. Cantu, *op. cit.*, p. 29.
17. Cooper, K.H. *The aerobics way.* New York: Evansand, 1977.
18. Getchell, *op. cit.*, p. 121.
19. Ellfeldt, L., & Lowman, C.L. *Exercises for the mature adult.* Springfield, Ill.: Thomas, 1973.
20. *Ibid.*, p. 108.
21. Simon, R.B. *Relax and stretch.* New York: Walker, 1973, p. 42.
22. Pipes, T.V., & Vodak, P.A. *The Pipes fitness test and prescription.* Los Angeles: Tarcher, 1978.
23. *Ibid.*, p. 85.
24. Kuntzleman, C.T. *The complete book of walking.* New York: Simon & Schuster, 1979, p. 138.
25. Borgman, *op. cit.*, p. 8.
26. Getchell, B., & Cleary, P. The caloric costs of rope skipping and running. *The Physician and Sports Medicine,* February 1980, *8,* 56–60.
27. Glasser, W. *Positive addiction.* New York: Harper & Row, 1976.
28. Geline, R.J. *The practical runner.* New York: Collier Books, 1978.
29. Bridge, R. *The runner's book.* New York: Scribner's, 1978.
30. Sheehan, G. *Dr. George Sheehan's medical advice for runners.* Mountain View, Calif.: World Publications, 1978.
31. Kuntzleman, *op. cit.*, p. 53.
32. DeVries, H.A. Electromyographic comparison of single doses of exercise and meprobamate as to the effects on muscular relaxation. *American Journal of Physical Medicine,* 1972, *51,* 130–141.
33. Fair, J., Rosenaur, J., & Thurston, E. Exercise management. *Nurse Practitioner,* 1979, *4,*13–18.
34. Kuntzleman, *op. cit.*, p. 161.
35. Anderson, J.L., & Cohen, M. *The West Point fitness and diet book.* New York: Rawson Associates, 1977, p. 171.
36. *Ibid.*, pp. 156, 162.
37. Eischens, R.R. Five easy steps for exercise regimen compliance: A new precise guide to running. *Behavioral Medicine,* June 1979, *2,* 14–17.
38. Getchell, *op. cit.*, p. 263.
39. Cantu, *op. cit.*, p. 78.
40. *Ibid.*, p. 80.
41. Cantu, *op. cit.*, pp. 134–151.
42. Kuntzleman, *op. cit.*, pp. 189–201.
43. Cantu, *op. cit.*, p. 138.
44. *Ibid.*
45. Nashelsky, G.M. *Redaptor guides for rehabilitation.* Hagerstown, Md.: Harper & Row, 1978.
46. Covalt, N.K. *Bed exercises for convalescent patients.* Springfield, Ill.: Thomas, 1968.
47. Stryker, R. *Rehabilitative aspects of acute and chronic nursing care* (2nd ed.). Philadelphia: Saunders, 1977.
48. Basmajian, J.V. *Therapeutic exercise* (3rd ed.). Baltimore: Williams & Wilkin, 1978.

# CHAPTER 11
# Nutrition and Weight Control

Adequate nutrition is a critical element in the nurturance of health. Not only is diet believed to play a major role in the prevention of disease but it also contributes to alertness and energy essential for full and productive living. Unfortunately, dietary inadequacies (malnutrition) in the guise of overnutrition or undernutrition plague 30 to 50 percent of Americans and are found at all socioeconomic levels. Affluent and poor alike often exhibit nutritional habits that are a direct threat to health and well-being.

The complexity of American life complicates the development and maintenance of health-promoting nutritional practices. It has been estimated that 30 percent of meals are eaten outside the home, and convenience foods constitute 60 percent of the American diet. Such foods are frequently high in fat, salt, and refined carbohydrates and low in fiber. By the fifth decade of life, one-third of the men and one-half of the women in the United States are more than 20 percent overweight.[1] This is not surprising, considering that the mean sugar consumption within the population is 125 pounds per person per year and that fats constitute 42 percent of dietary intake. The overconsumption of saturated fats, cholesterol, sugar, and salt has been linked to a number of chronic diseases that are the major causes of death and disability in the United States. Chronic diseases that fall into this category include cardiovascular disorders, hypertension, diabetes mellitus, cancer of the breast, and cancer of the gastrointestinal tract. Links with diet have been suggested for many other health problems.

Undernutrition is also a problem in many segments of the population despite excess caloric consumption among Americans. A dietary survey of low-income rural families in Iowa and North Carolina indicated that calcium intake is often inadequate, followed in frequency by deficiencies in vitamin A, vitamin C (ascorbic acid), and iron.[2] These deficiencies as well as inadequate nutritional habits that usually accompany them, are the precursors of many health problems in individuals of all ages.

Families often experience limited options in food choices as a result of cost or a confusing array of products for which nutrient content is unclear. The challenge of integrating healthful nutritional practices into individual and family lifestyle can be overwhelming.

275

Since the nurse is the health professional involved most often in extended contact with clients, he or she serves as a valuable resource to individuals, families, and communities in providing information and assistance in regard to nutrition and weight control. Dietary counseling should be an integral part of nursing practice in all settings. The professional nurse must be able to deal not only with therapeutic aspects of nutrition but also with nutrition as a critical element in healthy growth, illness prevention, and health promotion.

In Chapter 5 specific approaches to nutritional assessment were presented. Height and weight tables, growth standards for children, measurements of skinfold thicknesses, and use of a food diary to assess dietary patterns provide the nurse with valuable data for intervention. In this chapter, information on strategies for use with clients in promoting good nutrition and weight control will be presented.

## THE ROLE OF NUTRITION IN PREVENTION

The role of nutrition in prevention has been most vividly illustrated in relation to cardiovascular disease. The Framingham, Massachusetts, Heart Study conducted by the National Heart, Lung, and Blood Institute of more than 5,000 men and women between 30 and 62 years of age showed, particularly in males, a substantial increase in the incidence of coronary heart disease with serum cholesterol levels greater than 220 mg. Further studies indicated that 80 percent of heart disease victims were characterized by hyperlipoproteinemia, hypertension, and cigarette smoking.[3]

Hyperlipoproteinemia may be to some extent genetic or secondary to other diseases, such as diabetes, hypothyroidism, nephrosis, and obstructive liver disease, but is more frequently caused by environmental factors over which the individual has control, e.g., factors such as diet, alcohol intake, and sedentary lifestyle.[4] Both cholesterol and triglycerides (serum lipids) have been indicted in the health literature as contributing to the process of atherosclerosis, which leads to cardiovascular disease. Each results in a different type of lipoproteinemia.[5] While the body itself synthesizes cholesterol and triglycerides, dietary fat serves as an exogenous source of both. A 600-mg increase in cholesterol per 3000 calories can account for an 800-mg increase in serum cholesterol. For that reason, a decrease in total fat in the diet, particularly saturated fats and cholesterol, is recommended to prevent cardiovascular deterioration.

Modification of dietary habits recommended to decrease serum lipid levels and the associated threat of cardiovascular disease include the following:[6]

1. Decrease total fat intake to 30 percent of diet.
2. Decrease proportion of cholesterol and saturated fats (10 percent); increase proportion of polyunsaturated fats (20 percent) in diet (dietary cholesterol should not exceed 300 mg per day).
3. Reduce weight if obese.

**4.** Adjust carbohydrate intake to meet energy needs exactly (increase complex carbohydrates in proportion to highly refined sugars).
**5.** Decrease intake of alcohol.
**6.** Maintain but do not exceed adequate protein level.

A recent development in understanding the relationship between diet and cardiovascular disease has been the identification of five distinct types of lipoproteins: chylomicrons, very low-density lipoproteins, intermediate-density lipoproteins, low-density lipoproteins, and high-density lipoproteins. It appears that high-density lipoproteins predominate when triglyceride level is normal and actively retard the atherosclerotic process by transporting cholesterol out of tissue to the liver for breakdown. When triglycerides are elevated, low-density lipoproteins predominate, increasing the risk of cardiovascular disease by their transporting of cholesterol to tissues.[7] Total body weight and level of physical activity may also be related to the level of high-density proteins. Combining a diet low in saturated fats with participation in regular exercise appears to be a prudent approach to decreasing both serum cholesterol and triglyceride levels.[8]

While much controversy still surrounds the importance of dietary practices in the prevention of cardiovascular disorders, the preponderance of evidence supports both a direct and indirect relationship between diet and cardiovascular health. The professional nurse exercises good judgment in assisting clients to modify eating behaviors in order to decrease total fat intake, particularly the proportion of unsaturated fats in the diet.

The role, if any, of caffeine, a xanthine drug, in the etiology of cardiovascular disease has not been determined. While caffeine stimulates the sympathetic nervous system, increases cardiac and skeletal muscle contractility, increases excretory functions of the kidneys, increases respiration rate and depth, and stimulates the adrenal glands,[9] a definite link between coffee intake and cardiac disorders has not been identified. Preliminary studies briefly reviewed by Jean Mayer at a conference in Milwaukee on occupational health provide evidence that the combination of frequent smoking and high caffeine intake may synergistically increase the risk of cardiovascular disease.

Still another major chronic health problem in which diet is assumed to play a role is cancer. It has been estimated that diet is related to as much as 50 percent of the cancers in women and 33 percent of the cancers in men. Aspects of the diet that are suspect include intake of fats, vitamin deficiencies, surplus or deficiency of trace elements, degree of food processing, methods of food storage, techniques for food preparation, and food additives.[10] There is growing evidence that a high-fat diet contributes to the development of cancer of the colon, rectum, breast, and prostate gland.[11] While the mechanisms for explaining this apparent relationship have not been identified, it is possible that a high level of dietary fat and subsequent serum lipid elevation increases the activity of various carcinogens. It is interesting to note that a correlation of 0.64 between sugar consumption and incidence of breast cancer has also been reported.[12] Since many of these results have been obtained from animal studies or epidemiologic surveys of specific populations, the extent to which these findings can be generalized to the broader population has not been determined. Other studies have implicated the level of fiber, which is low in the American diet, as a possible precursor or risk factor for cancer of the colon and rectum. Research results on the impact of dietary fiber on health are less definitive than those on dietary fat.

The protective or preventive effects of vitamins and minerals have been addressed in cancer studies on animals. Some evidence exists that selenium (an antioxidant found in brewer's yeast, garlic, and liver), vitamin C, and vitamin E may provide protection against breast cancer. At present, these results are equivocal with much debate surrounding their validity.[13]

In light of current evidence on the link between diet and cancer, it appears that the prudent individual ought to decrease the amount of fat in the diet to 30 percent. That is the recommendation of the Senate Select Committee on Nutrition and Human Needs in the Dietary Goals for the United States. In addition, the intake of refined and processed sugars should be decreased, and the intake of complex carbohydrates and fiber increased.

At this point, the threat to health posed by chronic obesity will be mentioned; the subject will be discussed more fully under the section of this chapter on Weight Control. Studies have shown that the death rate among obese adults is 50 percent greater than that of normal-weight adults. Middle-aged males who are 30 percent overweight have four times as many myocardial infarctions as men of normal weight, and are seven times more likely to suffer a cerebrovascular accident.[14] Obesity is a health problem of epidemic proportions that the professional nurse will repeatedly encounter as she provides illness-prevention and health-promotion services to clients. Permanent modification of dietary behaviors must be the long-term goal for the client if excess weight is to be lost and the risk of obesity to health reduced.

## FACTORS INFLUENCING EATING BEHAVIOR

A wide variety of factors influence overt eating behavior. These factors can be classified as: biologic, psychologic, sociocultural, and environmental. The multicausal nature of eating behavior makes it highly complex and resistant to change. Eating behaviors are an integral part of individual and family lifestyle. Effective modification requires consideration of the factors that determine eating behavior and the use of appropriate change techniques. In order to select effective intervention strategies, the nurse must understand the determinants of eating behavior and their impact on nutritional status.

### Biologic Factors

Eating behaviors are determined biologically by nutrient requirements. Nutrients are the chemicals that are essential for proper body functioning. To date, approximately 50 macronutrients (e.g., fats, carbohydrates, and proteins) and micronutrients (e.g., vitamins and minerals) have been identified as essential for human growth and maintenance.[15] Nutrients have one or more of the following functions: (1) providing energy necessary for metabolic processes and movement, (2) providing structural components for bones and tissues, and (3) catalizing or regulating physiologic processes.

Nutrient needs of individuals vary according to metabolic rate, stage of growth, age, level of physical activity, excretory functions (menstruation, heavy perspiration), and reproductive functions (in women, i.e., pregnancy and lactation).

Metabolic rate is expressed as basal metabolism, that is, the number of kilocalories needed to maintain the body at rest. Basal metabolism rate declines sharply between 5 and 25 years of age and gradually thereafter. A rough guide for determining daily basal energy requirements for adults is to multiply ideal body weight by 10. For example, a woman weighing 120 pounds (recommended weight) would require 1200 calories to maintain body functions at complete rest. Obviously, activity increases the need for calories. Depending on the level of activity, caloric intake should be appropriately modified to maintain current weight or achieve desired weight.

During periods of rapid growth in childhood and adolescence, caloric and nutrient needs are increased. Throughout adulthood, nutrient needs remain relatively stable, but caloric needs gradually decline. The decrease in caloric needs generally reflects the lower basal metabolic rates of the elderly and decreases in activity because of physical limitations. Decreased energy requirements with aging may also reflect an increase in fat and a decrease in lean-tissue mass. Recommended caloric levels for individuals of different ages with moderate physical activity are presented in Table 11-1.

Energy requirements rather than nutrient needs appear to be the most salient biologic determinants of eating behavior. In general, individuals exhibit awareness and sensitivity to low energy levels. Fatigue, listlessness, and apathy can indicate a caloric intake that is inadequate to meet energy needs.

While overall nutrient requirements remain relatively stable throughout adult-

**TABLE 11-1   AVERAGE RECOMMENDED CALORIC INTAKE FOR MEN AND WOMEN OF DIFFERENT AGES: MODERATE ACTIVITY (in kilocalories)**

| Age | Men | | Women | |
|---|---|---|---|---|
| | MEAN | RANGE | MEAN | RANGE |
| 19–22 | 2900 | 2500–3000 | 2100 | 1700–2500 |
| 23–50 | 2700 | 2300–3100 | 2000 | 1600–2400 |
| 51–75 | 2400 | 2000–2800 | 1800 | 1400–2200 |
| over 75 | 2050 | 1650–2450 | 1600 | 1200–2000 |

hood, selected nutrients may have to be increased because of physiologic changes, e.g., diminished gastric secretions and decreased gastric motility that occur with aging. For example, decreased gastric secretions can result in limited absorption of iron, calcium, and vitamin $B_{12}$. Decreased gastric motility augments the need for foods high in fiber (fresh fruits, raw vegetables, whole grain breads, and cereals) and increases the importance of water consumption to promote regularity in bowel evacuation.

It should be noted that the hypothalamus is an important biologic determinant of eating behavior. The lateral nucleus of the hypothalamus is stimulated by hunger, initiating food-seeking behavior, while the ventromedial hypothalamus signals satiety and results in the urge to cease food consumption.[16] One theory of obesity is based on the malfunctioning of the hypothalamus in the biologic regulation of food intake.

### Psychologic Factors

Major psychologic factors that affect eating behavior include emotions, habits, self-esteem, perceptions of control, and perceived benefits of good dietary practices. People frequently engage in eating behavior because of the emotions of enjoyment, peace, and tranquility aroused. On the other hand, negative emotions, such as anger, frustration, and insecurity, can lead to disturbances in eating behavior (overeating or anorexia) that are indicative of a personal search for comfort, security, and nurturance through food intake.

Habits constitute another important determinant of eating behavior. A habit can be defined as a behavior that occurs often and is performed automatically or with little conscious awareness.[17] Habits are performed so frequently that many cues within the environment serve as signals for the behavior. They often result in a psychologic addiction to certain behaviors because they become a pervasive part of lifestyle. Such behaviors are known as consummatory because the response itself (eating) provides the reinforcement. People can also become psychologically addicted to the consequences of habitual behaviors such as the "energy spurt" experienced after the ingestion of highly refined sugars at midmorning (doughnuts or sweet rolls), late afternoon, or evening (snack foods). Habits can result in poor dietary practices because little or no conscious thought is given to eating behavior. Habits also depend on the availability of food stuffs that can be readily consumed without preparation. Fast foods that are high in fats and refined carbohydrates and low in protein, minerals, and vitamins often meet this requirement.

Level of self-esteem and nutrition knowledge have also been shown to be significantly correlated with eating behavior. Schafer[18] selected 116 married women under 36 years of age to test in relation to self-concept and diet quality. Self-concept was measured by ten adjective pairs selected from Gough and Heilbrim's adjective checklist, while diet quality was determined by the frequency of consumption and serving sizes for 67 different food items. Food items were converted to percentage of recommended daily allowances for six nutrients: protein, calcium, iron, vitamin A, thiamin, and ascorbic acid. Self-concept correlated 0.20 ($p < 0.01$) with diet quality, which is a low correlation but a statistically significant one. Consumption of "junk food" or empty calories was negatively correlated with self-concept ($-0.16$, $p < 0.05$). Previous involvement in nutritional courses correlated at 0.41 with self-concept.

Perceived control of nutritional status and belief in the benefits of good nutrition have also been shown to increase the quality of dietary behavior. In the Stanford three community study[19] discussed in detail in Chapter 7, a mass-media campaign informed citizens of two communities about the impact of a diet low in cholesterol and saturated fats on risk for cardiovascular disease. Results revealed that awareness of actions to be taken and the benefits of a low-fat diet within the target communities decreased the cholesterol and fat consumption among both men and women 20 to 40 percent.

### Sociocultural Factors

Ethnic and cultural backgrounds serve as important influences on eating behavior. Ethnic foods are a source of pride and identity for many groups. Ethnic foods often have deep emotional meanings for individuals because of their association with the "mother country" or because of fond childhood memories of holidays or special occasions on which particular foods were served. Recognition of and respect for individual food preferences is important for professional nurses in dealing with adults from a wide variety of cultural backgrounds. The nurse should become acquainted with food behaviors of different sociocultural groups in order to evaluate their beneficial, neutral, or harmful effects on health.[20]

Boykin[21] has made a number of helpful suggestions in dealing constructively with the food preferences of various ethnic and cultural groups:

* Food habits and preferences should be recognized.
* Consumption frequency for various ethnic foods should be ascertained.
* Positive attributes of ethnic foods should be recognized and reinforced.
* Nutrition information relevant to ethnic/cultural foods should be provided to clients.
* The client should be an active member of the dietary-planning team.
* Changes recommended in food preparation and consumption should be tailored as much as possible to ethnic/cultural patterns. Ethnic foods can serve as important sources of nutrients and as the basis for a well-balanced and nutritious diet. Every effort should be made by the nurse to incorporate ethnic/cultural food preferences in diet planning. Only when foods are clearly hazardous to health should clients be encouraged to make major changes in ethnic dietary habits.

### Environmental Factors

The major environmental factors influencing eating patterns appear to be accessibility, convenience, and cost. These factors can present barriers to positive nutritional practices during the action phase of health behavior. Seasonal variation in availability of foods such as raw vegetables and fresh fruits determines both accessibility and costs. The types of fruits and vegetables used by clients need to follow seasonal patterns in order to maximize nutrient quality and minimize cost. Use of frozen fruits and vegetables rather than canned during off-season is recommended to decrease the intake of sugar and salt. Home-frozen products can also be an important source of nutrients at reasonable cost.

Convenience foods constitute a significant portion of dietary intake in the American population. Unfortunately, the nutrient quality of many fast foods is questionable. Vending machines often have only foods high in fats and starch. If access to more nutritious foods is inconvenient, individuals often select the easiest option. Ease of preparation plays an important role in food selection. Quick and effortless preparation techniques appeal to many families because of busy work schedules. In addition, attractiveness of prepared foods is an important consideration. Assisting the client in selecting nutritious foods that are quickly prepared and esthetically appealing increases the likelihood of sustained changes in eating behavior.

With inflationary trends in the economy, cost of food is an important consideration for the majority of families. Sources of complex carbohydrates (fruits, vegetables, and grains) may exceed the cost of highly refined sugar products. Proteins also vary greatly in per unit cost. An important approach to optimizing nutritional quality of the diet at minimum cost is to calculate the per unit cost of given nutrients in food products. An example of a method for such calculations that is relatively easy for the client to use is presented in the next section of this chapter.

## HEALTH PROMOTION THROUGH POSITIVE NUTRITION PRACTICES

Many individuals engage in eating because of the pleasurable sensations experienced and the esthetic enjoyment of well-prepared and attractive foods. Interest in foods rather than concern about nutrients and health may largely determine patterns of food consumption. Visual appearance of foods as well as internal sensations of hunger provide powerful cues that initiate eating behavior. The mass media influence the types and variety of foods consumed through the presentation of information on various food products.

Meal planning is an important activity that facilitates preparation of well-balanced meals. In assisting clients with planning, the nurse must take into consideration food preferences, preparation time, purchasing practices, cost, and daily meal patterns (three or more meals per day). Variation in color, texture, and temperature are also important considerations to make meals attractive and appealing. Since meal planning and food preparation take place in the home, this provides an excellent environment for nutrition education. The nurse in using the home as a learning center capitalizes on environmental cues relevant to positive nutritional practices.[22]

### Guide to Good Eating

A simple guide to healthful eating for children, teenagers, and adults has been provided in Table 11-2. The milk group is a rich source of calcium, phosphorous,

## TABLE 11-2 GUIDE TO GOOD EATING: A RECOMMENDED DAILY PATTERN*

| Food Group | Recommended Number of Servings† | | | | |
| | CHILD | TEENAGER | ADULT | PREGNANT WOMAN | LACTATING WOMAN |
| --- | --- | --- | --- | --- | --- |
| Milk | 3 | 4 | 2 | 4 | 4 |

1 cup milk or yogurt OR calcium equivalent:

  1½ slices (1½ oz) cheddar cheese‡
  1 cup pudding
  1¾ cups ice cream
  2 cups cottage cheese‡

| | | | | | |
| --- | --- | --- | --- | --- | --- |
| Meat | 2 | 2 | 2 | 3 | 2 |

2 oz cooked, lean meat, fish, or poultry OR protein equivalent:

  2 eggs
  2 slices (2 oz) cheddar cheese‡
  1 cup dried beans, peas
  4 tbs peanut butter

| | | | | | |
| --- | --- | --- | --- | --- | --- |
| Fruit–Vegetable | 4 | 4 | 4 | 4 | 4 |

  ½ cup cooked or juice
  1 cup raw
  Portion commonly served, such as a medium-size apple or banana

| | | | | | |
| --- | --- | --- | --- | --- | --- |
| Grain | 4 | 4 | 4 | 4 | 4 |

Whole grain, fortified, enriched:

  1 slice bread
  1 cup ready-to-eat cereal
  ½ cup cooked cereal, pasta, or grits

*The recommended daily pattern provides the foundation for a nutritious, healthful diet. Amounts should be further modified by individual caloric needs.
†The recommended servings from the four food groups for adults supply about 1200 calories. The chart gives recommendations for the number and size of servings for several categories of people.
‡Count cheese as serving of milk or meat, not as belonging to both simultaneously.

protein, riboflavin, vitamin A, vitamin $B_{12}$, and vitamin D (if fortified). The meat group provides protein, B-complex vitamins, and minerals. Vegetable equivalents for meat, such as beans, dried peas, lentils, and nuts, do not contain significant amounts of vitamin $B_{12}$. The fruit and vegetable group provides vitamins A, C, E, K, and B-complex (except $B_{12}$), as well as minerals and fiber. Grains contain protein, B-complex vitamins, minerals, and fiber.[23] Appendix A, developed from a variety of information sources, presents an overview of the biologic importance, sources, deficiency symptoms, and toxicity levels of a wide variety of nutrients. Table 11-3 presents the National Research Council Recommended Daily Dietary Allowances as revised in 1979 for selected nutrients. The use of a variety of foods from each group and an adequate intake of water (the most basic human nutrient) assist in maintaining a desired level of nutrient quality within the diet.[24]

***Nutrient and Caloric Density.*** Important considerations in food selection are nutrient density and caloric density. Nutrient density refers to the content of specific nutrients in given amounts of food in relation to the kilocalories provided by that same amount.

$$\text{Nutrient density} = \frac{\text{Percent of RDA of nutrient provided by food}}{\text{Percent of mean energy requirements provided by food}}$$

Caloric density can be defined as the number of kilocalories provided per unit of food.[25] Fats, oils, and alcohol have the highest caloric density of all food substances, yet they are low in essential nutrients. The caloric density of fats is 9 kcal per gram and of alcohol 7 kcal per gram. Vegetables, fruits, milk products, and meat vary greatly in caloric density, while grain products are relatively similar for equivalent weights. Nutritive sweeteners, such as sugar, honey, corn syrup, fructose, and sorbitol, have comparable caloric densities, approximately 20 kcal per teaspoon. For this reason, fruit as a natural sweetener should be used as frequently as possible to decrease caloric intake and intake of highly refined sugar.

The nutrient and caloric densities of foods can be calculated from food-value tables, but the bioavailability of nutrients depends on the metabolic characteristics of the client, existing illnesses that may affect metabolic processes, the form of the nutrient present in food, and the presence or absence of other interacting nutrients. For example, "heme" iron available in meats is more bioavailable than is iron from vegetables. As another example, the presence of vitamin C increases the absorption of iron and the presence of vitamin D increases the absorption of calcium. The concept of bioavailability may be difficult for the client to grasp, but the nurse should be aware of these parameters in order to teach effective meal planning.

The seven nutrients, often referred to as index nutrients, that serve as the best overall indicators of diet and nutrient adequacy are calcium, iron, magnesium, vitamin A, vitamin $B_6$, pantothenic acid, and folacin. A rough estimate of the extent to which these nutrients are included in the diet can be obtained for any individual by nutritional analysis using manual or computerized tables of food composition.

***Loss of Nutrients in Food Preparation.*** Nutrients available to the client in foodstuffs can be lost through inadequate methods of preparation. Nutrients may be lost in the following ways:[26]

*Trimming (e.g., peeling potatoes, fruits, and vegetables)*
*Solution loss (particularly water-soluble vitamin C, B complex, and minerals)*

*Heat and exposure to air (e.g., in the case of carotene, vitamin C, thiamin, and folacin)*

Loss of nutrients can be avoided by decreasing the amount of water in which foods are cooked, decreasing the length of time foods are in water (i.e., by using a pressure cooker), avoiding the peeling or soaking of foods before cooking, refraining from adding salt to cooking water (draws out water-soluble nutrients), and decreasing food-cooking surface exposed to water by cutting food into large pieces.

*Maintaining Optimum Energy Balance.* For every 3500 excess kilocalories consumed that are not utilized for energy, one pound of fat is formed. This means that 100 unburned calories each day for 35 days will result in 1 pound of fat and in a 10-pound weight gain per year (350 days).[27] The same level of deficit in calories (100 per day for 35 days) can result in a 1-pound loss that, if continued over a year, would result in the loss of 10 pounds. The factors that determine energy balance include basal metabolism, level of physical activity, and food intake. Energy balance is maintained by burning all calories ingested. If excess calories are being consumed and undesirable weight gain is occurring, this can only be remedied by decreasing food intake or increasing exercise.

Some individuals express concern that if they exercise more, their appetite will increase. This has been found not to be true. Appetite is actually decreased following exercise because of lowered blood supply to the gastrointestinal tract. Few avid physical fitness enthusiasts wish to eat before exercising, since this makes physical activity more difficult and less comfortable. In addition, exercise may decrease stress and tension; as a result, there will be less frequent eating for nonnutritive purposes.[28]

## IMPORTANT NUTRIENTS

### Protein

The body's requirement for protein can be easily met if foods are properly combined to provide usable protein. Some foods, such as milk, milk products, eggs, and meat of all types, contain protein of high biologic value. Such proteins, sometimes called complete proteins, support growth. Other proteins, if used as the sole source of protein, can support life but not growth. They are referred to as partially complete or incomplete proteins.

Proteins are composed of amino acids. There are 22 amino acids, eight to nine of which are essential; that is, they must be ingested since they cannot be biologically synthesized. The essential amino acids are tryptophan, leucine, lycine, methionine, phenylalanine, isoleucine, valine, theonine, and histidine (for children). The bioavailability of protein depends on proper balance of essential amino acids. Amino acids can only be properly used when all of them are available at the same time.[29]

Meat, fish, poultry, and dairy products (complete proteins) contain good proportions of all essential amino acids, while vegetables and fruits (incomplete

## TABLE 11-3 RECOMMENDED DAILY DIETARY ALLOWANCES,* DESIGNED FOR THE MAINTENANCE OF GOOD NUTRITION OF PRACTICALLY ALL HEALTHY PEOPLE IN THE UNITED STATES, REVISED 1979

| | Age (years) | Weight (kg) | Weight (lb) | Height (cm) | Height (in.) | Protein (gm) | Water-Soluble Vitamins Vitamin C (mg) | Thiamin (mg) | Riboflavin (mg) | Niacin (mg N.E.)† | Vitamin $B_6$ (mg) | Folacin‡ (µg) | Vitamin $B_{12}$ (µg) |
|---|---|---|---|---|---|---|---|---|---|---|---|---|---|
| Infants | 0.0–0.5 | 6 | 13 | 60 | 24 | kg × 2.2 | 35 | 0.3 | 0.4 | 6 | 0.3 | 30 | 0.5§ |
| | 0.5–1.0 | 9 | 20 | 71 | 28 | kg × 2.0 | 35 | 0.5 | 0.6 | 8 | 0.6 | 45 | 1.5 |
| Children | 1–3 | 13 | 29 | 90 | 35 | 23 | 45 | 0.7 | 0.8 | 9 | 0.9 | 100 | 2.0 |
| | 4–6 | 20 | 44 | 112 | 44 | 30 | 45 | 0.9 | 1.0 | 11 | 1.3 | 200 | 2.5 |
| | 7–10 | 28 | 62 | 132 | 52 | 34 | 45 | 1.2 | 1.4 | 16 | 1.6 | 300 | 3.0 |
| Males | 11–14 | 45 | 99 | 157 | 62 | 45 | 50 | 1.4 | 1.6 | 18 | 1.8 | 400 | 3.0 |
| | 15–18 | 66 | 145 | 176 | 69 | 56 | 60 | 1.4 | 1.7 | 18 | 2.0 | 400 | 3.0 |
| | 19–22 | 70 | 154 | 177 | 70 | 56 | 60 | 1.5 | 1.7 | 19 | 2.2 | 400 | 3.0 |
| | 23–50 | 70 | 154 | 178 | 70 | 56 | 60 | 1.4 | 1.6 | 18 | 2.2 | 400 | 3.0 |
| | 51+ | 70 | 154 | 178 | 70 | 56 | 60 | 1.2 | 1.4 | 16 | 2.2 | 400 | 3.0 |
| Females | 11–14 | 46 | 101 | 157 | 62 | 46 | 50 | 1.1 | 1.3 | 15 | 1.8 | 400 | 3.0 |
| | 15–18 | 55 | 120 | 163 | 64 | 46 | 60 | 1.1 | 1.3 | 14 | 2.0 | 400 | 3.0 |
| | 19–22 | 55 | 120 | 163 | 64 | 44 | 60 | 1.1 | 1.3 | 14 | 2.0 | 400 | 3.0 |
| | 23–50 | 55 | 120 | 163 | 64 | 44 | 60 | 1.0 | 1.2 | 13 | 2.0 | 400 | 3.0 |
| | 51+ | 55 | 120 | 163 | 64 | 44 | 60 | 1.0 | 1.2 | 13 | 2.0 | 400 | 3.0 |
| Pregnant | | | | | | +30 | +20 | +0.4 | +0.3 | +2 | +0.6 | +400 | +1.0 |
| Lactating | | | | | | +20 | +40 | +0.5 | +0.5 | +5 | +0.5 | +100 | +1.0 |

|  | Age (years) | Weight (kg) | Weight (lb) | Height (cm) | Height (in.) | Protein (gm) | Fat-Soluble Vitamins Vitamin A (µg R.E.)|| | Vitamin D (µg)# | Vitamin E (mgα T.E.)** | Minerals Calcium (mg) | Phosphorus (mg) | Magnesium (mg) | Iron (mg) | Zinc (mg) | Iodine (µg) |
|---|---|---|---|---|---|---|---|---|---|---|---|---|---|---|---|
| Infants | 0.0–0.5 | 6 | 13 | 60 | 24 | kg × 2.2 | 420 | 10 | 3 | 360 | 240 | 50 | 10 | 3 | 40 |
|  | 0.5–1.0 | 9 | 20 | 71 | 28 | kg × 2.0 | 400 | 10 | 4 | 540 | 360 | 70 | 15 | 5 | 50 |
| Children | 1–3 | 13 | 29 | 90 | 35 | 23 | 400 | 10 | 5 | 800 | 800 | 150 | 15 | 10 | 70 |
|  | 4–6 | 20 | 44 | 112 | 44 | 30 | 500 | 10 | 6 | 800 | 800 | 200 | 10 | 10 | 90 |
|  | 7–10 | 28 | 62 | 132 | 52 | 34 | 700 | 10 | 7 | 800 | 800 | 250 | 10 | 10 | 120 |
| Males | 11–14 | 45 | 99 | 157 | 62 | 45 | 1000 | 10 | 8 | 1200 | 1200 | 350 | 18 | 15 | 150 |
|  | 15–18 | 66 | 145 | 176 | 69 | 56 | 1000 | 10 | 10 | 1200 | 1200 | 400 | 18 | 15 | 150 |
|  | 19–22 | 70 | 154 | 177 | 70 | 56 | 1000 | 7.5 | 10 | 800 | 800 | 350 | 10 | 15 | 150 |
|  | 23–50 | 70 | 154 | 178 | 70 | 56 | 1000 | 5 | 10 | 800 | 800 | 350 | 10 | 15 | 150 |
|  | 51+ | 70 | 154 | 178 | 70 | 56 | 1000 | 5 | 10 | 800 | 800 | 350 | 10 | 15 | 150 |
| Females | 11–14 | 46 | 101 | 157 | 62 | 46 | 800 | 10 | 8 | 1200 | 1200 | 300 | 18 | 15 | 150 |
|  | 15–18 | 55 | 120 | 163 | 64 | 46 | 800 | 10 | 8 | 1200 | 1200 | 300 | 18 | 15 | 150 |
|  | 19–22 | 55 | 120 | 163 | 64 | 44 | 800 | 7.5 | 8 | 800 | 800 | 300 | 18 | 15 | 150 |
|  | 23–50 | 55 | 120 | 163 | 64 | 44 | 800 | 5 | 8 | 800 | 800 | 300 | 18 | 15 | 150 |
|  | 51+ | 55 | 120 | 163 | 64 | 44 | 800 | 5 | 8 | 800 | 800 | 300 | 10 | 15 | 150 |
| Pregnant |  |  |  |  |  | +30 | +200 | +5 | +2 | +400 | +400 | +150 | †† | +5 | +25 |
| Lactating |  |  |  |  |  | +20 | +400 | +5 | +3 | +400 | +400 | +150 | †† | +10 | +50 |

*The allowances are intended to provide for individual variations among most normal persons as they live in the United States under usual environmental stresses. Diets should be based on a variety of common foods in order to provide other nutrients for which human requirements have been less well defined.
†1 NE (niacin equivalent) is equal to 1 mg of niacin or 60 mg of dietary tryptophan.
‡The folacin allowances refer to dietary sources as determined by *Lactobacillus casei* assay after treatment with enzymes ("conjugases") to take polyglutamyl forms of the vitamin available to the test organism.
§The RDA for vitamin B$_{12}$ in infants is based on average concentration of the vitamin in human milk. The allowances after weaning are based on energy intake (as recommended by the American Academy of Pediatrics) and consideration of other factors, such as intestinal absorption.
||Retinol equivalents. 1 retinol equivalent = 1 µg retinol or 6 µgβ carotene.
#As cholecalciferol. 10 µg cholecalciferol = 400 I.U. vitamin D.
**α tocopherol equivalents. 1 mg d α – tocopherol = 1 α T.E.
††The increased requirement during pregnancy cannot be met by the iron content of habitual American diets nor by the existing iron stores of many women; therefore the use of 30 to 60 mg of supplemental iron is recommended. Iron needs during lactation are not substantially different from those of nonpregnant women, but continued supplementation of the mother for 2 to 3 months after parturition is advisable in order to replenish stores depleted by pregnancy.
From Food and Nutrition Board, National Academy of Sciences, National Research Council. *Recommended dietary allowances, revised 1979.* Washington, D.C.: Government Printing Office.

proteins) may be low or missing some amino acids, thus limiting protein use. The amino acid present in the smallest amount (LAA) limits the bioavailability of others. For example, if a food contains 100 percent of the daily lycine requirement but only 20 percent of the methionine requirement, only 20 percent of the protein in that food is used as protein; the rest is used for fuel rather than for replenishing or building tissues. The following illustration of bioavailability vividly illustrates this point:[30]

|  | **Percent of Daily Protein Requirement (160-lb man)** |
|---|---|
| 2 poached eggs | 54% LAA |
| 2 pieces dry whole wheat toast | 10% LAA |
| Orange juice | 0% LAA |
| Total % of daily requirement | 64% |

Following the breakfast described, only 36 percent of the daily requirement of protein remains to be ingested. Thus, protein needs are easily met when incomplete proteins (whole-grain breads) are complemented by complete proteins (eggs) in the diet.

If incomplete proteins are the primary source of amino acids, as in a vegetarian diet, complementarity of proteins is particularly important. *Complementing proteins* is the term used for combining incomplete proteins with opposite amino acid strengths and weaknesses. For example, peanut butter or chili beans (high in lysine but low in methionine) can be served with whole wheat bread or corn bread (low in lysine but high in methionine). Balancing the amino acid strengths and weaknesses of foods can result in good biologic availability of proteins.

The cost of protein foods can also pose a problem for clients. The cost of adequate nutrition can be decreased by serving small portions of fish, poultry, or lower-grade, less tender cuts of meat that are cooked slowly to tenderize and enhance flavor. Milk, eggs, and vegetable sources of protein may be used as substitutes for meat products, but consumption of some red meat is desirable to obtain vitamin $B_{12}$.

As a cost comparison example, 4 ounces of lean ground beef supplies approximately 20 grams of protein, while 3.5 hot dogs must be eaten for the same amount of protein. Williams and Justice[31] have developed a guide for calculating protein costs (Figure 11-1). Foods that are good sources of protein are listed along with the amount that contains 14 grams, or one-fourth to one-third of RDA. The number of grams of protein in a one-pound edible portion of food has been taken from tables of food composition and divided by 14, giving a factor that, when multiplied by price per pound of the target food, gives the cost of 14 grams of protein. Remember that 14 grams constitute approximately 17 to 25 percent of the RDA for children between 1 and 10 years of age; 32 percent of the RDA for women; and 25 percent of the RDA for men. By use of the multiplication factors with current retail price of foods, protein costs can be calculated.

| Item | Serving Size to Provide 14 gm Protein | Multiplication Factor | Current Retail Price per Pound | Cost of 14/gm Protein |
|---|---|---|---|---|
| Dry beans | 1 cup cooked | 0.128 | × _____ | = _____ |
| Peanut butter | 3½ tbs | 0.123 | × _____ | = _____ |
| Eggs | 2 eggs | 0.269 | × _____ | = _____ |
| Bologna | 4–5 slices (if 18 slices/lb) | 0.255 | × _____ | = _____ |
| Beef liver | (6–7 servings/ lb) | 0.155 | × _____ | = _____ |
| Milk | 1¾ cup | 0.881 | × _____ | = _____ |
| Dry milk | 9 tbs dry | 0.086 | × _____ | = _____ |
| Cottage cheese | (4–5 servings/ lb) | 0.227 | × _____ | = _____ |
| Hamburger | (5–6 servings/ lb) | 0.172 | × _____ | = _____ |
| Ocean perch, fillet, frozen | (6 servings/lb) | 0.160 | × _____ | = _____ |
| Tuna fish | (3 servings to a 6–oz can) | 0.128 | × _____ | = _____ |
| American pro- cessed cheese | 2½ slices (if 16–18 slices/ lb) | 0.133 | × _____ | = _____ |
| Chicken, whole | (4 servings/lb) | 0.244 | × _____ | = _____ |
| Ham, whole | (4–5 servings/ lb) | 0.228 | × _____ | = _____ |
| Pork sausage links | 6 links (if 16 links/lb) | 0.329 | × _____ | = _____ |
| Frankfurters | About 2½ (if 10/lb) | 0.247 | × _____ | = _____ |

**FIGURE 11-1.** Guide for calculating protein costs. To figure the cost per pound for large eggs, multiply ⅔ times the price per dozen; for milk, divide the cost per gallon by 8.6; for dry milk, calculate the cost of 5 quarts of reconstituted milk; and for tuna, multiply 2⅔ times the cost of a 6-ounce can (continued on next page). (*Reprinted with permission from Williams, F. L., & Justice, C.L. A ready reckoner of protein costs. Journal of Home Economics, 1975, 67, pp. 20–21. With permission.*)

| Item | Serving Size to Provide 14 gm Protein | Multiplication Factor | Current Retail Price per Pound | Cost of 14/gm Protein |
|---|---|---|---|---|
| Pork chops, with bone | (4 servings/lb) | 0.239 | × _____ | = _____ |
| Bacon, sliced | 5½ slices (if 20 slices/lb) | 0.403 | × _____ | = _____ |
| Sirloin steak, choice grade | (4⅓ servings/ lb) | 0.229 | × _____ | = _____ |
| Rib roast of beef | (4–5 servings/ lb) | 0.227 | × _____ | = _____ |
| Round pot roast | (6–7 servings/ lb) | 0.158 | × _____ | = _____ |

**FIGURE 11-1**   (continued).

**Fats**

Fats are essential for the absorption of fat soluble vitamins and serve as an energy source. In the average American diet, fats compose roughly 42 percent of total caloric intake. Fats are needed in limited amounts; a total of 30 percent fat in the diet is recommended, with 10 percent being saturated fats and 20 percent unsaturated fats. Intake of meats high in saturated fats, such as beef and pork, can be avoided if fish, poultry, or veal are used frequently. In addition, low-fat or skim milk and low-fat dairy products can be substituted for those higher in fat content. Consumption of butter, eggs, shell fish, and other high-cholesterol sources should be limited. Animal fats are generally saturated, while vegetable sources of fat are unsaturated. Cholesterol consumption should not exceed 300 mg per day.

Abraham et al.[32] have shown that changes occur in total serum cholesterol from youth to old age. Median level of 18- to 24-year old males and females is approximately 180 to 190 mg per 100 ml. In men, levels rise sharply from 25 to 44 years of age and stabilize at 230 to 235 mg per 100 ml from 45 to 74 years. In women, the rise is steepest after 45 years of age, reaching a median of approximately 250 mg per 100 ml by 65 to 75 years of age. Upon autopsy following accidental death, studies have shown that in individuals with a cholesterol level of 180 mg per 100 ml or below, little atherosclerosis is present, while in individuals with a serum cholesterol above 220 mg per 100 ml, definite atherosclerotic changes have occurred.

The American Heart Association has made the following suggestions for controlling cholesterol and total fat intake:[33]

*To control your intake of cholesterol-rich foods:*
— *Eat no more than three egg yolks a week, including eggs used in cooking. Commercial egg substitutes or egg whites may also be used.*
— *Limit your use of shellfish and organ meats.*

*To control the amount and type of fat you eat:*
— *Eat 6 to 8 ounces of lean meat, fish or poultry daily. (Fish, poultry and veal are low in saturated fat, so should be eaten more frequently than beef, lamb or pork.)*
— *Choose lean cuts of meat, trim visible fat, and discard the fat that cooks out of the meat.*
— *Avoid deep fat frying; use cooking methods that help to remove fat—baking, boiling, broiling, roasting, stewing.*
— *Restrict your use of "luncheon" and "variety" meats like sausages and salami.*
— *Instead of butter and other cooking fats that are solid or completely hydrogenated, use liquid vegetable oils and margarines that are rich in polyunsaturated fats.*
— *Instead of whole milk and cheeses made from whole milk and cream, use skimmed or low fat milk and cheeses.*

**Carbohydrates**
The main function of carbohydrates is as an energy source for metabolic processes and activity. While 46 percent of the current American diet consists of carbohydrates, the Dietary Goals of the United States recommend an increase to 58 percent, with changes made in the types of carbohydrates consumed. In the average American diet, 18 percent of the carbohydrate intake consists of refined and processed sugars having high caloric density but low nutritional value. The Senate Select Subcommittee on Nutrition and Human Needs has suggested that this be reduced to 10 percent and that complex carbohydrates and naturally occurring sugars be increased to 48 percent of caloric intake. Fruits, vegetables, and whole-grain cereals and breads are sources of complex carbohydrates that are much richer in vitamins and minerals than are foods containing highly processed sugars. Suggestions for changing the nature of carbohydrate intake include the following:

• Carbonated beverages should be replaced with fruit juices or ice water.
• Fruit should be substituted for high-caloric desserts.
• Dried and fresh fruits used as natural sweeteners.
• Snacks should consist of fruit, raw vegetables, whole-grain breads or cereals, cheese (low-fat skim), milk (low-fat or skim), fruit juices, or nuts (unsalted).

### Vitamins

Vitamins and minerals serve many functions within the human body, as is indicated in Appendix A. Since vitamin A is stored in the liver, a good source of this vitamin each day or every other day is sufficient. Vitamin D, like vitamin A, is stored in the body, so large supplemental doses should be avoided. Vitamin C and the B-complex vitamins are not stored; therefore, several sources of these important vitamins should be consumed daily. Insofar as bioavailability is concerned, there is no apparent difference between natural and synthetic vitamins. However, if an adequate diet is maintained, supplements should not be necessary except in clinically apparent deficiencies.

### Sodium

Numerous minerals are critical to proper functioning of the body; information on many of them will be summarized in Appendix A. Sodium is the only mineral discussed in this chapter in more detail. The level of sodium intake has been related to systolic and diastolic blood pressures, even though the cause of hypertension is unknown. Therefore, in a prudent diet, even in the absence of hypertension, moderate salt restriction is recommended. Guidelines for restricting salt include:

- Do not add salt to foods at the table.
- Use herbs, spices, and lemon in place of salt or monosodium glutamate.
- Do not use baking soda as an antacid.
- Use fresh or frozen vegetables as opposed to canned vegetables, which may be high in salt.
- Avoid foods prepared in brine, such as ham, bacon, pickles, corned beef, and sauerkraut.
- Restrict use of carbonated low-calorie beverages, which often contain sodium saccharin.
- Do not add salt during cooking.
- Avoid snack foods with visible salt, such as pretzels, potato chips, and cheese curls.

Salt substitutes can be used to enhance the flavor of food if, after allowing a period of adjustment to low-sodium foods, the client finds such foods unpalatable.

### Fiber

Fiber is not a nutrient but plays an important role in the diet. Fiber is important to the efficient functioning of the gastrointestinal tract. A high-fiber diet has been suggested by some studies as being important in the prevention of colon and rectal cancer because it facilitates the movement of waste products out of the body before toxic products have a chance to accumulate. The difference in fiber between whole grains and processed grains can be seen in Figure 11-2. When grain is refined, little more than the endosperm is left. This refined product is primarily

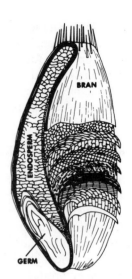

*Whole grain.* May be eaten as is (e.g., brown rice) or may be flaked into whole-grain cereal (e.g., oatmeal) or ground into whole-grain cereal or flour.

*Endosperm.* (refined white grains contain little else.) Mainly starch and protein.

*Germ.* High in vitamin E, many B vitamins, minerals, and protein; a source of polyunsaturated fat.

*Bran.* High in fiber, many B vitamins, and minerals.

**FIGURE 11-2.** Nutrient content of whole and refined grains. *(Reprinted with permission from Suitor, C. W., & Hunter, M. F. Nutrition: Principles and application in health promotion. Philadelphia: Lippincott, 1980, p. 15. With permission.)*

starch and protein and lacks many of the vitamins and minerals found in whole grains. Both because of their fiber and nutrient content, whole grains are an important part of a nutritious diet.

## FOOD ADDITIVES

In modern society, food additives are necessary to retard spoilage and prevent deterioration of quality. However, additives are also used for other purposes, such as to improve nutritional value, to enhance consumer acceptability, and to facilitate preparation. Currently, food processors can add more than 10,000 chemicals to food products. Types of additives include preservatives, acids, alkalies, buffers, neutralizers, moisture-content controls, coloring agents, flavorings, physiologic-activity controls, bleaching and maturing agents/bread improvers, processing aids, and nutrition supplements.[34]

By law, labels of many products must list the manufacturer, packer, and distributor, and the amount of each ingredient, and they must present the ingredients in order according to predominance. U.S. RDA may also be listed. However, for more than 300 standard foods (products made according to standard recipes issued by the federal government), including ice cream, catsup, and mayonnaise, no ingredients need be listed. Even when ingredients are listed, information on the products is often insufficient in and of itself to guide knowledgeable food selection.

Not only are potentially carcinogenic additives used in preparation of foods, e.g., nitrosamines in bacon and saccharin in low-calorie carbonated beverages, but unintentional food additives such as pesticides and other agricultural chemicals may appear in foods. A great deal of research must be done on the safety of large numbers of food additives. While studies are under way, the synergistic, cumulative, and long-term effects of many additives will only be determined after years of use and exposure within human populations.

## FOOD–DRUG INTERACTIONS

A word needs to be said about the interaction of foods and drugs. Foods and drugs can interact, increasing the absorption of some foods and drugs and decreasing the absorption of others. The rate of absorption or the total level of absorption of drugs or nutrients may be affected. For example, crackers, dates, jelly, and other carbohydrates may slow down the rate of absorption of analgesics such as Tylenol and limit their effectiveness in reducing pain. Milk, eggs, cereals, and dairy products can inhibit the absorption of iron. Antibiotics such as tetracycline are less readily absorbed when milk, dairy products, or iron supplements are taken. As a final example, prune juice, bran cereal and high-fiber foods can increase intestinal emptying time to the point where drugs such as digoxin cannot be adequately absorbed.[35]

Some medications increase the need for nutrients. Interesting findings have resulted from intensive studies of women on oral contraceptive medications. It appears that such medications lower levels of folacin, vitamin $B_6$, pyridoxine, riboflavin, and ascorbic acid in women; there is a need for further exploration of this and other food–drug interactions.

## WEIGHT CONTROL

It has been estimated that two out of every five Americans in the United States are 20 percent or more overweight.[36] At least 60 to 70 million individuals weigh more than they should for optimum health. In terms of prevention (health protection), maintaining recommended weight appears to have a powerful impact. Men 45 to 55 years of age appear to increase mortality rate by 1 percent for each pound that they are overweight.[37] The incidence of cardiovascular disease, hypertension, diabetes mellitus, and cancer, major causes of disability and death, is higher among the obese.

Obesity is generally defined as being 20 percent or more overweight by standard height and weight tables. While a large amount of muscle mass in individuals can make these tables inaccurate, they represent the most accessible and convenient way of determining obesity. Since obesity almost always results in excessive amounts of nonessential subcutaneous fat, measurement of skinfold thicknesses has also been used as a convenient and nonintrusive measure of obesity.[38] Both of these approaches to assessment have been discussed in Chapter 5 on Health Assessment.

While the physical basis for obesity is relatively simple and straightforward, that is, the ingestion of more calories than needed for energy expenditure, the actual causes of obesity are complex. Proposed causes of obesity include:

1. Heredity.
2. Cognitive factors (e.g., unrealistic personal standards and expectations)
3. Affective factors (e.g., emotional problems such as anxiety, boredom, and feelings of powerlessness).
4. Interpersonal factors (e.g., family problems, difficulties with fellow workers or colleagues).
5. Sociocultural factors (food selection, food preparation, and food consumption practices).
6. Environmental factors (e.g., salient cues for eating behavior and level of environmental sensitivity).

At this point, results of numerous studies suggest that it is more important to deal with personal, social, and environmental influences, rather than biochemical causes of obesity. Research has yielded little definitive information on biochemical etiology except in relation to a limited number of metabolic disorders.

Types of obesity have been classified to facilitate description of the problem and application of appropriate treatment strategies. Specific types include juvenile or adolescent-onset obesity (chronic obesity), adult-onset obesity (acute or chronic), reactive obesity (acute, sudden weight gain), and obesity secondary to a metabolic disorder.[39] Prevention is always the approach of choice since treatment of obesity after it develops has met with limited success. Juvenile-onset obesity appears to be the type most resistant to treatment.

The primary goal of interventions for obesity is the permanent alteration of eating patterns and behavior rather than weight loss only. The term *dieting* should be avoided since this has a negative connotation. Actually, adopting more healthful eating behaviors is directed toward increasing rather than decreasing the pleasures derived from eating. New awareness of taste, texture, and form of foods allows the individual to participate to the fullest in the eating experience, totally involving gustatory, visual, olfactory, and tactile senses. Eating that promotes optimum health can be fulfilling, self-actualizing and totally enjoyable.

## POSITIVE EFFECTS OF MAINTAINING RECOMMENDED WEIGHT

The individual who maintains desired weight has taken a major step in decreasing risk for many chronic health problems. The Framingham study sponsored by the National Heart, Lung, and Blood Institute found that a 15-percent loss in weight among males corresponded to a 10-percent drop in systolic blood pressure and a slightly lower percentage drop in diastolic blood pressure.[40] Many hypertensive individuals become normotensive through weight loss. Not only does weight loss decrease the risk of chronic disease, it has been shown to increase self-esteem, perceptions of control, and feelings of social desirability and acceptance. Individuals of normal weight are more active than their obese counterparts, and this further promotes health and decreases risk for health problems.

Maintaining weight has also been shown to result in a more consistent level of serum cholesterol. Frequent fluctuations in weight may be detrimental to health since serum cholesterol is elevated during weight loss. Frequent elevations predispose individuals to more rapid progress of atherosclerosis. Adipocytes are the fat cells within the body that increase in lipid content with weight gain. In the obese, the size of fat cells can increase from 50 to 100 percent. Weight reduction is achieved through decrease in size of cells. As increased byproducts of fat metabolism enter systemic circulation, precautions must be taken to prevent their deposit in the lining of vessels and their detrimental effects to internal organs such as liver and kidneys. Stability of weight can prevent many of these potential hazards.

## POINTS TO CONSIDER BEFORE INITIATING A WEIGHT-REDUCTION PROGRAM

The individual who desires to lose more than 20 pounds should have a medical history, physical examination, blood lipid and glucose analysis, and electrocardiogram before beginning a weight-loss program. Also, careful assessment of current dietary habits is essential in order to develop an individualized, effective program.

Other points to consider include the following:[41]

- Has the person maintained a stable weight for a period of time?
- Does the person have a history of repeated failure in either achieving or maintaining weight loss?
- Are there weight-reduction measures that offer the individual a good chance of success?
- Is the person well adjusted to his or her weight or strongly motivated to change?
- Are there health conditions that make weight reduction a high priority?
- If change is desired, are expectations realistic?
- Will weight loss and weight maintenance be compatible with continuance of valued social relationships?

These considerations are important in estimating the client's chances for success in weight loss. Studies have shown that individuals who derive the greatest benefits from a weight reduction program exhibit adult-onset rather than adolescent-onset obesity, report few previous attempts to achieve weight loss, cite numerous reasons for wanting to lose weight, and are more adept at self-reinforcement.[42] These tentative guidelines should be judiciously applied by the nurse to estimate each client's potential for successful weight loss.

## GENERAL GUIDELINES FOR HEALTHY WEIGHT LOSS

It is critical that health be maintained during periods of weight loss. Inappropriate approaches to changing eating patterns can threaten nutritional, psychological, and physical health status. The following guidelines should be followed:[43]

- Diet should be deficient in calories only, not in nutrients.
- Diet should be realistic.
- Foods should be used in the diet rather than vitamins, weight-loss pills, or prepared liquids.
- The diet should supply all vitamins and minerals needed for proper body functioning.
- No more than 2 to 3 pounds should be lost per week.
- Adequate fiber should be ingested for proper functioning of the GI tract.
- Enough fat should be ingested to supply the essential fatty acid, linoleic acid.
- Food servings should be small.
- A wide variety of high-nutrient foods should be included.
- Regular meals should be eaten and snacks avoided.
- A gradual decline in weight is desirable and more likely to be permanent than is rapid weight loss.
- Taking personal control is important; eating habits can be changed.
- Eating nutritious and attractive low-calorie foods should be made a way of life.

A sample of a good, nutritious weight-loss plan is provided in Table 11-4. Caloric and nutrient intake should be modified according to current age, weight, sex and health status of the client. The sample daily weight-loss plan provides 1200 calories, maintenance calories for a person weighing 120 lbs. The reader is referred to other excellent texts on nutrition for further specific information.[44-46]

## BEHAVIORAL APPROACHES TO CHANGING EATING BEHAVIOR

The presentation of a comprehensive overview of behavioral strategies for the promotion of weight loss is beyond the scope of this chapter. Many appropriate approaches for behavior change have already been discussed in Chapter 9. An attempt will be made here to summarize the behavioral approaches to weight loss that have been reported in professional literature. All behavioral approaches focus on either the antecedents or consequences of eating behavior as the points for professional intervention or self-control by the client. Meaningful application of strategies to change eating behaviors requires consideration of the client's personality, lifestyle, and environment if chances for success are to be optimized. Long-term and short-term goals should be carefully selected to provide a framework for behavior change that is realistic yet structured.

Nutrition education is an integral part of all behavioral approaches to weight

---

**TABLE 11-4    SAMPLE OF A ONE-DAY MENU: NUTRITIOUS WEIGHT-LOSS PLAN, PROVIDING 1200 CALORIES**

---

Breakfast
  1 serving fruit high in vitamin C
  1 serving enriched or whole-grain cereal
  1 serving whole wheat bread
  1 teaspoon liquid corn oil margarine
  ½ cup skim milk

Lunch
  2 slices whole wheat bread or 1 cup cooked enriched pasta
  1 teaspoon liquid corn oil margarine
  1 slice cheese
  1 serving vegetable or salad
  1 serving fruit
  ½ cup skim milk

Dinner
  Meat, fish, or poultry, 3½ oz
  Half a freshly cooked potato
  1 serving vegetable high in vitamin A
  1 serving other vegetable or salad
  1 teaspoon liquid corn oil margarine or salad dressing
  1 serving fruit

---

Reprinted from McGill, M., & Pye, O. *The no-nonsense guide to food and nutrition.* New York: Butterick, 1978, p. 215. With permission.

control. Clients must have information to use in understanding and structuring dietary practices and in assessing the potential effects of behavior change. Educational activities may be designed for individuals or groups, or a combined approach may be used. Families of clients should be included in nutrition education efforts.

The following five behavioral approaches to weight control have been used with clients and are reported in the literature to be effective for short-term weight loss:

1. Self-monitoring
2. Operant conditioning
   • Aversive conditioning and punishment
   • Self-reinforcement
   • Reinforcement by therapist
   • Reinforcement by significant others
   • Contingency contracting
   • Coverant conditioning

3. Classical conditioning
   • Covert sensitization
4. Stimulus control
   • Cue reduction
   • Cue expansion
5. Exercise

With the plethora of approaches available for intervention, the nurse should select the approach or combination of approaches that best fits each individual client.

**Self-Monitoring**

Most obese people are not aware of why they overeat, how much they eat, or how frequently they eat. Awareness can be increased by use of food diaries and frequency graphs of eating behavior. Through self-monitoring, the client may become more aware of internal cues that initiate eating behavior as well as cues that indicate satiety. Bellack[47] compared the effects of two different types of self-monitoring on weight loss. One group used premonitoring (recording food intake before consumption) while a second experimental group used postmonitoring (recording food after consumption). The premonitoring group was superior to both the postmonitoring group and the control group in weight loss.

It is possible that premonitoring makes eating less of an automatic behavior. Food intake is more carefully considered and planned. Gaining conscious awareness of eating behavior so that actions are more deliberate and under personal control can facilitate weight loss. However, few studies have shown major changes in weight with monitoring alone. It appears that this approach must be combined with others if it is to be effective. It is also possible that the studies that have shown little effect from monitoring have used postmonitoring rather than premonitoring, thus decreasing the possible effectiveness of monitoring activities.

**Operant Conditioning**

Positive reinforcement of desirable eating behaviors has been used successfully in a variety of studies. One thing that appears to be clear is that aversive conditioning through use of negative reinforcement or punishment is much less effective than conditioning of eating behaviors through positive reward or reinforcement. Mahoney, Moura, and Wade[48] had subjects either reward themselves for weight loss or fine themselves for weight gain from money that they had deposited to be used in that way. Individuals who rewarded themselves for weight loss rather than fined themselves for failure to lose weight were more successful.

In a subsequent study, Mahoney[49] compared a self-monitoring treatment with self-reward for weight loss. He also compared self-reward for weight loss with self-reward for positive changes in eating behavior. Self-reward was more effective than self-monitoring (premonitoring) and self-reward for changes in eating behavior was more effective than self-reward for weight loss in terms of pounds. This indicates the importance of proper selection of the target behavior to maximize the effects of positive reinforcement techniques.

Bellack[50] demonstrated the superiority of self-reinforcement to self-monitoring in promoting weight loss. Self-reinforcement has a number of advantages over reinforcement by the nurse or significant others. Reinforcement can be immediately contingent on appropriate eating behavior since the source of action and reward are the same. In addition, self-reward gives the individual a means of controlling his or her own behavior, thus supporting independence, autonomy, improved self-concept, and perceptions of control.

Saccone and Israel[51] studied seven treatment groups, each with different target behaviors to be reinforced (eating behavior versus weight loss) and differing sources of reinforcement (experimenter versus significant other). They found that the greatest weight loss occurred in the group reinforced by a significant other for positive changes in eating behavior. Family members or significant others are likely to be aware of effective sources of reward and environmental contingencies of reinforcement because of intimate contact with the client. Use of family members in applying reinforcement contingencies for behavioral change provides a continuing support sytem for the client.

In operant conditioning, rewarding new behaviors that are incompatible with health-damaging behaviors (in this case unhealthy eating patterns) assists in extinguishing undesirable behaviors. New behaviors to be learned as substitutes for health-damaging behaviors should be activities that the client enjoys performing and that are readily accessible to the client. For instance, the desire to eat a midday snack could signal the client to call a friend for a telephone visit, go bike riding, or go for a walk. If feelings of frustration provoke eating behavior, learning to relax through imagery, deep breathing, or use of systematic relaxation can be helpful as a replacement behavior for eating. In addition, the client learns to cope more effectively with stressful situations so that there is less need to eat as a coping strategy.

Shaping is an important concept in the application of positive reinforcement to change eating behavior. In shaping, progressive approximations of the desired behavior are rewarded. Initial reinforcements may be given for skipping one between-meal snack or even for cutting down on the amount eaten for a snack or for improving the quality of the snack selected (e.g., for choosing fruit or raw vegetables). Gradually, the client can be move toward omitting between-meal snacks entirely if that is the new behavior that he or she has selected to develop.

Contingency contracting has been discussed in detail in Chapter 9. Its application to changing eating behavior has met with considerable success. Contracting makes explicit the parameters of behavior to be engaged in and the conditions or rewards that are to be expected upon fulfillment of the contract. While the promise of tangible reinforcement for changing eating behaviors is undoubtedly of considerable importance, the commitment to behavior change made by the client in contingency contracting also seems to be an important factor in accomplishing desired behaviors.

Lambert and Schwab[52] conducted an intensive nutrition campaign in two communities during a one-week period. Three weeks later a group of people in one community were asked to sign a pledge card to change a particular eating behavior of their choice. That is, they were asked to make a commitment to behavior change relevant to personal nutrition and diet. Of those who made a pledge to change, 67 percent had fulfilled their commitment 90 to 100 percent of the time after 1 week. Of the sample, 51 percent made a commitment to change an old behavior, while 46 percent made a commitment to adopt a new eating habit. After 1 week, a higher percentage of those who made a commitment to adopt a new behavior were more persistent (69 percent) than of those who made a commitment to change or discontinue an old behavior (52 percent). After 3 months, 59 percent of the individuals who signed a pledge were fulfilling that pledge over more than 50 percent of the time. In the control community exposed to the intensive information program on nutrition but not asked to plege, only 10 percent had actually changed a nutritional habit for the better. It appears that personal commitment plays a major role in persistence of dietary changes.

Conditioning covert behavior has been espoused as a logical approach to changing overt eating behavior since covert operants (coverants) precede actual operant behavior. For instance, the thought "I should eat an apple instead of a cookie" should be reinforced, since it is a thought that serves as a precursor or intervening variable for desired dietary behavior. By increasing the frequency of such positive thoughts through reinforcement, negative coverants such as "That sundae looks so creamy and delicious" may be decreased in frequency. Reinforcement for coverants can be tangible objects, experiences, praise by others, or self-praise. Since coverants are private events, self-reinforcement is usually more effective than is reinforcement by others to whom coverants have to be reported. Coverant conditioning represents a special instance of operant conditioning. Horan et al.[53] found that positive coverants used as reinforcers for desirable overt eating behaviors were more effective in sustaining positive behavior than was use of negative coverants. From the research conducted thus far, it appears that covert control of eating behavior can be combined with other strategies and may then act in a synergistic manner to facilitate effective weight loss.

### Classical Conditioning

Covert sensitization represents the classical conditioning of avoidance behavior to foods and food products. Generally, the client is asked to imagine an attractive meal containing foods that he or she likes that are high in (refined) carbohydrates or fats. The client is then asked to imagine as vividly as possible that he or she has just eaten the meal and is extremely ill and uncomfortable. By imagining various undesirable symptoms and feelings of illness and by doing this repeatedly, the sight of attractive foods of low nutritional value and high caloric content may cause an overt avoidance response. Actual objects of food may also be used for purposes of conditioning. The ultimate goal is to assist the client in developing an aversion to foods that are undesirable because of poor nutritional quality.

### Stimulus Control

Stimulus control consists of modifying the environment to decrease cues for eating behavior and increase cues for positive or neutral behaviors that are incompatible with eating. Schachter[54] proposed the ''external cue hypothesis,'' which states that the obese individual is more under the control of external cues for eating behavior than under internal cues. That is, eating behavior may be controlled by the frequency and availability of food rather than by hunger and satiation. McReynolds et al.[55] found that when two groups were compared, one receiving self-control instruction and the other receiving information about stimulus control, both groups exhibited comparable weight losses at the end of treatment. However, on both 3- and 6-month follow-up, the stimulus-control group was superior to the self-control group. These findings provide support for the importance of changing external as well as internal cues to facilitate change in eating behaviors.

Cues that trigger eating can be reduced. This is referred to as *stimulus reduction*. For instance, the client may reinforce eating only when it occurs in the dining room, i.e., in no other location within the house. This means that snacks cannot be eaten while the client is watching television in the family room, nor can food be consumed while the client is sitting in the kitchen making out a grocery list. By cue reduction or stimulus narrowing for eating behavior, food consumption comes under the control of a restricted number of stimuli that can be controlled and manipulated. Clients can also learn to respond to external food cues with behaviors that are positive but do not involve eating. Reading the paper, sewing, or knitting in environmental situations where food was usually eaten occupy the client with meaningful activity while preventing the occurrence of ingestion of food.

### Exercise

Physical activity is also a behavioral intervention that promotes expenditure of energy and can facilitate weight loss. Most obese individuals are less active than their normal-weight counterparts. Exercise is not only useful in burning excess calories; studies have suggested that it prevents the loss of protein from muscle that frequently occurs when dieting is accompanied by inactivity. The reader is referred to Chapter 10 for exercises appropriate for clients who are overweight.

## COMBINING BEHAVIOR APPROACHES TO WEIGHT CONTROL

Exercise is often used in combination with other behavioral interventions. Dahlkoetter et al.[56] compared the relative effectiveness of exercise versus eating habit change and both in combination on weight loss. Forty-four subjects were assigned to four groups: exercise, eating habit change, combination, or the control group. Each group met for eight 1-hour sessions. Results indicated significant improvements for all groups on body weight. The combined group of exercise and eating habit change showed the most progress in weight and body circumference measures. At the 8-week follow-up, only the combination group continued to lose weight. These results suggest the desirability of combining exercise and eating habit change in dealing with obesity.

Kelly[57] demonstrated the effectiveness of combining approaches to weight control in working with 53 male officers from the Boston Police Department. The officers participated in a 12-week program during which they did the following:

- Kept record of weight change (monitoring)
- Attended lectures on nutrients, stress, heart disease, food, energy, and respiratory disease (education)
- Engaged in light to moderate physical activity (exercise)
- Completed homework that included behavior modification assignments given at the end of each lecture (reinforcement contingencies)

Immediately following completion of the program, the 53 officers had a mean weight loss of 7.5 kg. One year later, when 26 of the officers responded to a follow-up questionnaire, mean weight loss maintained was 11.4 kg. At completion of the initial program, the mean weight loss for these 26 individuals had been 10.9 kg. Thirteen had lost a mean of 4.4 kg on their own; one maintained weight loss; 12 had a mean weight gain of 3.5 kg. None of the officers had returned to his original weight. Romanczyk et al.[58] initially found no difference between self-monitoring, relaxation training, self-control, and therapist reinforcement at the end of 4 weeks of treatment to change dietary habits. However, in a second experiment, self-monitoring was compared with a combination of behavioral treatments including all of the above. While both groups lost weight at the end of the treatment, the complex behavioral treatment was significantly more effective initially, at 3 months, and at 6-month follow-up.

In contrast, some studies have failed to support the superiority of combined approaches over single interventions. Abrahms and Allen,[59] in comparing the effectiveness of stimulus control, financial payoffs, and group pressure in weight reduction, found that stimulus control and monetary reward (contingency contracting) from the therapist were no more effective in achieving weight loss than was stimulus control alone.

Heckerman and Prochaska[60] reported a study of 43 young adults who were randomly assigned to one of four groups for behavioral modification of eating behaviors: standard self-control, self-control plus external control via contingency contracting, self-control plus additional internal control, or the no-treatment control group. The standard self-control program consisted of presenting nutritional information and behavioral principles, including self-monitoring, stimulus control, self-reinforcement, and social reinforcement. The self-control plus external reinforcement group received the standard self-control program with an external reinforcement system by way of a contingency contract. The self-control plus more internal control group received the standard package and additional attempts to increase personal control of eating behavior. All experimental groups differed from the no-treatment control group, but there were no significant differences among the experimental groups.

Failure to find differences between the groups may have been the result of a lack of match between the locus of control of the subjects and type of weight-loss program. Wallston et al.[61] found that externally oriented individuals were more satisfied with a group weight-reduction program where external sanctions and control were used while internally oriented individuals preferred an individualized program in which they could set their own goals.

Findings as to the differential effects of single versus combined behavioral approaches are equivocal at this point in time. Further research is needed to clarify the usefulness of single and combined interventions in assisting individuals with differing characteristics to change eating behaviors.

## BARRIERS TO CHANGING EATING BEHAVIORS

Obstacles or difficulties that may be anticipated during the action phase in changing eating behaviors include the following:

- Reaching a plateau
- Perception and balance problems with relatively rapid weight loss
- Premature cessation of newly acquired behaviors because of compliments on progress or negative reactions and ridicule of others
- Temptation to reward weight loss with food treats
- Failure to enlist the assistance of family or significant others in weight-loss program
- Lack of "booster sessions" with health professional during stabilization phase for newly acquired eating behaviors (first 6 months to 1 year)
- Heterosexual anxiety aroused by weight reduction and fear or apprehension concerning increased attractiveness to opposite sex
- Interpersonal difficulties with significant others because of physical changes and accompanying psychologic adjustments

If at all possible, the client should be alerted to these possible difficulties and preventive measures instituted to avert problems. Professional support of the client by the nurse and suggestions for constructively dealing with barriers when they arise will facilitate the client's efforts to eliminate or minimize obstacles that block attainment of desired nutritional goals.

## MAINTAINING WEIGHT LOSS

An important consideration in evaluating the effectiveness of any behavior change program directed at weight loss is the maintenance of weight or continued loss after cessation of the initial program. Hall[62] found that subjects participating in an organized weight-loss program had regained all treatment losses 2 years after cessation of the program. Harris and Bruner[63] report that their experimental and control subjects did not differ in weight loss after a period of 10 months. Beneke et al.[64] report more encouraging results, their subjects gaining a mean of 5.9

pounds after cessation of the behavioral treatment program but maintaining 66 percent of the treatment loss. Stunkard[65] has summarized this dilemma:

> *Most obese persons will not remain in treatment. Of those that remain in treatment, most will not lose weight and of those who do lose weight, most will regain it.*

This presents a major dilemma for health care professionals providing care to overweight clients and for the clients themselves. Not only are wide fluctuations in weight detrimental to health, but they are psychologically demoralizing. Feelings of hopelessness can result from unsuccessful attempts at weight reduction or from regaining weight that previously had been lost. Continued research and creative approaches to intervention are needed to provide more effective strategies for facilitating permanent weight loss.

## SUMMARY

An attempt has been made to present an overview of salient principles, concerns, and issues related to effective nutritional care. Since obesity is a health problem of epidemic proportions within the American population, special attention has been given to this difficulty. The reader is encouraged to consult the many references listed at the end of this chapter in order to acquire more information about nutritional care of clients. Promoting good nutrition is a critical concern in illness prevention and health promotion and an important dimension of competent self-care.

## REFERENCES

1. Cantu, R.C. *Toward fitness: Guided exercises for those with health problems*. New York: Human Science Press, 1980, p. 60.
2. Inano, M., & Pringle, D.J. Dietary survey of low-income rural families in Iowa and North Carolina. 2. Family distribution of dietary adequacy. Journal of the American Dietetic Association, 1975, *66*, 361–365.
3. Corey, J.E. Dietary factors in athersclerosis: Prevention should begin early. *Journal of School Health*, November 1974, *44*, 511–513.
4. Suitor, C.W., & Hunter, M.F. *Nutrition: Principles and application in health promotion*. Philadelphia: Lippincott, 1980, p. 350.
5. DHEW, NIH, National Heart, Lung and Blood Institute. *The dietary management of hyperlipoproteinemia*. DHEW Publ. No. (NIH) 76-110. Bethesda, Md.: Government Printing Office, 1976.
6. U.S. Senate Select Committee on Nutrition and Human Needs. *Dietary Goals for the United States*. Washington, D.C.: Government Printing Office, 1977.
7. Suitor & Hunter, *op. cit.*, p. 351.
8. Cantu, *op. cit.*, p. 42.

9.  Van Handel, P.J., & Essig, D. *Caffeine*. (Unpublished manuscript.) Muncie, Indiana, Human Performance Laboratory, 1980.
10. Scarpa, I.S., & Kiefer, H.S. (Eds.). *Sourcebook on food and nutrition* (1st ed.). Chicago: Marquis Academic Media, 1978, p. 23.
11. *Ibid.*
12. Fredericks, C. *Winning the fight against breast cancer: The nutritional approach.* New York: Grosset and Dunlap, 1977.
13. *Ibid.*, p. 59.
14. Cantu, *op. cit.*, p. 61.
15. Beal, V.A. *Nutrition in the life span.* New York: Wiley, 1980, p. 58.
16. Suitor & Hunter, *op. cit.*, p. 36.
17. Martin, R.A., & Poland, E.Y. *Learning to change: A self-management approach to adjustment.* New York: McGraw-Hill, 1980, p. 56.
18. Schafer, R.B. The self-concept as a factor in diet selection and quality. *Journal of Nutritional Education,* 1979, *11,* 37–39.
19. Stein, M.P., Farquhar, J.W., Maccoby, N., & Russell, S.H. Results of a two year health education campaign on dietary behavior: The Stanford three community study. *Circulation,* November 1976, *54,* 826–832.
20. Suitor & Hunter, *op. cit.*, p. 57.
21. Boykin, L.S. Soul foods for some older Americans. *Journal of the American Geriatric Society,* 1975, *23,* 380–382.
22. Kolasa, K., Wenger, A., Paolucci, B., & Bobbitt, N. Home based learning implications for nutrition educators. *Journal of Nutrition Education,* 1979, *11,* 19–21.
23. Suitor & Hunter, *op. cit.*, p. 12.
24. Nutrition Search, Inc. *Nutrition almanac* (rev. ed.). New York: McGraw-Hill, 1973.
25. Suitor & Hunter, *op. cit.*, p. 37.
26. *Ibid.*, pp. 123–124.
27. Kuntzlemann, C.T. *The complete book of walking.* New York: Simon and Schuster, 1979, p. 53.
28. Suitor & Hunter, *op. cit.*, p. 40.
29. *Ibid.*, p. 26.
30. *Nutrition almanac, op. cit.*, pp. 9–10.
31. Williams, F.L., & Justice, C.L. A ready reckoner of protein costs. *Journal of Home Economics,* 1975, *67,* 20–21.
32. Abraham, S., Johnson, C.L., & Carroll, M.D. Total serum cholesterol levels of adults 18 to 74 years, U.S. 1971–1974. DHEW Publ. No. (PHS) 78-1652. Washington, D.C.: Government Printing Office, 1978.
33. American Heart Association. *Eat well but eat wisely.* New York: The Association, 1973.
34. Winter, R. *A consumer's dictionary of food additives.* New York: Crown, 1978.
35. Wakefern Food Corporation. *Food–drug interactions: Can what you eat affect your medication?* Elizabeth, N.J.: The Corporation, 1978.
36. Kelly, K.L. Evaluation of a group nutrition education approach to effective internal control. *AJPH,* August 1979, *69,* 813–816.
37. Abramson, E.E. *Behavioral approaches to weight control.* New York: Springer, 1977.
38. Gain, S.M., & Clark, D.C. Trends in fatness and the origins of obesity. *Pediatrics,* 1976, *57,* 443–456.
39. Suitor & Hunter, *op. cit.*, p. 274.
40. Cantu, *op. cit.*, p. 62.
41. Suitor & Hunter, *op cit.*, p. 274.
42. Abramson, *op. cit.*, p. 40.
43. McGill, M., & Pye, O. *The no-nonsense guide to food and nutrition.* New York: Butterick, 1978.

44. Suitor & Hunter, *op. cit.*
45. Beal, *op. cit.*
46. *Sourcebook on food and nutrition, op. cit.*
47. Bellack, A.S. A comparison of self-reinforcement and self-monitoring in a weight reduction program. *Behavior Therapy,* 1976, *7,* 68–75.
48. Mahoney, M.J., Moura, N.G.M., & Wade, T.C. Relative efficacy of self-reward, self-punishment, self-monitoring techniques for weight loss. *Journal of Consulting Clinical Psychology,* 1973, *40,* 40–47.
49. Mahoney, M.J. Self-reward and self-monitoring techniques for weight control. *Behavior Therapy,* 1974, *5,* 48–57.
50. Bellack, *op. cit.*
51. Saccone, A.J., & Israel, A.C. Effects of experimenter versus significant other–controlled reinforcement and choice of target behavior on weight loss. *Behavior Therapy,* 1978, *9,* 271–278.
52. Lambert, V.E., & Schwab, L.O. Can we change our food habits? *Journal of Home Economics,* 1975, *67,* 33–34.
53. Horan, J.J., Baker, S.B., Hoffman, A.M., & Shute, R.E. Weight loss through variations in the coverant control paradigm. *Journal of Consulting Clinical Psychology,* 1975, *43,* 68–72.
54. Schachter, S. Some extraordinary facts about obese humans and rats. *American Psychologist,* 1971, *26,* 129–144.
55. McReynolds, W.T., Lutz, R.N., Paulsen, B.K., & Kohrs, M.B. Weight loss resulting from two behavior modification procedures with nutritionists as therapists. *Behavior Therapy,* 1976, *7,* 283–291.
56. Dahlkoetter, J., Callahan, E.J., & Linton, J. Obesity and the unbalanced energy equation: Exercise versus eating habit change. *Journal of Counseling and Clinical Psychology,* 1979, *47,* 898–905.
57. Kelly, *op. cit.*
58. Romanczyk, R.G., Tracey, D.A., Wilson, G.T., & Thorpe, G.L. Behavioral techniques in the treatment of obesity: A comparable analysis. *Behavioral Research and Therapy,* 1973, *11,* 629–640.
59. Abrahms, J.L., & Allen, G.J. Comparative effectiveness of situational programming, financial payoffs and group pressure in weight reduction. *Behavior Therapy,* 1974, *5,* 391–400.
60. Heckerman, C.L., & Prochaska, J.O. Development and evaluation of weight reduction procedures in a health maintenance organization. In Stuart, R.B. (Ed.), *Behavioral self-management: Strategies, techniques and outcomes.* New York: Brunner/ Mazel, 1977, pp. 215–229.
61. Wallston, B.S., Wallston, K.A., Kaplan, G.D., & Maides, S.A. Development and validation of the health locus of control (HLC) scale. *Journal of Consulting Clinical Psychology,* 1976, *44,* 580–585.
62. Hall, S.M. Behavior treatment of obesity: A two-year follow-up. *Behavior Research and Therapy,* 1973, *11,* 647–648.
63. Harris, M.B., & Bruner, C.G. A comparison of a self-control and a contract procedure for weight control. *Behavior Research and Therapy,* 1971, *9,* 347–354.
64. Beneke, W.M., Paulsen, B., McReynolds, W.T., Lutz, R.N., & Kohrs, M.B. Long-term results of two behavior modification weight loss programs using nutritionists as therapists. *Behavior Therapy,* 1978, *9,* 501–507.
65. Stunkard, A.J. The management of obesity. *New York State Journal of Medicine,* 1958, *58,* 79–87.

# CHAPTER 12
# Stress Management

*Stress* is a popular term in modern society. Thousands of articles and books have been written on the subject, yet the complexity of the concept continues to baffle the best scientific minds. Selye, a pioneer in stress research has defined stress as "the nonspecific response of the body to any demand made on it."[1] The body's response to stress involves the nervous, endocrine, and immunologic systems, which in turn affect all organ systems. Stress is an all-too-common human experience that over time can produce health-damaging effects.

In nursing literature, stress produced by the experiences of illness and hospitalization has been the most frequent focus of investigation. Less attention has been given to the mechanisms by which reactions to everyday life events affect neurohormonal functions, often resulting in recurrent and prolonged stress. While the nurse in the hospital setting may actively manage sources of social, biologic, and psychologic stress for the patient who is acutely ill, the major responsibility for preventing the effects of stress rests with the client. Stress management is a critical aspect of self-care. Consequently, nurses must assume responsibility not only for assessing stress levels and coping strategies of clients but also for providing counseling and instruction in various approaches to managing stress.

As an example of what nurses can do in this area, the author provides training in progressive relaxation and biofeedback to clients with hypertension as part of a comprehensive hypertension program within the community. Clients contract individually with the author for the 13- to 16-week program. Details of the author's private practice will be provided in a later section of this chapter.

Two other nurses actively involved in providing training in stress management to clients include Helen Nakagawa of Seattle, Washington, and Arlene Putt of Tucson, Arizona. Through use of biofeedback and other techniques these clinicians assist clients in learning how to prevent the psychophysiologic effects of stress that are detrimental to health.

As a context for the discussion of stress management, various conceptualizations of stress will be presented. In addition, what is currently known about the mechanisms that mediate stress will be summarized briefly.

Selye breaks the stress response down into eustress and distress. Eustress is an agreeable and healthy experience in which, as stress increases, health and

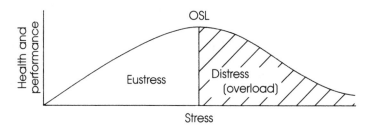

**FIGURE 12-1.** Optimum stress level (OSL) and effects of overload on health and performance (From Hans Selye).

performance also increase. Distress is a disagreeable and pathogenic state in which, as stress increases, health and performance decrease.[2] Stress overload is considered to be the cause of distress. The relationship between eustress and distress is pictured in Figure 12-1. According to Selye, the optimal stress level for any individual is the point on the stress continuum where performance and health are maximized. Selye proposed that eustress and distress are not qualitatively different; they are only quantitatively different.

Internal and external manifestations of stress are referred to by Selye as the General Adaptation Syndrome (GAS) or the ''fight or flight'' response. Specific physiologic or behavioral changes that occur are presented in Table 12-1. In modern society, the ''fight-or-flight'' response serves few useful functions since distress seldom results from direct physical threat. The major sources of distress experienced by individuals today are interpersonal relationships (communication) and performance demands (action). Since communication and action represent two basic human processes, the potential for stress is always present.

It is the belief of this author that eustress and distress represent positive and negative states of tension respectively and that *the two states are qualitatively as well as quantitatively different*. Positive tension (actualizing tendency) is a force for growth, maturation, fulfillment, and increasing complexity. Positive tension is created primarily through self-initiated activity or through response to environmental stimuli that are novel, varied, or puzzling. Positive tension is synonymous with intrigue or challenge. On the other hand, negative tension (stabi-

---

**TABLE 12-1  FLIGHT-OR-FIGHT RESPONSE**

| | |
|---|---|
| Dilatation of pupils | Increased muscle tension |
| Increased respiratory rate | Increased gastric motility |
| Increased heart rate | Release of adrenalin |
| Peripheral vasoconstriction | Increased blood glucose level |
| Increased perspiration | Raising of body hair |
| Increased blood pressure | Cold and clammy hands |

lizing tendency) is the primary force for adaptation, with the body responding adversely to a lack of or excessive stress. The qualitative difference between positive and negative tension is depicted in Figure 12-2. Within this chapter, the term *stress* denotes states of negative tension. Stress management entails the control of distress rather than eustress. Prevention of distress or states of negative tension is critical to maximize health and prevent illness.

## MEDIATION OF STRESS

In order to plan effectively for stress management, the health professional must understand the neuroendocrine pathways currently believed to mediate stress. Neuroendocrine pathways responsible for the stress response are presented in Figure 12-3. The early work of Papez[3] and McLean[4] indicate that emotional states or responses are correlated with electrophysiologic activity in the limbic system of the brain. This activity is then transmitted to the sympathetic network of the autonomic nervous system, the hypothalamus, the pituitary gland, the adrenal cortex, and the adrenal medulla, resulting in release of corticoids, norepinephrine, and epinephrine. Thus, limbic signals are converted to autonomic and hormonal processes through the transducing machinery of the hypothalamus and pituitary.[5] Hormones released into systemic circulation appear to be responsible for the myriad effects observed in human beings experiencing stress.

## APPROACHES TO STRESS MANAGEMENT

Sources of stress or negative tension experienced in modern living can be classified into four basic categories:

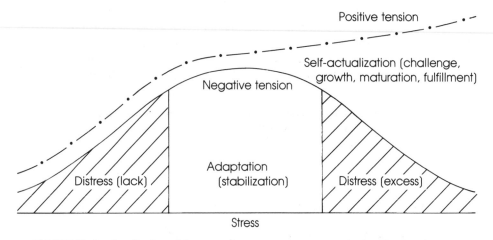

**FIGURE 12-2.** Qualitative differences between positive and negative tension.

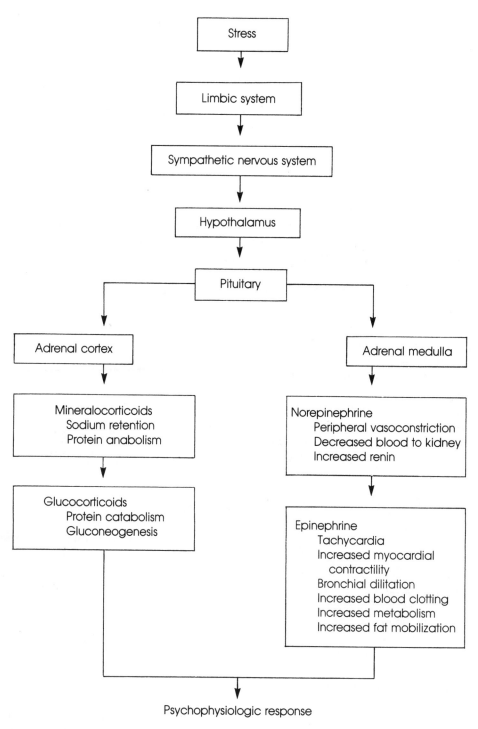

**FIGURE 12-3.** Neuroendocrine pathways that mediate response to stress. *(Adapted from Smith, M.J.T., Selye, H. Reducing the negative effects of stress. AJN, 79, November 1979, p. 1954).*

- *Adaptation* — increased energy demands required for adjustment to change.
- *Frustration* — impediment of progress toward a desired goal or inhibition of desired behavior.
- *Excessive stimulation* — increased environmental, interpersonal, or physical sensory input resulting in prolonged arousal of sympathetic nervous system. If prolonged, can lead to exhaustion.
- *Lack of stimulation* — insufficient sensory input, resulting in discomfort and boredom.

At any point in time, an individual may be subjected to one or more sources of stress. Multiple stressors combine synergistically, resulting in a nonspecific response to cumulative stress. The nurse and client together must assess the level of existing stress and the sources of stress and then determine the appropriate point(s) for intervention to achieve stress reduction.

The primary points for intervention in stress management consist of the following:

- Minimizing the frequency of stress-inducing situations
- Psychologic preparation to increase resistance to stress
- Counterconditioning to avoid physiologic arousal resulting from stress

Each point of intervention will be discussed in this chapter, and appropriate self-regulatory strategies will be described. Major attention will be given to counterconditioning techniques that can be used by the client to "turn off" physiologic responses to stress when tension-producing situations cannot be avoided.[6]

### Minimizing the Frequency of Stress-inducing Situations
In a technologic society, the need for adjustment to externally imposed change is continuous. The work of Holmes and Rahe[7] has indicated the importance of "life change" as a risk factor for illness and the impact of change on the level of health. The statistical probability of becoming ill is greater following a period of high life change than after a period of few life changes. Stressful events can include changes in family relationships, work setting, or geographic location. Adaptation reflects the human stabilizing tendency in response to environmental change. In addition, adaptation keeps physiologic and psychologic parameters within ranges compatible with continuing existence.

How does the client deal with the continuing need to adjust yet avoid the destructive effects of negative tension states? Approaches to assisting clients in preventing stressful situations include (1) habituation, (2) change avoidance, (3) time blocking,[8] (4) time management, and (5) environmental modification.

*Habituation.* Habit explains much of the behavior about which we have to exercise little conscious thought. Many behaviors are accomplished automatically through routines or stabilized behavior patterns. Routines reduce physical and psychologic energy needed for those tasks where few behavioral options are available. Habituation results in resistance to change and thus serves as a stabilizing force. The importance of routines and the threat imposed by their disturbance can be easily seen among hospitalized patients. A major source of stress during hospitalization is the disturbance of usual patterns of living. Every activity takes more energy than is required in the patient's natural setting because it must be done differently. Therefore, during periods of high stress, routines should be supported by health personnel in order to conserve energy that can be reallocated to deal directly with stressful events.

*Change Avoidance.* During periods of high life change and resulting negative tension states, any unnecessary changes should be avoided. As an example, if a family is experiencing the illness of one of its family members and a subsequent job loss, this may not be the time to consider geographic relocation, pregnancy, or any other major change in lifestyle. Negative tension created by multiple changes is synergistic. Each time a distressing change occurs, the potency of previous changes for upsetting stability is increased. Deliberately postponing changes that result in negative tension assists clients in dealing more constructively with unavoidable change and prevents the need for multiple adjustments all at one point in time.

Any changes that are made in lifestyle during periods of high or moderate stress should be self-initiated and provide challenge to the client rather than threat. Increasing positive sources of tension that promote growth and self-actualization can offset the deleterious effects of negative tension. For instance, learning to play tennis, to swim, or to dance may provide an enjoyable challenge to counterbalance stress.

*Time Blocking.* Girdano and Everly[9] have suggested a time-blocking technique that sets aside specific time for adaptation to various stressors. This block of time may be daily, weekly, or monthly. It offers clients time to focus on a specific change and develop strategies for adjustment. For instance, if a family member has just been diagnosed as diabetic, time must be set aside to meet the new needs of that individual and to learn more about the care and support that family members can provide. Acquisition of new information and thoughtful planning makes a specific change easier to adapt to and allows time for the expression of feelings and emotions that may hinder adjustment. Nurses as health professionals can be a rich resource of information and assistance as clients integrate unavoidable changes into their lifestyle. The major advantage of time blocking is that it insures that important goals or concerns will be addressed and critical tasks accomplished. This can reduce the sense of time urgency, the level of anxiety, and associated feelings of frustration and failure.

*Time Management.* After clients have used the clarification techniques described in Chapter 6 to identify their values and goals as part of comprehensive health counseling, prioritized goals can serve as a framework for time management. Overcommitment to others or unrealistic expectations of oneself is a frequent source of stress. Excess stimulation or overload can be avoided by learning to say "no" to those activities that do not result in accomplishment of prized personal goals. Overload results in frustration and loss of satisfaction from the work accomplished since one can seldom expend one's best efforts under strain and pressure.

Another important approach to time management is the reduction of a task into smaller parts. A task as a whole may appear as an overload; however, if the task is broken down into smaller segments, accomplishment becomes feasible. An example of this for a client may be learning several effective conditioning exercises before learning a complete conditioning routine, or developing skill with a conditioning routine before beginning a walk-jog activity. To take the whole health-promoting behavior as one task may be overwhelming. Breaking it down into component parts allows mastery and feelings of competence.

Avoiding overload by delegating responsibilities to others and enlisting their assistance is also important. The delegation of responsibilities must be realistic based on the abilities of others so that delegated tasks can be accomplished without excessive supervision. Making use of the skills of others and recognizing their ability to perform assigned tasks provides freedom from the expectation of having to be "all things to all people."

Just as overload can be avoided, periods of low levels of stimulation that produce negative tension can also be anticipated and prevented. Time can be used wisely by planning activities that increase positive tension and promote growth. For example, the salesperson who spends a great deal of time driving between business appointments seldom finds the long trips relaxing. Experiences of boredom are common. This may be the time when audiotapes can be used to present new ideas or assist in the development of new skills. Boredom or sensory monotony can be addressed effectively through adequate planning. Periods of potential negative tension can be replaced with experiences of positive tension that facilitate growth, health, and well-being.

*Environmental Modification.* Changing the environment is the most extensive approach to minimizing the frequency of stress-inducing situations. Job-related stresses may be avoided by carefully identifying experiences and personalities that are abrasive or stress-producing and minimizing contact to the extent possible. Changing the physical work environment may be difficult unless the client moves to a new position or a new company, but the immediate interpersonal environment can be modified considerably by planning interaction patterns. Committee membership in groups that are stress inducing might be better delegated to someone else who experiences less stress from the activity or who obtains enjoyment from participation.

Stress often results when the clients set themselves up for frustration by lack of assertiveness in structuring the immediate work environment. Clients have more control over their work situation than they may realize. Assisting the client in optimally using that control to avoid stress and subsequent physiologic arousal is an important role of the professional nurse in comprehensive health counseling. If a job change is required by the client to decrease stress, new employment possibilities should be analyzed to make sure that stress-phenomena similar to those already encountered are not an inherent part of the new employment setting.

### Psychophysiologic Preparation to Increase Stress Resistance
Resistance to stress is achieved through psychologic and physical conditioning. Such preparation is an important intervention point in stress management. Psy-

chologic conditioning consists of (1) enhancing feelings of self-esteem, (2) increasing assertiveness, and (3) developing goal alternatives. The major approach to physical conditioning for stress resistance is physical exercise, described in Chapter 10 of this book. Approaches to psychologic conditioning will be briefly described below.

*Enhancing Self-Esteem.* While self-esteem as a personality trait is developed over time, studies have shown that the level of self-esteem can be changed. Several methods have been suggested by Girdano and Everly[10] for achieving a positive image of self. One approach is positive verbalization. In using this technique, clients identify positive aspects of self or personal characteristics that they value highly. Each characteristic, one per day, is placed on a 3 × 5" index card, and the cards are placed in a conspicuous place. Each card should be read several times a day. This technique helps clients to become comfortable with positive thoughts about themselves and decreases the amount of time spent in self-devaluation. Identifying positive characteristics of the self can also focus attention on attributes that are admired by others. Increased self-awareness of positive characteristics and their presence in conscious thought will result in more frequent behavior that reflects these attributes and more positive responses from significant others.

*Increasing Assertiveness.* Substituting positive assertive behaviors for negative passive ones can increase personal capacity for psychologic resistance to stress. Assertiveness is the appropriate expression of oneself, one's thoughts, and one's feelings and can result in greater personal satisfaction in living. Assertiveness is more constructive than aggression and deals more effectively than aggression with most problems encountered in the course of living. Many books and articles have been written on assertiveness training. Assertiveness allows individuals to share their perceptions and feelings with others in a way that facilitates rather than inhibits personal and/or group productivity. Several suggestions for becoming more assertive that clients ought to be encouraged to use include the following:

- Making a deliberate effort to greet others and call them by name
- Maintaining eye contact during conversations
- Commenting on the positive characteristics of others
- Initiating conversation
- Expressing opinions
- Expressing feelings
- Disagreeing with others when holding opposing viewpoints
- Taking initiative to engage in a new behavior or learn a new activity

The webs and constraints that entangle human beings are frequently self-constructed and disappear easily when efforts are made to become more open, assertive, and self-fulfilling. While it is possible for clients through use of simple techniques to become more assertive, very passive and reserved clients might well benefit from more comprehensive assertiveness training by a competent instructor or counselor. The nurse can assist clients in locating such resources for personal development.

*Developing Goal Alternatives.*[11] Clients must be aware not only of the goals that they have set but why accomplishment of those goals is rewarding. Similar sources of reward or reinforcement may be possible through accomplishment of alternative goals. For example, a client's wished-for advancement within his or her current work situation may not materialize. If the primary reasons for wanting advancement are recognition and increased income, these rewards may be achieved by accomplishing similar goals. Recognition can come through community or organizational involvement and additional monies may be generated through wise investments. Flexibility on the part of the client permits achievement of desired outcomes through several different approaches. As a result, lack of success in initial attempts to reach goals becomes much less ominous because of the probability of success in similar tasks. The format for assisting clients to develop a goal alternative system is presented in Figure 12-4.

The nurse can assist the client in dealing more constructively with stress by using the above strategies. Other approaches that may be used include desensitizing the client to stressful situations and helping the client gain greater control over daily experiences and personal lifestyle.

---

Step 1: What is the desired goal? _____

Step 2: Is this goal immediately obtainable?
  _____ No   STOP! Why are you doing this exercise?
  _____ Yes

Step 3: What is (are) the obstacle(s) that keep(s) you from obtaining this goal?

  _____

  _____

  _____

Step 4: Can this obstacle be removed within a reasonable time period?

  _____ No   _____ Yes   If any reasonable methods exist by which you may obtain your goal by removing the obstacle, use them.

Step 5: Consider your desired goal. Take some time and make a list of the specific rewards or desirable characteristics that make that goal desirable to you. Now go back and give each one of those desirable characteristics a score indicative of how important each one is to you. A score of 1 would be the lowest; 10, the highest. Do this very carefully; it is very important.

---

**FIGURE 12-4.** Format for identification of a goal alternative system. (*From Girdano, D., & Everly, G., Controlling Stress and Tension: A holistic approach, pp. 131–132. Reproduced by permission of Prentice-Hall, Inc. Englewood Cliffs, N.J.*)

| Rewards | Points |
|---|---|
| _____ | _____ |
| _____ | _____ |
| _____ | _____ |
| _____ | _____ |

Step 6: Are there any other reasonable ways to obtain those *same* rewards listed in Step 5?

_____ Yes
List alternatives,
then try them out:

_____

_____

_____

_____

_____ No
If you have arrived at this point, it seems apparent that *all* of those desirable characteristics listed in Step 5 are currently unobtainable. Therefore, instead of feeling sorry for yourself, make a list of alternatives that are *possible* and have at least some of the same desirable characteristics as the original goal. Select the behavior that results in the highest-point score possible. This alternative is your best one because it is most similar to your original behavior, based on the points assigned in Step 5.

| Alternatives | Points |
|---|---|
| _____ | _____ |
| _____ | _____ |

**FIGURE 12-4** (continued).

### Counterconditioning to Avoid Physiologic Arousal

Control of physiologic responses to stressful events through counterconditioning techniques is receiving increasing attention within the health community as an approach to stress management. The fact that one can control the autonomic nervous system, which had been thought to be under unconscious control, has been discovered only in recent years through classical conditioning experiments. The goal of counterconditioning is to replace muscle tension and heightened sympathetic nervous system activity produced by stress with muscle relaxation and increased parasympathetic functioning. The three interventions most frequently used to assist the client in accomplishing this are relaxation training, biofeedback, and imagery. Each of these approaches to stress management will be discussed here within the context of the author's private practice.

The clients that the author sees have essential hypertension, are monitored within the hypertension program of the county health department, have a private physician, and are interested in relaxation and biofeedback as an approach to hypertension control. Participation in the program is voluntary. The program is 13 to 16 weeks in length, with 6 months of follow-up.

For the first four weeks, clients are seen individually for purposes of assessment. Information is gathered on client history, therapeutic regimen, and lifestyle. In addition, the Modified Health Locus of Control (MHLC) Scale, Health Value Scale, Speilberger State-Trait Anxiety Scale, Twenty Things I Love to Do, Signs of Distress, and Stress Charting* are completed by clients. Systolic and diastolic blood pressure (resting) and muscle tension (forearm and forehead) are measured at each visit. Muscle tension is measured by an electromyogram (EMG). In addition, goals of the client for the relaxation program are discussed and clarified. Identifying client expectations and the reality of such expectations is an important activity during initial sessions.

During the second phase of the program, clients attend three group-training sessions in which the physiologic effects of stress are discussed and training in progressive relaxation is initiated. The rationale for progressive relaxation and an overview of the approach used by the author in working with clients is presented below.

***Progressive Relaxation through Tension–Relaxation Techniques.*** Edmund Jacobson, who began his work on relaxation as early as 1908 at Harvard University, proposed that relaxation decreases voluntary muscle activity and activity within the sympathetic nervous system while increasing parasympathetic functioning.[12] There has been an increasing accumulation of evidence in the scientific literature that supports Jacobson's findings that tension levels can be reduced through use of relaxation skills. Relaxation appears to be a way of turning off the body's response to the sympathetic nervous system and of actually decreasing neurohormonal changes that take place in reaction to the experience of negative tension states.[13]

Relaxation is thought to result in the following changes:

- Decrease in the body's oxygen consumption
- Lowered metabolism
- Decreased respiration rate
- Decreased heart rate
- Decreased muscle tension
- Decreased premature ventricular contractions
- Decreased systolic and diastolic blood pressures
- Increased alpha brain waves

The relaxation procedures that the author uses are an adaptation of the basic procedures presented by Bernstein and Borkovec.[14] Reclining lawn chairs or

---

*See Chapter 5 for description of these instruments.

lounge chairs arranged in a very pleasant, quiet, sound-proofed room where lighting can be dimmed to a low level provides an optimum setting for group relaxation training. External noise is particularly disturbing to clients who are just beginning relaxation training since the ability to maintain inner awareness or consciousness and to block out external stimuli is a skill developed over time.

Before each session, tight clothing should be loosened, glasses removed, shoes removed, and a comfortable position assumed in the chair. Relaxation should never be taught with clients lying flat. Although this is a common position assumed for rest and sleep, it often results in muscle strain in upper back and neck along with drowsiness, which interferes with training. A reclining position or sitting position is most appropriate. The reclining position recommended by the author for relaxation training of clients is depicted in Figure 12-5.

At the beginning of each session, clients are encouraged to focus on their own breathing as the air moves gently in and out. The purpose of this focusing activity is to increase awareness of self and the often imperceptible functions of the human body. The author guides clients through the relaxation maneuvers one by one. The relaxation sequence is progressively modified throughout the three sessions as indicated below.

SESSION I. Following the focusing activity, clients are moved slowly through tension and relaxation cycles for each of the major muscle groups listed in Table 12-2, maintaining tension for 8 to 10 seconds and releasing tension instantaneously on cue. The entire tension–relaxation cycle should be repeated twice during the

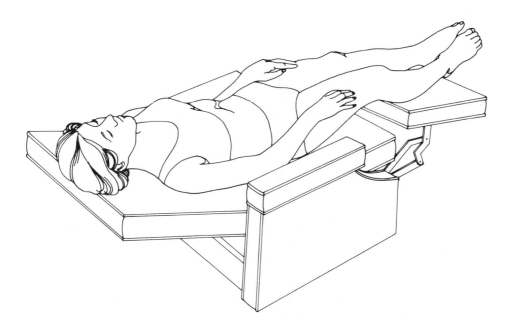

**FIGURE 12-5.** Appropriate reclining position for relaxation training.

**TABLE 12-2 FIFTEEN MUSCLE GROUP SEQUENCE FOR TENSION–RELAXATION CYCLE**

| Muscle Group | Abbreviated Instructions |
|---|---|
| 1. Right hand and forearm | Make a fist. |
| 2. Right upper arm | Pull elbow tightly into side. |
| 3. Left hand and forearm | Make a fist. |
| 4. Left upper arm | Pull elbow tightly into side. |
| 5. Forehead | Wrinkle brow. |
| 6. Upper cheeks and nose | Squint eyes and wrinkle nose. |
| 7. Lower cheeks and jaws | Place teeth together and make a "forced" smile. |
| 8. Neck and throat | Pull chin toward chest. |
| 9. Chest, shoulders, and upper back | Take a deep breath. Push shoulder blades toward each other. |
| 10. Upper abdomen | Pull stomach in and hold. |
| 11. Lower abdomen | Bear down against the seat of the chair. |
| 12. Right upper leg | Push down against the foot of the chair. |
| 13. Right lower leg and foot | Point toes toward head and body. |
| 14. Left upper leg | Push down against the foot of the chair. |
| 15. Left lower leg and foot | Point toes toward head and body. |

first session to increase clients' awareness of the differences in body sensations during tensed and relaxed periods. The tension–relaxation instructions should be given very slowly, allowing clients to enjoy the feelings of relaxation they are experiencing.

The guidance provided by the nurse is critical for successful relaxation. A detailed description of the many pertinent considerations is beyond the scope of this book. The reader is referred to other sources for additional information.[15-17]

SESSION II. After the first group session, training tapes are used by clients at home to facilitate daily practice of relaxation techniques. Clients are also requested to keep a schedule of the frequency and length of time that relaxation is practiced. A self-report sheet is provided. This report is turned in at the beginning of each session. During the first part of the second session, the fifteen muscle group tension–relaxation cycle is again reviewed and practiced. In the second half of the session, a relaxation procedure is taught to the group that combines the fifteen muscle groups into seven muscle groups (Table 12-3).

During the seven-muscle group sequence, the client may report that he or

**TABLE 12-3   SEVEN MUSCLE GROUPS FOR TENSION–RELAXATION CYCLE**

| Muscle Group | Abbreviated Instructions |
|---|---|
| 1. Right hand, forearm, and upper arm | Make a fist and pull elbow tightly into side. |
| 2. Left hand, forearm, and upper arm | Make a fist and pull elbow tightly into side. |
| 3. Forehead, upper cheeks and nose, lower cheeks and jaws | Wrinkle brow; squint eyes; wrinkle nose; place teeth together and make a "forced" smile. |
| 4. Neck and throat | Pull chin toward chest. |
| 5. Chest, shoulders, back, upper and lower abdomen | Take a deep breath; push shoulder blades toward each other; pull stomach in and bear down. |
| 6. Right upper leg, lower leg, and foot | Push down against the foot of the chair and point toes toward head and body. |
| 7. Left upper leg, lower leg, and foot | Push down against the foot of the chair and point toes toward head and body. |

she did not achieve as deep relaxation as with the fifteen-muscle-group sequence. This is to be expected. Encourage clients to practice using seven-muscle groups, assuring them that they will develop increasing comfort and skill with the procedure as they engage in home practice. During the second week of practice, clients are encouraged to "think through" the relaxation procedure and do their own coaching. A "prompt sheet" on the sequence of the seven-muscle groups is sent home with them for reference. This is intended to move clients toward independent practice of relaxation rather than encouraging reliance on the nurse or the coaching tape as a means of providing relaxation cues.

SESSION III. During the first part of the third session, self-report sheets on frequency and time of practice are again collected. Clients are encouraged to talk about any difficulties that they are having. Some common problems that clients report include:

- Overly rapid self-pacing through the relaxation sequence
- Distraction by environmental noise
- Difficulty keeping attention on own monologue
- Interruption of distracting thoughts during relaxation
- Residual tension in some muscles after tension–relaxation

The problem of overly rapid self-pacing can usually be solved by encouraging clients to slow down internal speech or coaching pace. Phrases like "I feel calm,"

''I feel very relaxed,'' and ''My arms/legs feel heavy'' can be interspersed throughout self-instruction. To avoid distraction by environmental noise, a time of day should be chosen when the client is alone and without interruption. This may be at home in the evening or in the office during the day. Encouraging family members to join in the relaxation practice sessions may be another way of minimizing environmental distractions.

Distraction from self-instructions for relaxation and interruption of extraneous thoughts can be curtailed if the client focuses on the physical sensations experienced during relaxation and on the character of his or her own breathing.

If the client is experiencing any remaining tension after one tension–relaxation cycle in a particular muscle group, the tension–relaxation sequence should be repeated. Generally, after tensing and relaxing a second time, residual tension is considerably diminished.

During the last half of the third session, a relaxation procedure for four muscle groups is taught. While tensing smaller groups of muscles may result in little risk for hypertensive clients, tensing large groups of muscles may significantly increase blood pressure. Therefore, clients with relatively high systolic and diastolic blood pressures should not progress to the four-muscle-group tension–relaxation cycle. Instead, counting down or recall (to be described in the following sections) should be used. For clients with only mild hypertension, the seven muscle groups can be combined into four muscle groups as shown in Table 12-4.

Once clients have learned to achieve deep relaxation using the four muscle groups, the entire relaxation procedure, including focusing and tension–relaxation cycles should not take any longer than 10 to 12 minutes. The object of shortening the procedure is not speed per se but greater flexibility for the client in using relaxation at any time in a variety of settings.

**TABLE 12-4   FOUR MUSCLE GROUPS FOR TENSION–RELAXATION CYCLE**

| Muscle Group | Abbreviated Instructions |
| --- | --- |
| 1. Entire right and left arms | Make fists with both hands and pull both elbows tightly into sides. |
| 2. Muscles of face, neck, and throat | Wrinkle brow; squint eyes; wrinkle nose; place teeth together; make a ''forced'' smile; pull chin toward chest. |
| 3. Chest, shoulders, back, upper and lower abdomen | Take a deep breath; push shoulder blades toward each other; pull stomach in and bear down. |
| 4. Entire right and left legs | Push down against the foot of the chair with both feet and point toes toward head and body. |

*Progressive Relaxation without Tension.* While tension–relaxation techniques result in high levels of voluntary muscle relaxation, clients must be taught how to relax without first tensing muscles. Such techniques are taught to clients by the author during individual sessions. They include relaxation through recall, relaxation through counting down, and relaxation through imagery. The major advantage of these techniques is that tension is no longer required. This is particularly important for clients with hypertension, where, as previously indicated greater elevations in pressure may be caused by prolonged or extensive muscle tensing. Deep relaxation without tension is the goal for the hypertensive client.

RELAXATION THROUGH RECALL. In this approach, the client is asked to focus on feelings of tension experienced in each of the four muscle groups used in Session III. With increased sensitivity to muscle sensations, the tension in a particular muscle group should be recognized. The client is asked to recall feelings of relaxation previously experienced in that part of the body and to allow the target muscle group to become similarly relaxed. The sequence for the four muscle groups is the same as the tension–relaxation sequence. The suggestions of relaxation should continue for 30 to 45 seconds for each muscle group. If recall is ineffective at first, the seven- or four-muscle-group tension–relaxation cycle can be repeated, followed immediately by recall to make the sensations of tension and relaxation more vivid. Transition from tension–relaxation techniques to use of recall may be a difficult step for some clients, yet with practice clients can master this self-control technique.

Phrases that can be repeated to facilitate relaxation through recall are listed in Table 12-5. These phrases have been suggested by Elmer and Alyce Green as a result of work in biofeedback at the Menninger Foundation. Such phrases result in physiologic imagery that can decrease both sympathetic nervous system activity and tension in voluntary muscles.

RELAXATION THROUGH COUNTING DOWN. The countdown procedure initially focuses on each of the seven or four muscle groups used previously. The client is encouraged to relax each muscle group progressively as the count proceeds from 10 down to 1. When the client has practiced and become skilled with this procedure, total body countdown can be used: relaxing the entire body while silently counting down from 10 to 1. This is a particularly useful procedure for the office or when facing stressful social situations. In 2 to 3 minutes, the skilled client can achieve total body relaxation while in a sitting position with eyes open and focused on a specific object. This is one of the shortest procedures through which relaxation can be accomplished. Mini-relaxation sessions several times throughout the day can promote generalization of relaxation training to everyday life.

RELAXATION THROUGH IMAGERY. The client may find that passively concentrating on pleasant scenes or experiences from the past can greatly facilitate relaxation. Recalling the warmth of the sun, the feeling of warm sand, the sensations of a gentle breeze, the vision of palm trees swaying, or sounds of ocean waves may be comfortable and pleasant for clients. Such recall can promote muscle relaxation.

**TABLE 12-5 RELAXATION-PROMOTING PHRASES**

1. I feel quiet.
2. I am beginning to feel quite relaxed.
3. My feet feel heavy and relaxed.
4. My ankles, my knees, and my hips feel heavy.
5. My solar plexus and the whole central portion of my body feel relaxed and quiet.
6. My hands, my arms, and my shoulders feel heavy, relaxed, and comfortable.
7. My neck, my jaws, and my forehead feel relaxed. They feel comfortable and smooth.
8. My whole body feels quite heavy, comfortable, and relaxed.
9. I am quite relaxed.
10. My arms and hands are heavy and warm.
11. I feel quite quiet.
12. My whole body is relaxed and my hands are warm—relaxed and warm.
13. My hands are warm.
14. Warmth is flowing into my hands. They are warm, warm.
15. I can feel the warmth flowing down my arms into my hands.
16. My hands are warm, relaxed, and warm.
17. My whole body feels quiet, comfortable, and relaxed.
18. My mind is quiet.
19. I withdraw my thoughts from the surroundings and I feel serene and still.
20. My thoughts are turned inward and I am at ease.
21. Deep within my mind, I can visualize and experience myself as relaxed, comfortable, and still.
22. I am alert, but in an easy, quiet, inward-turned way.
23. My mind is calm and quiet.
24. I feel an inward quietness.

Each client will vary in those scenes or images that result in actual changes in muscle tension (EMG). For some clients, visualizing specific colors, shapes, or patterns will be as effective as visualizing landscapes or scenes. The important point for the nurse to emphasize to the client concerning use of imagery is that feelings and sensations that accompany specific visualizations should be the primary dimensions for focus, rather than visual detail.

If the clients initially have difficulty in using imagery or visualization for relaxation, the nurse may use one of the following techniques:

- Have the client with eyes closed visualize a particular room of his or her house (livingroom, bedroom, kitchen), focusing on colors, shapes, and specific objects. The client's mind should wander about the room and he or she should describe verbally what is seen in as much detail as possible.
- Have the client focus on a particular piece of clothing that is a personal favorite. The client should describe in detail the color, texture, design, and trim of the clothing and how it feels when worn (e.g., soft, loose, fitted, light, warm).

As individuals become more vivid in descriptions of concrete objects, their ability to use less concrete imagery for purposes of relaxation should increase. Use of imagery can be an important and pleasant adjunct to other relaxation techniques described.

Increasingly, research on relaxation techniques indicates the usefulness of such approaches in the prevention and treatment of a variety of stress-related diseases. Relaxation also has been shown to increase feelings of energy, vitality, and self-control. However, like any other skill, continued use and practice of approaches to relaxation is essential if clients are to experience maximal prevention and health-promotion benefits from their use.[18]

**Biofeedback.** During individual sessions following group relaxation training, the author assists clients in acquiring greater skill in relaxation through providing biofeedback regarding level of muscle tension (EMG) and/or skin temperature. A general discussion regarding use of biofeedback for stress management is presented below; however, a detailed discussion of the many biofeedback modes and how to use them in working with individual clients is beyond the scope of this book.

Biofeedback has in recent years offered the possibility for awareness and control of processes previously thought to be under unconscious rather than conscious control. Biofeedback can be defined as a process in which a person learns reliably to influence physiologic responses that are not ordinarily under voluntary control. The four basic operations in biofeedback are as follows:[19]

1. Detection and amplification of bioelectric potentials
2. Conversion of bioelectrical signals to easy-to-process information
3. Feedback of information to the client
4. Voluntary control of target response through learning based on feedback

The foundations of biofeedback hinge on a very simple idea: Clients need to be provided with information about what is going on inside their bodies, since bodily functions cannot be controlled unless information about them is available to the controller.[20] A wide range of autonomic processes can be controlled through response to feedback. Some of the physiologic parameters that have been controlled or modified through feedback include the following:

- *Heart rate* — acceleration and deceleration
- *Heart rhythm* — occurrences of premature ventricular contractions
- *Blood pressure* — systolic and diastolic
- *Peripheral vascular responses* — skin surface temperature
- *Muscle tension* — muscle contractility
- *Alpha wave activity* — as recorded in the electroencephalogram
- *Galvanic skin response* — resistance of skin to passage of electrical current
- *Sexual response* — increased or decreased sexual arousal

Biofeedback is an important modality for facilitating stress management. The ultimate goal is establishing self-regulation that allows the client to control autonomic responses. A permanent change in the target response is desired following training. While biofeedback instrumentation facilitates learning during the training period, the client must learn to read and interpret body signals without the aid of equipment and to function effectively in modifying responses. That is, relaxation rather than tension (fight-or-flight response) should result when stress occurs. It is the belief of the author that relaxation when taught prior to the use of biofeedback provides the client with specific skills for controlling body responses.

The mechanism for biofeedback is illustrated in Figure 12-6. Electrophysiologic studies indicate that every perception of external events (OUTS) has associated electrical activity in both conscious and unconscious central nervous system structures, those involved in both emotional and mental responses. The

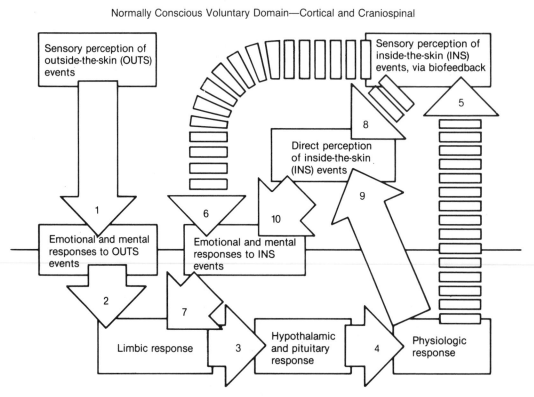

**FIGURE 12-6.** Simplified operational diagram of "self-regulation" of psychophysiologic events and processes. *(From Green, E., Green, A., Norris, P. Self-regulation training for control of hypertension.* Primary Cardiology, *March 1980, p. 129. With permission.)*

limbic system is considered primarily unconscious, although neural pathways lead from limbic structures directly to cortical region, providing some contact with conscious centers. Emotional states and visceral processes are correlated with electrophysiologic activity in the limbic system. The limbic system is connected to the hypothalamus, where limbic signals are converted to autonomic and hormonal processes through the transducing capacities of the hypothalamus and pituitary. It is a relatively new idea, that one can detect what is going on inside the skin (INS) and change it voluntarily in a direction of choice. However, when an individual is given continuous auditory or visual feedback of physiologic information, a new mental-emotional response can be learned. The new response is followed by an appropriate limbic response that combines with, modifies, or replaces the original response. Subsequently, changes occur in the patterns of hypothalamic firing and pituitary response; the physiologic state is altered, and this change is fed back via the monitor to the conscious cortex.[21]

Two specific feedback modalities used by the author in her practice will be discussed: electromyograph feedback and skin-temperature feedback. These modalities are frequently used in the clinical setting and appear most relevant for the kinds of clients that nurses would be seeing for stress management; that is, clients learning relaxation as a means of health promotion, prevention, or treatment of stress-related disorders.

ELECTROMYOGRAPH (EMG) FEEDBACK. Early experimental work in this area was conducted by Basmajian, using needle electrodes. Subjects learned to control the rate of firing of various motor units within muscles.[22] EMG is now used to train clients to lower tension in whole muscle groups. The most frequent sites of training are the forearm and the forehead (frontalis muscle). The mechanism is that of voluntary muscle control, as opposed to autonomic conditioning as in temperature training. The forearm is easier to train than the frontalis muscle, so it is often recommended for beginning sessions. Once muscle control is achieved in the forearm, training can be moved to the frontalis. It is generally believed that the frontalis muscle is a good indicator of the overall state of body tension.

The EMG measures the amount of electrical discharge in the muscle fibers and quantifies muscle contraction in microvolts, showing this value on a meter as an auditory or visual display. Once the client is aware of what his or her level of muscle tension is, he or she can begin to work on bringing about change. Changes in muscle tension levels can be brought about primarily in two ways: by relaxation or by use of imagery.

EMG feedback has been shown to be effective in treating many stress-related disorders, such as chronic back pain, tension headaches, and essential hypertension. It can also be used for muscle reeducation (increasing muscle tension) in clients with cerebrovascular accidents and other central nervous system insults.[23]

The results of EMG training reported by clients in a variety of settings are very impressive. They have reported experiencing decreased muscle strain and discomfort, decreased feelings of mental stress, anxiety, and tension, increased feelings of personal control, increased energy, and enhanced feelings of health and well-being. Positive changes in physiologic parameters (e.g., muscle tension, heart rate, and diastolic and systolic blood pressure) are supported in the literature. Further research is needed before the parameters of clinical usefulness are established for this biofeedback modality.

SKIN-TEMPERATURE FEEDBACK. Historically, the major thrust for use of temperature control as a therapeutic modality came through the work of Elmer and Allyce Green in their laboratory at the Menninger Foundation. They developed the use of temperature training for treatment of migraine headache.[24] More recently, the Greens have used temperature training successfully in the treatment of hypertension, lowering both systolic and diastolic pressures.[25] Temperature training has also been used successfully in treatment of Raynaud's and Buerger's diseases, where spasms of peripheral arteries cause coldness of extremities.

Peripheral skin temperature is regulated by vasomotor control mechanisms. The body responds to external temperature changes through a thermoregulatory response by constriction or dilation of the smooth muscles around the peripheral blood vessels. With decreases in environmental temperature, these vascular changes allow increased blood flow to internal organs and maintenance of constant core temperature. Biochemical factors influencing skin temperature are alcohol, tobacco, histamine, epinephrine, lactic acid, and carbon dioxide. Psychologic factors influencing skin temperature include emotional stress, anxiety, and environmental stimuli. Activation of the sympathetic nervous system and subsequent neurohormonal changes result in smooth muscle constriction around the peripheral vessels and decreased skin temperature. Thus, an increase in skin temperature can reflect decreased sympathetic nervous sytem activity.[26]

Heat flow constitutes an indirect measure of blood flow. In temperature training, a thermistor is attached to the finger, and visual or auditory feedback is used to indicate temperature change. Initial readings, which can range from 75 F to 96 F, can give a clue as to the potential effectiveness of temperature training for any given client. Fuller[27] has indicated that if initial finger temperature readings are above 90 F (32.2 C), the potential for raising temperature is limited compared to when initial readings are between 75 F (23.8 C) and 90 F (32.2 C).

Quiet internal states produced by relaxation or imagery (visualization of warming sensations in the extremities) appear to decrease sympathetic nervous system activity and cause peripheral dilation. This change is reflected in increased finger temperature, which provides helpful feedback to the client.

The effectiveness of temperature training in decreasing physiologic responses to stress must be further evaluated through carefully designed clinical research. To date, systematic studies support the potential usefulness of this technique in self-management of hypertension, migraine headache, and other circulation disorders.

## SUMMARY

A number of different approaches for assisting clients in managing stress have been presented in order to familiarize the reader with the range of strategies available. Some approaches suggested are relatively unstructured while others are more formally defined and/or require instrumentation. The decision regarding which strategies to use must be made collaboratively by the client and the nurse. This decision should be based on the characteristics of the client, sources of stress experienced by the client, and his or her general patterns of response to stressful events. The reader is encouraged to consult the references at the end of this chapter for further information on relaxation training and biofeedback. The nurse must acquire skill with these intervention modalities before use with clients.

## REFERENCES

1. Selye, H. Introduction. In Wheatley, D. (Ed.), *Stress and the heart*. New York: Raven Press, 1977.
2. *Ibid.*, p. 3.
3. Papez, J.W. A proposed mechanism of emotion. *American Medical Association Archives of Neurology and Psychiatry*, 1937, *38*,725–743.
4. McLean, P.D. Psychosomatic disease and the "visceral brain": Recent developments bearing on the Papez theory of emotion. *Psychosomatic Medicine*, 1949, *11*,338–353.
5. Green, E.E., Green, A.M., & Norris, P.A. Self-regulation training for control of hypertension. *Primary Cardiology*, March 1980, *6*,126–137.
6. Sutterley, D.C. Stress and health: A survey of self-regualtion modalities. *Topics in Clinical Nursing*, April 1979, *1*,1–21.
7. Holmes, T.H., & Rahe, R.H. The social readjustment rating scale. *Journal of Psychosomatic Research*, 1967, *11*,213–218.
8. Girdano, D., & Everly, G. *Controlling stress and tension*. Englewood Cliffs, N.J.: Prentice-Hall, 1979.
9. *Ibid.*, p. 128.
10. *Ibid.*, p. 146.
11. *Ibid.*, p. 129–133.
12. Bernstein, D.A., & Borkovec, T.D. *Progressive relaxation training: A manual for the helping professions*. Champaign, Ill.: Research Press, 1973.
13. Cautela, J.R., & Groden, J. *Relaxation: A comprehensive manual for adults, children, and children with special needs*. Champaign, Ill.: Research Press, 1978.
14. Bernstein & Borkovec, *op. cit.*, pp. 25–32.
15. Cautela & Groden, *op. cit.*, pp. 1–35.
16. Jacobsen, E. *Anxiety and tension control*. Philadelphia: Lippincott, 1964.
17. Bernstein & Borkovec, *op. cit.*, 1–56.
18. *Ibid.*, pp. 52–70.
19. Blanchard, E.B., & Epstein, L.H. *A biofeedback primer*. Reading, Mass.: Addison-Wesley, 1978, pp. 7–9.
20. Gaarder, K.R., & Montgomery, P.S. *Clinical biofeedback: A procedural manual*. Baltimore: Williams and Wilkins, 1977.
21. Green, Green & Norris, *op. cit.*, p. 128.
22. Basmajian, J.V., Baeza, M., & Fabrigar, C. Conscious control and training of individual spinal motor neurons in normal human subjects. *Journal of New Drugs*, 1965, *5*,78–85.
23. Fuller, G.D. *Biofeedback: Methods and procedures in clinical practice*. San Francisco, Biofeedback Press, 1977.

24. Sargent, J., Green, E.E., & Walters, E.D. The use of autogenic feedback training in a pilot study of migraine and tension headaches. *Headache*, 1972, *12*,120–124.
25. Green, Green & Norris, *op. cit.*, pp. 126–137.
26. *Ibid.*, p. 47.
27. Fuller, *op. cit.*, p. 138.

# CHAPTER 13
# Social Support and Health

The nurse responsible for assisting clients of all ages in maintaining and improving health cannot ignore the importance of social networks as the context for personal health behaviors. The social network in which the client resides can facilitate or thwart efforts directed toward health protection and/or health promotion. Since social networks can be made more responsive to client needs, the role of the nurse in assisting clients to assess, strengthen, and develop social support systems will be addressed in this chapter.

## SOCIAL NETWORKS

Social networks consist of those persons or groups with whom clients maintain contact and have some form of social bond.[1,2] Social networks generally consist of family (traditional or nontraditional), neighbors, friends, fellow workers, and other acquaintances with whom the person interacts through work, organizational/political activities, travel, or leisure.[3] Social networks often serve as the interface between individuals and their environment, thus exerting powerful influence on how individuals think, act, and react. A personal social network differs in distinct ways from an organized network (e.g., social group or work group). In an organized group, component individuals make up a larger social whole with common aims, interdependent roles, and a distinct subculture. In a network, only some, not all component individuals have social relationships with one another. The extent to which persons within a social network know each other determines the connectedness of the network.[4] Figure 13-1 contrasts the connectedness of individuals within a hypothetical social network as opposed to those in a hypothetical work group. The frame of reference for each diagram is a single individual (Jane).

### Characteristics of Social Networks
Social networks have a number of important characteristics of which the nurse should be aware. Key characteristics of social networks include:[5-7]

**331**

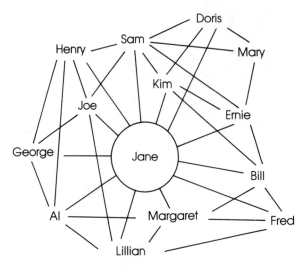

**Work Group**

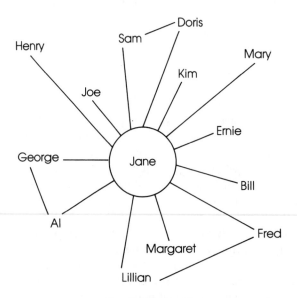

**Social Network**

——— = relationship or
        acquaintance

**FIGURE 13-1.** Comparison of "connectedness" (density) of organization versus social network. In the work group, it is possible that everyone would know each other. In the social network, individuals seldom know all other persons in the network.

- Size—the number of people identified as belonging to a specific social network. Generally, in order to be included in the network, an ongoing personal relationship must exist that results in some contact at least once a year.
- Density—the number of dyadic relationships that exist among members of the network.
- Homogeneity—members sharing common demographic, personal, or social characteristics.
- Intensity—the amount of time spent in contact, emotional intensity, and intimacy (mutual confiding), and the degree of reciprocity characterizing relationships.
- Content—the type(s) of behaviors characterizing relationships. The following types of behaviors have been identified:
  Assistance—seeking help or aid from individuals in order to meet own needs.
  Value similarity—congruity between desired end states (goals) and/or means for achieving desired end states.
  Concern—extent of altruistic or caring (affective) emotions directed toward individuals.
  Trust—using individuals as confidants for sharing information of a private or intimate nature.
  Desired interaction—personal affinity or attraction to individuals for interaction/communication and physical proximity.
  (Relationships may have one or more content areas. Generally, the larger the number of content areas, the stronger the dyadic ties.)
- Dispersion—the ease with which network members can make face-to-face contact.
- Duration—the length of time relationships within network have been in existence. Mean length of time may be most representative of network history.
- Directionality—the extent of movement of component members toward common goal(s).

The above characteristics may be applied to any social network in order to describe it in detail. Assessment and diagramming of social networks provide critical information for determining the adequacy of support available to clients.

### Functions of Social Networks
Social networks can serve a number of functions for individuals. Social networks may serve any or all of the following three functions:[8]

- Support—actions or behavior on the part of individuals within the network that assist the focal person in meeting personal goals or in dealing with the demands of a particular situation. Support can be tangible or intangible.
  Tangible support—money or active assistance.
  Intangible support—encouragement, personal warmth, love and/or emotional support.

- Advice—information or guidance on how to achieve a certain goal or complete a certain task.
- Feedback—provision of evaluative statements regarding how expectations or requirements for reaching specific goals are being met. Provides information on how well individuals are performing.

Individuals within a social network often serve more than one of the above functions. Generally, the more functions each person in a social network serves, the more supportive the network is to the target member.

## SOCIAL SUPPORT

Social support can be defined as the subjective feeling of belonging, of being accepted, loved, esteemed, valued, and needed for oneself, not for what one can do for others.[9] Support is provided to any individual by a specific group of persons who constitute his or her social support system. A social support system is the set of personal contacts through which an individual maintains social identity, receives emotional support, material aid, information, and services, and makes new social contacts.[10] The support system represents an enduring pattern of continuous or intermittent ties that play a significant role in maintaining psychologic and physical integrity of the individual over time. Communication and mutual obligations characteristic of support systems meet the needs of members for succorance, nurturance, and affiliation. Social support systems are not static but dynamic, evolving, or changing throughout a person's life span. They provide security for individuals by sustained membership and active involvement in a definite human group.[11]

Five types of social support systems relevant to health have been identified and described in the literature: natural support systems, peer support systems, religious organizations or denominations, organized support systems of care-giving or helping professionals, and organized support groups not directed by health professionals. In most instances, the family (natural support system) constitutes the primary support group. Families, in order to provide appropriate support, must be sensitive to the needs of family members, establish effective communication, respect the unique needs of members, and establish expectations of mutual help and assistance. Family structures may be traditional in nature or nontraditional (e.g., unrelated adults, siblings, etc.).

Peer support systems consist of informal care givers who function as generalists or specialists in meeting the needs of others. Generalists are characterized by wisdom in human relations, knowledge about community care-giving systems, and gregariousness. They make contacts easily and enjoy being involved with other people. They maintain a reputation of helpfulness because of support provided to others. Informal care givers who are specialists generally have encountered an experience of major impact in their own life and achieved successful adjustment and/or growth. Because of extent of insight, their advice is sought primarily in relation to one specific area of concern. Examples include the avid runner, the health food enthusiast, the widow, or the parents of a retarded child. Successful achievement or coping is the primary credential of the informal care giver who is viewed as a specialist.

Religious organizations or denominations constitute the oldest community support systems evident today. Churches or religious groups represent a congregation of individuals which hold regular meetings, share joint allegiance to theology, a common value system, a body of traditions, and a set of guidelines for living. Even highly mobile individuals may find a ready support system in the local denomination or church.

A third type of support system is composed of care-giving or helping professionals with a specific set of skills and services to offer clients.[12] The professional support system is seldom the first source of help for an individual. Family and close friends or peers are sought out initially for advice and support. It is often only when this source of help is unavailable, interrupted, or exhausted that health professionals enter the support scene.

Organized support systems not directed by health professionals include voluntary service groups and mutual help groups. Voluntary service groups provide assistance to individuals who are in need or for some reason are unable to provide services for themselves. Self-help groups attempt to effect change in behavior of members (Alcoholics Anonymous, TOPS, Recovery, Inc.) or promote adaptation to a life change (a chronic health problem, terminal illness, or disabled family member).[13]

All support systems of a given individual are synergistic. In combination, they represent the social resources available to him or her to facilitate stability and self-actualization.

### Functions of Social Support Groups

The functions of social support groups in promoting and protecting health have been conceptualized in two ways as depicted in Figure 13-2. Social groups can contribute to the maintenance of health by decreasing the likelihood of life change and its concomitant stress or by "buffering" the effects of life change, thus decreasing the potential for illness. Buffers are protective social processes that control interpretation of events and emotional responses to them.[14]

Personal and contextual factors that mediate the impact of life events include:[15] (1) personal resiliency, (2) openness to alternative coping strategies, (3) interpersonal relationships and ties to sources of support within the family and community,[16] (4) the kind of life event occurring, and (5) the degree of stress induced.

Resources for dealing with life events are of two main types: psychologic resources (self-esteem, adequacy of coping in major life roles, and personal competence) and social resources (the number of persons within social network viewed as resources; the amount, frequency, and duration of interaction with these in-

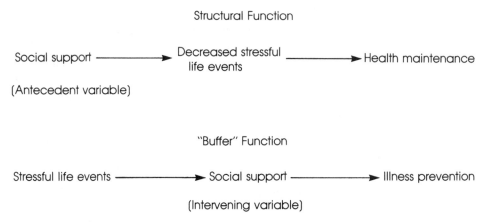

FIGURE 13-2. Possible impact of social support on health status.

dividuals; the degree of intimacy and dependability).[17] Generally, mobilization of personal resources occurs first, followed by mobilization of the social support network. Both types of resources serve a protective or facilitative function by (1) modifying interpersonal or environmental conditions, (2) perceptually controlling the meaning of an experience, and (3) promoting appropriate emotional arousal.

The extent of integration of a given individual within his or her social support system is a critical factor in mediating the impact of life events.[18] On the whole, poor social integration appears to be a more prevalent condition among individuals in the low-income group than among persons at other socioeconomic levels. Stress may also be greater in this group and extent of total supportive resources less. This can make members of this group more vulnerable to the negative effects of occupational and domestic stress.[19] People with undifferentiated or minimal social support systems exhibit poorer coping behavior and emotional stability than do those with well-developed, mutually supportive relations.

The relationship between socioeconomic class and pathologic stress reactions has two possible explanations. The first is the social selection theory. That is, individuals with coping difficulties suffer from financial exigencies and distresses that result in their attaining and maintaining lower class status. Their lack of coping abilities results in their natural selection into the lower class. Alternative explanations are referred to as social causation theories. The essence of such theories is that the stress from community or neighborhood life is different in intensity and quality from that found in other class environments and the potential for meaningful support is lower, resulting in a high number of pathologic reactions to stressful situations.[20]

The primary functions of social support groups are to augment personal strengths of members and facilitate mastery of the environment.[21] Support groups appear to protect and promote health by meeting the needs of a given individual for enduring interpersonal relationships that provide the following:[22]

- Love and affection
- Intimacy that facilitates self-expression
- Validation of personal identity and worth
- Satisfaction of nurturance and dependency
- Assistance with life tasks and activities of daily living
- Help in handling emotions and controlling behavior
- Refuge or sanctuary for rest and recuperation
- Support in achieving inherent and acquired human potential

Within a support aggregate, the individual is dealt with as a unique person. There is heightened sensitivity to personal needs that are deemed worthy of respect and satisfaction. The support group also plays an important function in providing accurate feedback. Through collecting and storing cues about the outside world, support groups offer guidance and direction in interpreting reality. In general, support groups can be characterized as follows:[23]

- They share common social concerns
- They provide intimacy
- They prevent isolation
- They respect mutual competencies
- They offer dependable assistance in crises
- They serve as referral agents
- They provide mutual challenge

### Support During Crises

During a crisis period, support groups take on added significance. They increase in the incidence of supportive behavior for the target individual and relieve the stress and strain of social roles temporarily through role complementarity and role adjustment.[24] The individual is assisted in mobilizing psychologic resources as well as attaining material resources to deal with the crisis situation. Increased access to both tangible and intangible resources is usually important during a crisis. Unfortunately, low socioeconomic groups may have little access to both. A high level of stress during crises and lack of social support may in combination threaten health and increase the potential for illness.

A number of support groups strategically located within the community that serve both structural (health promotion) and buffering (preventive) functions are critical to health and well-being. The family, fellow workers, church, and cohorts in recreational activities often constitute such groups. For most individuals, the family serves as the pivotal or primary support group. The term family will be used to refer to both traditional and nontraditional primary group structures. This fundamental source of support is supplemented by other groups that serve a secondary rather than a primary support function. The family and community will be given special attention as sources of social support in the following sections of this chapter.

### Family as the Primary Support Group

For most individuals, work and family roles provide the infrastructure of social integration. The family serves an important function during early childhood in orienting individuals to values, beliefs, and behavior styles through social experiences and interaction patterns. These early learning experiences exert continuing influence on behavior throughout life. Resources of the family that can be instrumental in providing support include:

- Family traditions
- Value systems
- Child-rearing practices
- Methods of discipline
- Emotional climate
- Curiosity and exploratory behavior
- Patterns of creative behavior
- Recreational pursuits
- Material and economic resources
- Time and money management skills
- Sense of identity and purpose
- Sharing and cooperation
- Coping strategies

Disruption of structural properties of families, such as broken homes because of death, separation, or divorce, have been shown to correlate with increased risk of both physical and emotional disorders.

The emotional support environment within the family of origin has been shown to be curvilinearly related to psychologic problems in later adulthood. Too much warmth and overinvolvement on the part of the parents can engulf the child leaving him or her unable to meet and master life's problems. Too little warmth results in feelings of rejection, powerlessness, lack of worth, and despair. Both support and stress are usually present to some extent in all families. The important consideration is the balance achieved.[25] Figure 13-3 depicts two possible combinations of stress and support that may typify any given family. Assessment of support characteristics of families allows the nurse to account more fully for a given client's level of health and adjustment. Lack of support by family members can interact with sources of stress synergistically, creating a high level of individual vulnerability. On the other hand, high-quality emotional support and task-oriented assistance from the family can provide a social context in which the client can grapple successfully with the problems of living.[26]

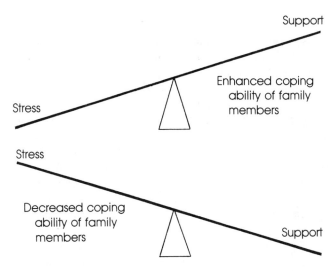

**FIGURE 13-3.** Family as a source of support/stress.

### The Community as a Support Group

The characteristics of a community have a direct bearing on the level of well-being of individuals and families that reside therein. The quality of social inter-action and the life experiences of residents can contribute positively to health or negatively to social disorganization and overt illness. Stability within a community tends to promote close-knit ties among residents that mitigate the effects of crises on community members. Stable communities are characterized by value similarity, mutual assistance, mutual trust, and concern for members.

Minority groups frequently lack the backup support of the community since they may be out-of-phase with the predominant culture, social support systems, and community services. Because of differing values and ethnic background, members of minority groups can become socially isolated within a community having few, if any, supportive relationships. In interacting with members of minority groups, the professional nurse should be particularly sensitive to the extent of social support available to them. The nurse in her caring role as a health professional may need to personally supplement this support as well as link the minority person with appropriate networks within the community.

### REVIEWING SOCIAL SUPPORT SYSTEMS

It is important for clients to be aware of sources of social support available to them. Several approaches will be suggested in this chapter for reviewing the social support networks of clients. One or more of the suggested approaches can be useful in giving both client and nurse increased insight into existing support resources.

**Support Systems Review**
Glaser and Kirschenbaum[27] have suggested a straightforward approach to be used in reviewing sources of social support for clients. In the support systems review the client is asked to list those individuals that provide personal support (financial, emotional, and/or intellectual). The client is then asked to indicate whether the supportive others are family members, fellow workers, or social acquaintances. By next identifying those individuals that have been sources of support for 5 years or more, the client gains increased awareness of the stability of personal support systems. After examining current sources of support, the client and the nurse can mutually determine the adequacy of support. If inadequate, decisions should be made concerning what can be done to enhance existing social support networks. Figure 13-4 provides a sample support system review for a hypothetical client. Following review of the client's social support systems, the following additional questions can be explored:

- In what areas do you need more support: financial, emotional, intellectual?
- Who within your present support system might provide that support but is not already providing it?
- What other individuals could become a part of your support system?
- What could you do specifically to add the people whom you believe you need in your support system?

Answers to these questions suggest actions that the client could take to expand sources of personal support.

---

List those individuals below who provide financial, emotional, or intellectual support to you. Indicate the type of support provided by placing the appropriate letter next to each name. *F* = financial support, *E* = emotional support, and *I* = intellectual support. Any individual may provide more than one type of support. Next, indicate whether the supportive other is a family member *(FM)*, fellow worker *(FW)*, or social acquaintance *(A)*. Finally, after each person who has been a source of support for *5 years* or more, place the number *5*.

| | | | |
|---|---|---|---|
| John | F, E, I, FM (husband), 5 | Nancy | E, A |
| Peter | E, FM (son), 5 | Larry | E, I, A |
| Carmen | E, FM (daughter), 5 | Arlene | E, I, A |
| Helen | E, FM (mother), 5 | Duane | I, A, 5 |
| Ted | E, FM (father), 5 | Elaine | I, A, 5 |
| Audrey | E, FM (cousin), 5 | Margaret | E, I, FW |
| Andrew | E, I, FM (cousin), 5 | Marlene | E, I, FW |
| Jane | E, I, A | Frances | I, FW |
| David | E, I, A | Rose | I, FW |
| Tom | I, A, 5 | Karen | I, FW |
| Elsa | E, I, A, 5 | Theresa | I, FW |
| Jack | E, A | Diane | I, FW |

**FIGURE 13-4.** Support systems review.

The individuals identified on the previous page should be grouped in the following way:

## Sources of Emotional Support

| FAMILY | WORK | SOCIAL GROUP |
|---|---|---|
| John | Margaret | Jane |
| Peter | Marlene | David |
| Carmen | | Elsa |
| Helen | | Jack |
| Ted | | Nancy |
| Audrey | | Larry |
| Andrew | | Arlene |

## Sources of Intellectual Support

| FAMILY | WORK | SOCIAL GROUP |
|---|---|---|
| John | Margaret | Jane |
| Audrey | Marlene | David |
| Andrew | Frances | Tom |
| | Rose | Elsa |
| | Karen | Larry |
| | Theresa | Arlene |
| | Diane | Duane |
| | | Elaine |

## Sources of Financial Support

| FAMILY | WORK | SOCIAL GROUP |
|---|---|---|
| John | | |

## Sources of Support for More than 5 Years

| FAMILY | WORK | SOCIAL GROUP |
|---|---|---|
| John | | Tom |
| Peter | | Elsa |
| Carmen | | Duane |
| Helen | | Elaine |
| Ted | | |
| Audrey | | |
| Andrew | | |

**FIGURE 13-4** (continued).

**Mutual Support Patterns**

A second approach to reviewing social support networks has been described by Simon et al.[28] The format for this approach to assessing mutual support patterns is presented in Figure 13-5. The client is asked to identify those individuals who have been to his or her home for a meal or visit within the past 3 months. The client is also asked to list those individuals who have invited him or her to their house within the same time period. With the client as the point of reference, persons within the support network are coded in the following way: similar religion (*SR*) or different religion (*DR*), similar age (*SA*) or different age (*DA*), similar ethnic background (*SE*) or different ethnic background (*DE*), and predominantly similar values (*SV*) or different values (*DV*). The client is to place an *H* by those individuals that he or she was happy to see when they came and an *X* by those individuals whom the client does not look forward to seeing again.

---

List below in the left-hand column those individuals who have visited your home during the past 3 months. In the right-hand column, list those individuals whose home you have visited during the past 3 months. Then code each individual in the following way:

FM = Family Member
FW = Fellow Worker
 A = Social Acquaintance

SR = Similar Religion
DR = Different Religion
SE = Similar Ethnic Background
DE = Different Ethnic Background
SV = Similar Values
DV = Different values

 H = Individuals that I was happy to see when they came or that I believe were happy to see me
 X = Individuals that I was not particularly happy to see or that were not particularly happy to see me

| Persons Who Have Visited My Home | Persons Whose Homes I Have Visited |
|---|---|
|  |  |

**FIGURE 13-5.** Mutual support patterns. (*Reprinted by permission of A & W Publishers, Inc. from* Values Clarification: A handbook of practical strategies for teachers and students, *revised edition by Sidney B. Simon, Leland W. Howe, and Howard Kirschenbaum. Copyright © 1972, 1978. Hart Publishing Co., Inc.*).

Identify below those persons with whom you have one or more similarities and whom you were happy to see. These individuals are likely to provide the core of your extended family or social support system. Consider what you can do specifically to further strengthen these relationships to enhance the social support available to you.

**FIGURE 13-5** (continued).

Through this review, clients can identify individuals within their support networks with whom they have mutual interests and backgrounds as well as mutually supportive relationships. The nurse can provide appropriate follow-up for this exercise by discussing with the client ways in which mutuality of caring relationships can be strengthened.

### Emotional-Support Diagram

Sources of emotional support can also be diagrammed in such a way that strength of support is readily apparent. Figure 13-6 presents a sample emotional-support diagram that is coded to indicate strong, moderate, and weak sources of support, as well as current conflicts with supportive individuals. The length of each line can be used to indicate geographic proximity to the client. This approach is particularly appropriate for the individual who needs a more visual presentation of his or her emotional-support system in order to take action effectively to sustain or enhance emotionally satisfying relationships.

### Accepting and Giving Emotional Support

Caplan et al.[29] have presented an approach for determining the extent to which clients can both give and receive emotional support. This questionnaire is presented in Figure 13-7, with only minor modifications. The questionnaire was initially developed in order to evaluate social support and its impact on adherence to medical regimens. However, the tool can also be used for the general purpose of determining the extent of mutual emotional support within a given client's social network. The following areas are addressed: number of friends and social visits, emotional support from significant others, and ability to give emotional support. The questionnaire is interesting and easy to fill out, yet it provides a great deal of helpful information for the client and the nurse to use as a basis for

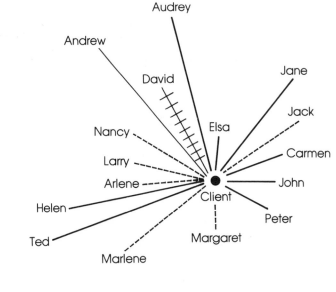

Audrey

Andrew

David

Jane

Jack

Nancy   Elsa

Larry   Carmen

Arlene   John
Client

Helen

Peter

Ted   Margaret

Marlene

Legend: ―――――― Strong emotional support

――――― Moderate emotional support

-------- Weak emotional support

+|+|+|+ Relationship in which conflict currently exists

**FIGURE 13-6.** Emotional-support diagram.

actions to enhance sources of personal support at home, at work, or in the community.

### Dyadic Support or Marital Adjustment

An important part of emotional support is that provided in the husband–wife relationship. The degree of marital adjustment can set the tone for the support climate that the entire family experiences. While many tools are available to measure both marital and sexual adjustment, the short questionnaire presented here provides a general indication of marital adaptation (Figure 13-8). The questions included are taken from *The Adaptation Potential for Pregnancy Scale* developed by Nuckolls[30,31] for assessing the extent of social support available to women during pregnancy. The nature of the questions included in the scale permit their use as a general measure of marital adjustment or satisfaction. Since marital adjustment and happiness is a highly personal topic for clients, this questionnaire should be used with discrimination and the client assured of the confidentiality of the information. The nurse should be ready to listen to the client and provide support if use of the questionnaire is emotionally distressing.

For each of the questions below, fill in or circle the appropriate response.

A. *Number of Friends and Social Visits*

1. How many close friends do you have who live within 45 minutes travel?

   _____ FRIENDS

2. How many times have you visited with any of these close friends in the past

   4 weeks? _____ TIMES

B. *Social Support*

Please read what Mike and Jim are like. Then indicate the extent to which the following people are like Mike and Jim.

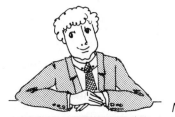

Mike      Jim

Mike is a warm, friendly person. When something concerns a person, Mike listens sympathetically and attentively. Mike gives people encouragement and praises people's efforts, no matter how small those efforts may be. Most of all, Mike is very understanding and accepting of others' feelings.

Jim is a cold, businesslike person. People rarely talk to Jim about their concerns, and when they do, he appears unsympathetic and inattentive. Jim shows his disappointment in people and their concerns. He rarely praises others' efforts. People often feel that Jim is not very understanding or accepting of their feelings.

How much does each of the following persons resemble Mike or Jim? CIRCLE ONE NUMBER FOR EACH ITEM.

1. Your immediate supervisor at work? If you have no boss or don't work check here ☐.

| Exactly or a lot like Mike | Somewhat like Mike | Halfway between | Somewhat like Jim | Exactly or a lot like Jim |
|---|---|---|---|---|
| 1 | 2 | 3 | 4 | 5 |

**FIGURE 13-7.** Receiving and giving emotional support (continued on next page).
(*From Caplan, R.D., Robinson, E.A., & French, J.R.* Adhering to Medical Regimens: Pilot experiments in patient education. *1976. © Institute for Social Research, University of Michigan, Ann Arbor, Mich.*)

2. *Your spouse* (if you are not married, rate your closest relative).

| Exactly or a lot like Mike | Somewhat like Mike | Halfway between | Somewhat like Jim | Exactly or a lot like Jim |
|---|---|---|---|---|
| 1 | 2 | 3 | 4 | 5 |

3. *Your best friend or acquaintance within 45 minutes of where you live.*

| Exactly or a lot like Mike | Somewhat like Mike | Halfway between | Somewhat like Jim | Exactly or a lot like Jim |
|---|---|---|---|---|
| 1 | 2 | 3 | 4 | 5 |

C. Supportive Behavior

How often did someone do each of the following for you *during the past week?*
CIRCLE ONE NUMBER FOR EACH ITEM.

| | Not at all | Once | Twice | Three times | Four or more times |
|---|---|---|---|---|---|
| 1. Showed warmth or friendliness toward you when you were troubled about something. | 0 | 1 | 2 | 3 | 4 |
| 2. Listened attentively to you when you needed to talk about something. | 0 | 1 | 2 | 3 | 4 |
| 3. Encouraged you or showed approval for something you did. | 0 | 1 | 2 | 3 | 4 |
| 4. Showed understanding when you felt upset or irritable. | 0 | 1 | 2 | 3 | 4 |

D. *Concern of Others*

*How much real concern about you and your well being* has been shown within the past week by each of the following people?
CIRCLE ONE NUMBER PER ITEM.

**FIGURE 13-7** (continued).

| | Almost none | A little | Some | A lot |
|---|---|---|---|---|
| 1. Your immediate supervisor? | 1 | 2 | 3 | 4 |
| 2. Your closest friend? | 1 | 2 | 3 | 4 |
| 3. Your spouse (if no spouse, a close relative or friend)? | 1 | 2 | 3 | 4 |
| 4. Your closest neighbor? | 1 | 2 | 3 | 4 |

E. *Giving Social Support*

How often did you *do* each of these activities during the past week?
CIRCLE ONE NUMBER PER ITEM.

| | Not at all | Once | Twice | Three times | Four or more times |
|---|---|---|---|---|---|
| 1. Showed warmth or friendliness toward someone when he or she was troubled by something. | 0 | 1 | 2 | 3 | 4 |
| 2. Listened attentively to someone who needed to talk about something that was bothering him or her. | 0 | 1 | 2 | 3 | 4 |
| 3. Encouraged or showed approval to someone who needed encouragement. | 0 | 1 | 2 | 3 | 4 |
| 4. Showed understanding with someone who felt upset or irritable. | 0 | 1 | 2 | 3 | 4 |

F. *Ability to Accept Social Support*

How *comfortable* do you usually feel about friends doing each of the following *for you?*
CIRCLE ONE NUMBER PER ITEM.

1. Showing warmth or friendliness toward you when you are troubled about something.

| Very Comfortable | Somewhat Comfortable | Somewhat Uncomfortable | Very Uncomfortable |
|---|---|---|---|
| 1 | 2 | 3 | 4 |

**FIGURE 13-7** (continued).

2. Listening attentively to you when you need to talk about something.

| Very Comfortable | Somewhat Comfortable | Somewhat Uncomfortable | Very Uncomfortable |
|---|---|---|---|
| 1 | 2 | 3 | 4 |

3. Encouraging you or showing approval for something you do.

| Very Comfortable | Somewhat Comfortable | Somewhat Uncomfortable | Very Uncomfortable |
|---|---|---|---|
| 1 | 2 | 3 | 4 |

4. Showing understanding when you fell upset or irritable.

| Very Comfortable | Somewhat Comfortable | Somewhat Uncomfortable | Very Uncomfortable |
|---|---|---|---|
| 1 | 2 | 3 | 4 |

G. *Trust in Others*

Generally speaking, would you say that
☐ most people can be trusted.

OR

☐ you can't be too careful in dealing with people.

Would you say that most of the time
☐ people try to be helpful.

OR

☐ they are mostly just looking out for themselves.

Do you think that most people
☐ would try to take advantage of you if they got the chance.

OR

☐ would try to be fair.

**FIGURE 13-7** (continued).

Review of social support systems can be an integral part of the action phase of health behavior. Through review, the client is assisted in recognizing current sources of support and in identifying barriers in social relationships that may thwart desirable health actions. The nurse must always be alert to client situations where social support is minimal or nonexistent. Extensive review of support systems may cause anxiety and depression for the client. In this case, a more informal, nonthreatening approach should be used.

Please indicate for each of the following scaled items, the response that best fits your current feelings about your marital relationship.

1. Has marriage been for you:

| Very | Quite | About | Somewhat | Extremely |
| happy | happy | average | unhappy | unhappy |

2. Do you consider your marriage a success in accomplishing the goals you want your marriage to achieve?

| Very | | | In many | Quite |
| definitely | Mostly | Somewhat | ways, no | unsuccessful |

3. Has your marriage brought you many disappointments?

| None | Almost | Only a | | Quite |
| at all | none | few | Some | a few |

4. What kind of an adjustment do you feel that you and your husband or wife have made to each other in marriage?

| Extremely | Very | | Somewhat | |
| good | good | Satisfactory | unsatisfactory | Poor |

5. Has your marriage brought you satisfactions that you could not have achieved otherwise?

| Very | | | | |
| many | Many | Some | Few | None |

6. Has marriage given you the personal satisfactions which you believe marriage should bring?

| To the | Very | | Very | |
| fullest extent | much so | Somewhat | little | Not at all |

**FIGURE 13-8.** Review of marital relationship (continued on next page). (*Adapted from The Potential for Pregnancy Scale in Nuckolls, K.B.,* Psychosocial assets, life crisis and the prognosis of pregnancy. *Doctoral dissertation, University of North Carolina at Chapel Hill, 1970. With permission.*)

7. Are you satisfied with the extent of emotional support provided to you by your husband or wife?

| Perfectly satisfied | Very well satisfied | Well satisfied | Satisfied | A little bit Dissatisfied | Very disatisfied |

8. Is sexual intercourse between you and your husband or wife a satisfying expression of love and affection?

| Always | Usually | Sometimes | Hardly ever | Never |

9. How would you describe your husband or wife for each of the following characteristics?

(A)

| Very easy-going | Fairly easy-going | Somewhat irritable | Very irritable |

(B)

| Placid and calm | Fairly placid | Sort of nervous | Very nervous |

(C)

| Very even temper | Fairly even temper | Quick temper | Uncontrollable temper |

(D)

| Very permissive | Sort of permissive | Sort of strict | Very strict |

10. To what extent would you be inclined to marry the same person again if you were unmarried?

| Very much | Quite a bit | Somewhat | A little bit | Not at all |

**FIGURE 13-8** (continued).

## SOCIAL SUPPORT AND HEALTH

The intent of this section is to provide the reader with an overview of completed research that has explored the relationship between social support and health or illness. Several key questions will be addressed in this section:

- What is the role of social support in promoting health?
- What role does lack of support play in increased susceptibility to illness or as a direct causative factor?
- What are the mechanisms by which social support exerts its impact on human health and well-being?

### Role of Social Support in Health Promotion

Before discussing the role of social support in the maintenance of individual health and well-being, it should be emphasized that this area is a relatively new field for exploration within the social sciences. While the amount of information available is limited, several studies that address the relationship between social support and positive health states will be cited.

In a study of 153 women Brim[32] explored the relationships between reported happiness or life satisfaction (a dimension of health) and five dimensions of social networks: concern, trust, value similarity, assistance, and desire for interaction. The pattern of correlations between these dimensions differed for married and unmarried women as illustrated in Figure 13-9. Married women considered value similarity as the most important dimension of support relationships; unmarried women gave less importance to value similarity. Assistance available from the relationship and concern evidenced on the part of the other were significantly correlated with happiness or life satisfaction for unmarried women. It is possible that the tangible assistance and continuing concern generally experienced by married women from their husbands made this dimension of social support less important to them. On the other hand, single women who had no one readily available to rely on were more aware of the need for assistance with life tasks and for show of concern on the part of individuals close to them.

While this study does not directly address health per se, happiness and life satisfaction are important dimensions of health that need to be considered in any holistic approach to health assessment. The study results provide information helpful to the professional nurse in understanding the dimensions of human support relationships generally important to married and single women. Additional data are needed on married and single men.

In a study of 280 adults 63 years of age and older, Lowenthal and Haven[33] investigated the impact on morale of a confidant. In old age, decreased social interaction and loss of social roles occur frequently. The investigators were interested in whether a confidant could maintain morale in spite of decreased social participation. The positive effects of a confidant were evident in that loss of social roles and decreased social participation produced significantly less loss of morale or depression if a confidant was available than if such a person was unavailable.

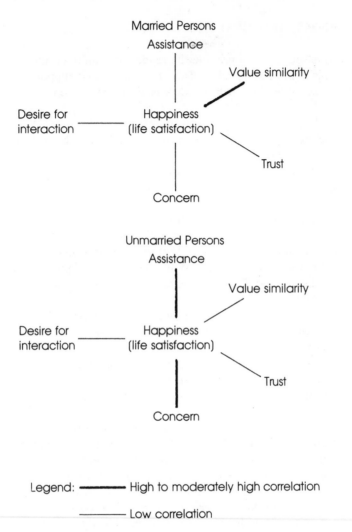

**FIGURE 13-9.** Strength of relationship to expressed happiness and life satisfaction for five dimensions of social support networks.

Women were more likely to report confidants than men, and the usual confidants were spouse, child, or friend. A study by Blau[34] further supports these findings in that older individuals who were married or employed with considerable associated activity had higher morale than did the elderly who were unmarried and/or unemployed.

In studying the experience of widowhood, Walker et al.[35] found that during the initial stage of bereavement, needs of the new widow were met by strong ties within a small but dense social support network that provided high levels of empathy. However, it was interesting to note that in the stage of psychosocial readjustment following the initial bereavement period, the needs of widows changed, making the support system that had fulfilled needs at the onset inappropriate or maladaptive. The small, dense network with strong ties maintained the identity of the widow during the initial loss crisis but entrapped the widow when she sought to change her identity and adjust to a new lifestyle. The small group seemed to offer a limited set of normative expectations, restricted information, and few new social contacts. Transition to new social roles was better served by interacting with individuals who had bridging relationships to other groups in addition to the target group. If there were individuals who were part of other social groups, the likelihood was increased that widows would meet compatible people with potential for strong tie relationships.

From these findings, it is difficult to predict an optimum support network for any client. However, it appears evident that every individual needs both intimate ties within a primary group and less intimate ties with individuals in other groups that can expand horizons and offer new social possibilities.

### Role of Support in Prevention

The role of social support in prevention has been demonstrated by the findings of a number of studies. The "buffer" effect of social support appears to be instrumental in the prevention of both physical and psychologic disorders.

Nuckolls[36] explored the relationship between social support, life change, and complications of pregnancy. A large number of variables were measured in order to determine the extent of social support available to more than 150 pregnant women. Measures of social support included the quality of marital relationships, extent of interaction with extended family, and level of adjustment within the community. The extent of life change experience was determined from responses to the social readjustment rating scale.

While neither extent of life change nor support resources alone predicted ease of pregnancy, those women with high life change and also high support scores had only one-third the complications of women with many life changes and low support scores. In other words, individuals who had high life stress but little social support had three times the difficulties of women with strong support. The study provides evidence for the "buffer" effects of strong social relationships. In spite of life change, support appeared to prevent untoward reactions (complications) during pregnancy.

In a study that explored the relationship between social support and illness symptoms, Gore[37] studied 100 rural and urban, married, blue-collar workers who had suffered job loss. The mean age of the men was 49 years, with average employment seniority of 20 years. These men were compared to a control group of 74 men employed in comparable jobs in four other companies. The focus of the study was on the effect of social support in moderating the health consequences of unemployment. Social support was measured by 13 items covering the individual's perception of wife, relatives, and friends as supportive; frequency of activities outside the home with the above individuals; and perceived opportunities to engage in social activities that were satisfying and allowed him to talk about his problems. The health outcomes measured were level of serum cholesterol, illness symptoms, depression, and self-blame.

The rural men were more supported than were urban men, possibly because of the ethnic cohesion of the rural area and the economic threat posed to the entire community by the massive layoffs. The mean cholesterol level dropped over time following the layoff except for men who were unemployed and unsupported at the time of the last interview. The number of reported illness symptoms was higher initially after job loss than at later interviews, but social support did not have a significant effect on this variable.

Perceived economic deprivation was significantly associated with depression *only* for those men who were unsupported. In addition, the majority of men who exhibited self-blame were among the unsupported. It appeared from this study that social support buffered the severity of physiologic and psychologic responses to unemployment. While unemployment resulted in loss of instrumental accomplishments important to self-worth, self-esteem appeared to be maintained through supportive relationships with significant others.[38] Social support also appeared to play a key role in sustaining mental health despite job loss.

The work of de Araujo et al.[39] showed a remarkable interaction between social support and life change[40,41] in respect to the need of adult asthmatics for steroid therapy. Table 13-1 depicts this relationship. Individuals with high life change and low social support required at least three times the daily dosage of steroids compared to any of the other groups in order to maintain control of their respiratory problems. It is possible that support buffered the deleterious effects of life change by decreasing physiologic reactivity or increased compliance with other aspects of asthma control as a result of the expectations of significant others. Regardless of the exact explanation, support appeared to decrease the need for steroids.

The potential impact of stressful events on mental status and the occurrence of overt psychiatric disorders have been studied by a number of investigators.[42,43] Life change does appear to result in stress that can be the initiating or

---

**TABLE 13-1  AVERAGE DAILY STEROID DOSAGE IN MILLIGRAMS PER DAY FOR PATIENTS WITH ASTHMA, BY LIFE-CHANGE SCORE AND SOCIAL SUPPORT (BERLE INDEX)**

| Life-Change Score | Social Support | |
| --- | --- | --- |
| | High | Low |
| High | 5.6 (12) | 19.6 (11) |
| Low | 5.0 (10) | 6.7  (4) |

The number of individuals is given in parentheses. The other number gives the average dosage in milligrams per day.

exacerbating factor in mental illness. Dohrenwend and Dohrenwend[44] found a significant correlation between life change and ratings of psychologic impairment in urban adults. Schwab and Schwab[45] found that frequency of contact with friends correlated significantly with rated psychologic impairment. That is, the fewer the social contacts with significant others, the higher the probability of mental impairment or difficulties. This suggests that social support can be instrumental in maintaining mental health and in preventing the catastrophic effects of life stress.

The findings of Tolsdorf[46] support those of Schwab and Schwab in that he found in comparing medical and psychiatric patients that medical patients had a higher number of mutually reciprocal relationships than did psychiatric patients. Psychiatric patients engaged in more unilateral relationships where they received more from others than they gave and received support from fewer persons than did the medical patients studied. The medical patients appeared to share more of themselves with others so that people could be genuinely helpful. They also used the advice of others and used the support provided by others more effectively than did psychiatric patients.

Lin et al.[47] in studying the Chinese-American population within the United States found that social support correlated $-0.36$ with psychiatric symptoms, while stressful life events correlated at $0.21$. Social support rather than life change was a stronger predictor of extent of psychiatric symptoms. This gives credence to the idea that social support rather than life change may be the key variable in the prevention of illness or in the amelioration of distressing physical and psychologic symptoms.

### Social Support and Health Behavior

The question must be raised concerning the extent to which support networks affect observed health behavior. It is well known that significant others function as an important lay referral system for individuals making decisions to seek professional care for health promotion, illness prevention, or care in illness. The priority given to health-related needs often depends on the previous experience of significant others with the same problem or dilemma. The individual passes through the lay referral system not only during the decision phase, concerning whether to seek care, but also during the action phase. Physician and nurse behavior, diagnosis, prescriptions for medication, and life changes recommended by the professional care system are discussed with others. Concurrence by the lay referral system often determines the extent to which advice or counseling by health professionals will affect self-care.

When a client is a member of a subculture that differs markedly from that of the health professionals available, an extended lay-referral and consultant structure may be available that actually retards action to seek professional care. Folk practices, religious incantations, or other rituals that do not have therapeutic value may be applied before health professionals are consulted.

In subcultures that approximate that of health professionals available, the lay system is usually truncated or does not exist at all. Contact with health personnel is generally made early in the course of a problem or concern.

Larger social networks are more likely to have individuals with similar illness experiences who might be consulted for empathy and advice than are smaller networks. Walker *et al.*[48] emphasized the importance of bridging relationships with other personal networks. Such bridging relationships as depicted in Figure 13-10 widen the possibility of information input from a variety of sources. In studying the lay referral system of pregnant women, Walker found that 33.3 percent of the individuals that underutilized prenatal care did not have a friend in whom they confided outside their own family, while only 23 percent of the users lacked such a confidant or friend. The user of prenatal care was more likely to seek advice from her husband or a friend than from other relatives. Under-utilizers more frequently consulted other relatives for advice. It appeared that users of prenatal care had a larger lay referral system that included other sources of information in addition to relatives. They sought care earlier and used prenatal services more frequently.

Compliance with therapeutic regimen has also been shown to correlate with extent of social support received from significant others. Only one of 22 articles

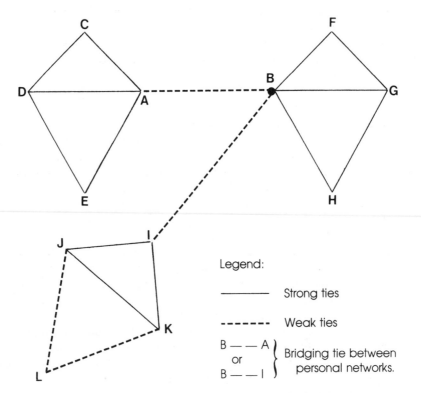

**FIGURE 13-10.** Bridging ties to other networks can increase health information potentially available. *(Adaptation of diagram from Granovetter, M.S. The strength of weak ties. American Journal of Sociology, 1973, 78, 1360.)*

in which social support was measured failed to substantiate the positive relationship between social support and compliance.[49] Caplan *et al.*[50] found that support from the spouse of patients on a hypertension-treatment regimen was associated with low levels of depression related to the health problem. Social support from other sources had no reported effect.

The importance of support from spouse was also apparent in the study by Heinzelmann and Bagley[51] of 239 men participating in a physical-exercise program. Although few men reported joining the program because of pressure from their wives, 80 percent of the men with wives exhibiting positive, supportive attitudes toward the program had good adherence. Only 40 percent of the men with wives exhibiting neutral or negative attitudes established a good record for participation in the program.

The importance of social support in facilitating health protection is also evident from the work of Pratt.[52] In studying a large group of married couples, he found that couples with traditional conjugal relationships (unequal power in decision making, strong sex-role differentiation, and low companionship) had poorer preventive health behaviors when socioeconomic status was controlled than did couples with more egalitarian conjugal relations.

A final study to be cited in this section is that of Langlie,[53] who studied the relationship between social group characteristics and direct and indirect risk behavior of individuals. Her primary concern was whether variations in preventive health behavior were a result of differences in personal health beliefs or characteristics of social groups with which the individual was affiliated. The direct risk behaviors studied were driving behavior, pedestrian behavior, smoking, and personal hygiene. The indirect risk behaviors studied were seat-belt use, medical checkups, dental care, immunization, diagnostic screening, exercise, and nutrition. The health belief variables employed in the study were perceived vulnerability, perceived benefits, perceived barriers or costs, salience of health, and attitudes toward providers. Social network variables studied were neighborhood socioeconomic status, family socioeconomic status, conjugal structure (single, egalitarian/wife works, traditional/wife does not work), kin interaction, nonkin interaction, and religious affiliation.

The Health Belief Model variables of perceived susceptibility and salience of health had little predictive power in this study. Social network variables were related to the extent of indirect risk behavior but not to direct risk behavior. Persons who were Protestant, above the mean in neighborhood and family socioeconomic status, and had frequent interaction with nonkin were more likely to have higher than average preventive health behavior related to indirect risk factors. Individuals who consistently participated in preventive behaviors related to direct and indirect risk behavior had higher socioeconomic status, interacted more frequently with nonkin, had more positive attitudes toward providers, were older, and were more likely to be female than were nonparticipants. It also appeared that individuals with social groups exhibiting norms close to that of health professionals were more likely to provide information on how to prevent disease and where to go for various health services.

While many retrospective studies have been done to determine the impact of social support on health behavior, prospective studies are needed in which networks of social support are identified and differences between health-promotion and illness-prevention behaviors are observed. The results from early studies appear promising, but additional research is needed to delineate more clearly the impact of social support on health and the salient dimensions of support that exert the greatest impact on well-being.

### Help-seeking Behavior

In studying help-seeking behavior among adults, Brown[54] observed that help seeking in coping with life stresses was the rule rather than the exception. Of the individuals in his study who sought help, 48 percent sought help from their social network, thus substantiating the importance of the lay referral system; 12 percent reported using formal systems of professional assistance; and 40 percent reported using both. Those people most likely to seek help were individuals with resources already available to them, rather than individuals with sparse resources. Those individuals who did not report seeking help with life change or crisis fell into two separate and distinct groups representing opposite ends of a continuum: (1) those who possessed the most social and psychologic resources and felt that they could handle the problem themselves and (2) those individuals with poor personal and social resources who felt that no one was available, that seeking help required too much effort, or that seeking help would draw attention to their problems and result in personal embarrassment.

It appeared that the social group was the first point of contact for help. Following contact with the social group, if further help was needed it was sought from self-help groups and/or professional care providers. Social networks of family and friends influenced the nature of help-seeking in the following ways:[55]

- They buffered the impact of stress which obviated the need for additional help.
- They precluded the need for professional assistance through provision of instrumental and affective support.
- They acted as screening and referral agents to professional services.
- They transmitted attitudes, values, and norms about help seeking.

The degree to which a target life event is perceived as stressful or threatening influences the extent of help-seeking behavior. Interestingly, help-seeking behavior decreases with age, is more prevalent among whites than among blacks, and is generally sought from family and friends, depending on the nature of the problem, before professionals are consulted. Young, well-educated, white, middle-class females are the individuals most likely to seek professional assistance when faced with a life crisis.

### Self-help Groups

This chapter would not be complete in exploring social support networks if self-help groups were not included in the discussion. While family and friends generally serve as primary sources of support, self-help groups are an important source of assistance within most communities. Examples of self-help groups include Mended Hearts, Compassionate Friends, Weight Watchers, and Physical Fitness Clubs. Characteristics of self-help groups include a critical mass sufficient to form a group, a form of publicity or recruitment to attract appropriate members, and a central goal or activity that gives the group purpose and sustains the psychologic investment of its members. The question has been raised as to why individuals use self-help groups rather than other resources such as professional services. Two hypotheses have been offered: (1) Self-help groups arise in society to fulfill a need for services not being offered, or (2) self-help groups arise because of disappointment with the inadequate assistance or lack of meaningful resources within the community.

Self-help groups have been found to share the following common characteristics:[56]

- Membership consists of those who share a common condition, situation, heritage, symptom, or life experience.
- The group is self-regulating and self-governing, emphasizing peer solidarity rather than hierarchical governance.
- Members advocate self-reliance and require intensive commitment and responsibility.
- The group has a code of precepts, beliefs, and practices.
- Members maintain a face-to-face or phone-to-phone support network.
- The more experienced members provide anticipatory guidance.
- Members provide empathy for each other.
- The group provides specific guidance in dealing with a dilemma or life problem.
- Members can suggest practical ways for handling day-to-day problems.

In studying 20 self-help groups, Levy[57] identified the following four types of self-help groups by purpose: behavioral control or conduct reorganization, stress coping and support, survival orientation, and personal growth or self-actualization. The process operating within the groups appeared to be behaviorally and cognitively oriented.

Behaviorally oriented processes included:

- Direct and vicarious social reinforcement for the development of desirable behaviors and the elimination of troublesome behaviors
- Training, indoctrination, and support in the use of various kinds of self-control behaviors
- Modeling of methods of coping with stresses and changing behaviors
- Providing members with agenda of actions they can engage in to change the social environment

Cognitively oriented processes were the following:

- Removal of members' mystification over their experience and increase expectancy for change and help by providing them with a rationale for their problems or distress and for the group's way of dealing with it
- Provision of normative and instrumental information and advice
- Expansion of the range of alternative perceptions of members' problems and circumstances and of the actions they might take to cope with their problems
- Enhancement of members' discriminative abilities regarding the stimulus and event contingencies in their lives
- Support for change in attitudes toward self, one's own behavior, and society
- Social comparison and consensual validation leading to reduction or elimination of members' uncertainty and sense of isolation or uniqueness regarding their problems and experiences
- The emergence of an alternative or substitute culture within which members can develop new definitions of their personal identity and new norms upon which they can base their self-esteem

In all, 28 different support or help-giving activities that the group used for mutual assistance of members were identified. The nine help-giving activities that were most frequently used included positive reinforcement, self-disclosure, sharing, mutual affirmation, empathy, morale building, personal goal setting, explanation, and catharsis.[58]

Self-help groups are a valuable source of support within many communities. Their records of success in assisting millions of individuals in coping with a variety of different life experiences attest to their continuing viability as an integral part of community health resources.

## ENHANCING SOCIAL SUPPORT SYSTEMS

The importance of social support for health promotion and illness prevention has been addressed within this chapter. A review of current systems is important before the identification of how an individual client's support system can be further enhanced and strengthened. General suggestions for enhancing support systems include the following:

- Increasing frequency of contact with individuals with whom the client desires stronger personal ties
- Building ties with individuals who share common life values
- Mutual goal-setting with significant others to achieve common directions in actions and efforts
- Providing additional encouragement, personal warmth, and love to significant others
- Supporting coping efforts of significant others in dealing with life experiences
- Enhancing personal identity and self-esteem of persons within support network
- Providing increased intimacy to promote self-expression

- Dealing constructively with conflict between oneself and support-group members
- Increasing reciprocity and mutality of interpersonal relationships
- Offering assistance more frequently to individuals within personal social network to show concern and promote trust
- Increasing personal capacity to accept emotional support and love
- Seeking counseling as needed to enhance marital adjustment
- Making use of self-help groups or the extended family as a source of support
- Making use of the nurse and other health professionals as community support resources
- Making use of the church or religious affiliation as a source of emotional and spiritual support
- Capitalizing on ties to a number of social groups in order to expand horizons for new growth opportunities

Many references are available in the areas of parenting, marital relationships, social assertiveness, interpersonal relationships, and self-help groups that the reader should consult for additional information on building strong bonds within social networks. A number of references appear at the end of this chapter. In attempting to enhance personal support networks, clients should be encouraged to identify specific goals to be achieved. By focusing on one or two changes at a time relevant to goals of highest priority, clients can often markedly alter the breadth and depth of social support available to them.

## SUMMARY

With the important role that social support appears to play in the health and well-being of clients, the nurse cannot provide holistic care without considering the social context within which the client resides. Social support groups appear to be highly significant in the promotion of health and in assisting clients to cope with stressful life experiences. The extent to which life change threatens well-being and health may well depend to a large extent on the support available from significant others. Additional research is needed in order to understand more fully the mechanisms underlying the structural and buffering functions of social support groups in relation to human health.

## REFERENCES

1.  Brim, J. Social network correlates of avowed happiness. *Journal of Nervous and Mental Disease*, 1974, *158*,432–439.
2.  Tolsdorf, C. Social networks, support and coping: An exploratory study. *Family Process*, 1976, *15*,407–417.
3.  Liem, R., & Liem, J. Social class and mental illness reconsidered: The role of eco-

nomic stress and social support. *Journal of Health and Social Behavior,* June 1978, *19,*139–156.

4. Bott, E. *Family and social networks.* London: Tavistock, 1971.
5. Brim, *op. cit.,* p. 434.
6. Walker, K.N., MacBride, A., & Vachon, M.L.S. Social support networks and bereavement. *Social Science and Medicine,* 1977, *11,*35–41.
7. Tolsdorf, *op. cit.,* p. 408.
8. *Ibid.*
9. Moss, G.E. *Immunity and social interaction.* New York: Wiley, 1973.
10. Walker, MacBride, & Vachon, *op. cit.,* pp. 35–37.
11. Cobb, S. Social support as a moderator of life stress. *Psychosomatic Medicine,* 1976, *38,*300–314.
12. Liem & Liem, *op. cit.,* pp. 139–156.
13. Lieberman, M.A., & Borman, L.D. *Self help groups for coping with crisis.* San Francisco: Jossey-Bass, 1979.
14. Chen, E., & Cobb, S. Family structure in relation to health and disease. *Journal of Chronic Diseases,* 1960, *12,*544–567.
15. Brown, G., Birley, J., & Wing, J. Influence of family life on the course of schizophrenic disorders: A replication. *British Journal of Psychiatry,* 1972, *121,*241–258.
16. Antonovesky, A. Conceptual and methodological problems in the study of resistance resources and stressful life events. In Dohrenwend, B.S., & Dohrenwend, B.P. (Eds.), *Stressful life events: Their nature and effects.* New York: Wiley, 1974, pp. 245–258.
17. Brown, B. Social and psychological correlates of help seeking behavior among urban adults. *American Journal of Community Psychology,* 1978, *6,*425–439.
18. Lin, N., Ensel, W.M., Simeone, R.S., & Wen, K. Social support, stressful life events and illness: A model and an empirical test. *Journal of Health and Social Behavior,* June 1979, *20,*108–119.
19. Brown, G. Meaning, measurement and stress of life events. In Dohrenwend, B.S., & Dohrenwend, B.P. (Eds.), *Stressful life events: Their nature and effects.* New York: Wiley, 1974, pp. 217–243.
20. Dohrenwend, B.S. Social status and stressful life events. *Journal of Personality and Social Psychology,* 1973, *28,*222–235.
21. Caplan, G. *Support systems and community mental health: Lectures on concept development.* New York: Behavioral Publications, 1974, p. 7.
22. *Ibid.,* p. 5.
23. McKinley, J.B. Social networks, lay consultation and help-seeking behavior. *Social Forces,* March 1973, *51,*275–292.
24. Baker, G.W., & Chapman, D.W. *Man and social disaster.* New York: Basic Books, 1962, p. 212.
25. Petroni, F. Significant others and sick role behavior: A much neglected sick role contingency. *Sociological Quarterly,* Winter 1969, *10,*32–41.
26. Liem & Liem, *op. cit.,* p. 151.
27. Glaser, B., & Kirschenbaum, H. Using values clarification in a counseling setting. *Personnel and Guidance Journal,* May 1980, *59,*569–575.
28. Simon, S.B., Howe, L.W., & Kirschenbaum, H. *Values clarification: A handbook of practical strategies for teachers and students.* New York: Hart, 1972.
29. Caplan, R.D., Robinson, E.A., & French, J.R. *Adhering to medical regimens: Pilot experiments in patient education and support.* Ann Arbor: Research Center for Group Dynamics, Institute for Social Research, University of Michigan, 1976.
30. Nuckolls, K.B. *Psychosocial assets, life crisis and the prognosis of pregnancy.* Doctoral dissertation, University of North Carolina at Chapel Hill, 1970. *Dissertation Abstracts International,* 1970, *31,* 2796B. (University Microfilms No. 70-21, 219)
31. Nuckolls, K.B. Psychosocial assets, life crisis and the prognosis of pregnancy. *American Journal of Epidemiology,* 1972, *95,*431–441.

32. Brim, *op. cit.,* pp. 432–439.
33. Lowenthal, M.F., & Haven, C. Interaction and adaptation: Intimacy as a critical variable. *American Sociological Review,* 1968, *33,*20–30.
34. Blau, Z.S. *Old age in a changing society.* New York: New Viewpoints, 1973.
35. Walker, MacBride, & Vachon, *op. cit.,* pp. 35–41.
36. Nuckolls, 1970, *op. cit.*
37. Gore, S. The effect of social support in moderating the health consequences of unemployment. *Journal of Health and Social Behavior,* 1978, *19,*157–165.
38. Moss, G.E. *Immunity and social interaction.* New York: Wiley, 1973.
39. de Araujo, G., van Arsdel, P.P., Holmes, T.H., & Dudley, D.L. Life change, coping ability and chronic intrinsic asthma. *Journal of Psychosomatic Research,* 1973, *17,*359–363.
40. Holmes, T., & Masuda, M. Life change and illness susceptibility. In Dohrenwend, B.S., & Dohrenwend, B.P. (Eds.), *Stressful life events: Their nature and effects.* New York: Wiley, 1974.
41. Rahe, R. Subjects' recent life changes and their near-future illness reports: A review. *Annals of Clinical Research,* 1972, *4,*393–397.
42. Meyers, J., Lindenthal, J., & Pepper, M. Life events and psychiatric impairment. *Journal of Nervous and Mental Disease,* 1971, *152,*149–157.
43. Vinokur, A., & Selzer, M. Desirable versus undesirable life events: Their relationship to stress and mental distress. *Journal of Personality and Social Psychology,* 1975, *32,*329–337.
44. Dohrenwend, B.S., & Dohrenwend, B.P. (Eds.). *Stressful life events: Their nature and effects.* New York: Wiley, 1974.
45. Schwab, J., & Schwab, R. The epidemiology of mental illness. Paper presented at the American College of Psychiatrists, Sixth Annual Seminar for Continuing Education of Psychiatrists, New Orleans, 1973.
46. Tolsdorf, *op. cit.,* pp. 412–417.
47. Lin *et al., op. cit.,* pp. 111–119.
48. Walker *et al., op. cit.,* p. 36.
49. Haynes, R.B., & Sackett, D.L. *A workshop/symposium: Compliance with therapeutic regimens—Annotated bibliography.* Department of Clinical Epidemiology and Biostatistics, McMaster University Medical Center, Hamilton, Ontario, 1974.
50. Caplan *et al., op. cit.,* p. 6.
51. Heinzelmann, F., & Bagley, R.W. Response to physical activity programs and their effects on health behavior. *Public Health Reports,* 1970, *85,*905–911.
52. Pratt, L. Conjugal organization and health. *Journal of Marriage and the Family,* 1972, *2,*85–95.
53. Langlie, J.K. Social networks, health beliefs and preventive health behavior. *Journal of Health and Social Behavior,* September 1977, *18,*244–260.
54. Brown, B. Predicting patterns of help-seeking in coping with stress in adulthood. Doctoral dissertation, University of Chicago, 1979. (Unpublished.)
55. Lieberman & Borman, *op. cit.,* p. 121.
56. *Ibid.,* p. 14.
57. Levy, L. Processes and activities in groups. In Lieberman, M.A., & Borman, L.D. (Eds.), *Self help group for coping with crisis.* San Francisco: Jossey-Bass, 1979.
58. *Ibid.,* pp. 260–263.

# Part IV
# SOCIOPOLITICAL STRATEGIES FOR PREVENTION AND HEALTH PROMOTION

Changes in individual behavior must be complemented by changes in group health practices and changes in the environment if personal health is to be maximized. The importance of altering collective behavior and the environment to support personal health practices will be discussed in Chapter 14. Social change can expand the range of health-protecting and health-promoting behaviors available to clients and decrease opportunities for health-damaging behavior. The extent to which social change can be imposed is an important ethical question that must be considered. However, failure to work for a better society and environment in which to live results in "victim blaming" and frustration for persons seriously attempting to achieve improved personal lifestyles.

In Chapter 15 economic issues related to illness prevention and health promotion will be discussed. Costs and benefits are critical factors to consider in the delivery of all types of health services. Studies relevant to the potential cost effectiveness of illness-prevention and health-promotion efforts will be presented.

Finally, the major ideas proposed in the book will be summarized in Chapter 16, and productive directions for the future will be charted. The need for further research to test the descriptive models of health-protecting behavior (Health Belief and Modified Health Belief Models) and health-promoting behavior (Health Promotion Model) will also be addressed.

# CHAPTER 14
# Illness Prevention and Health Promotion Through Social and Environmental Change

Health is both an individual and a social responsibility. Personal change in and of itself may be only partially effective in improving health status without concomitant changes in the social, organizational, and environmental circumstances in which people live. It is becoming increasingly apparent that both behavioral and environmental factors play a role in the etiology of major chronic health problems. Since personal health practices are only one of the determinants of health, a comprehensive approach to health promotion requires that attention be given to the environmental, cultural, and social constraints imposed on clients in their quest for health. Personal health services must be coordinated with national and local community health initiatives in order to deal effectively with problems that threaten human health or retard movement toward more desirable health states.

The possible choices that a client can make and the range of health behaviors available are dependent on the values of the society in which he or she lives, as well as on personal knowledge, values, and attitudes. As indicated in the proposed Health Promotion Model, expectations of significant others within the community, family patterns of behavior, health-promoting options available, and prior experience with health-promoting options all influence or modify predisposition to engage in health-related behaviors. In addition, barriers to health-promoting actions as well as cues for specific health behaviors often arise from the external environment. Therefore, any strategy for health promotion that focuses only on individual behavior change will be doomed to failure without simultaneous efforts to alter collective behavior and the environment.

Vuori[1] has commented on the importance of developing a "value atmosphere" within society that allows the use of societal means such as legislation,

**367**

production policies, and price control to influence the health behavior of populations positively. In order to accomplish this, it is his belief that health education must be an integral part of the educational system of the nation as well as a service offered within the health care system. Internalization of positive health values occurs most effectively during early childhood, long before the medical care system has made much, if any, significant educational impact on the individual. Therefore, parents, early socialization groups, and the educational system bear the major responsibility for health teaching. It is only as values change toward increased priority for health among large segments of society that an environment can be created that supports choices conducive to health-promoting life patterns rather than health-damaging lifestyles.

The intricate interplay between the individual and society in the quest for health was well stated in a paper presented by Gustave Weigel[2] at the Center for the Study of Democratic Institutions in 1958:

> *Man is not for society but society for man. This does not mean that society exists to grant man the objects of his caprice and uncriticized impulses. The individual has rights which society cannot nullify, and the commonwealth has rights which it cannot abdicate. All historical malaise comes from the failure of either the individual to respect the rights of the collectivity, or the collectivity's tyrannical suppression of the rights of the individual.*

The mutuality that exists between the efforts of individuals and society in promoting health mandates a multidimensional approach to improving the health status of any population. Health-promotion efforts within the larger society can support and enhance personal health behaviors by increasing the range of health-promoting options available, by decreasing opportunities for health-damaging behaviors, and by assisting the public to discern the difference between them. It is this larger arena of social and environmental factors that the present chapter will address. Primary focus will be given to interpersonal and situational factors that impact on personal health care as well as to barriers and cues within the environment that influence health behaviors.

## COMMUNITY APPROACHES TO CHANGING BEHAVIOR

The realities of the home, work, and community environments must be dealt with in developing prevention and health-promotion programs directed at lifestyle change. The reference groups and environment in which individuals live out their daily existence can either support or inhibit personal protective/promotive-health efforts. Given the high potential for impact of significant others and the social collective on individual behavior, a number of arguments can be made for community-based programs. The strengths of such programs include the following:[3]

*Permit the development of programs that are applicable to the "real world" in which people live.*

*Increase intervention power due to enhanced opportunity for diffusion and social support.*

*Allow the development of programs with wider impact than services targeted to individuals or small groups in circumscribed clinical settings.*

*Reduce costs.*

*Permit conclusions to be drawn through program evaluation that are applicable to populations with a wide range of demographic characteristics.*

The theoretical S-curve of diffusion of a new health practice resulting from community intervention is compared with the usual individual adoption curve in Figure 14-1. The benefits of altering collective behavior can be seen in examining

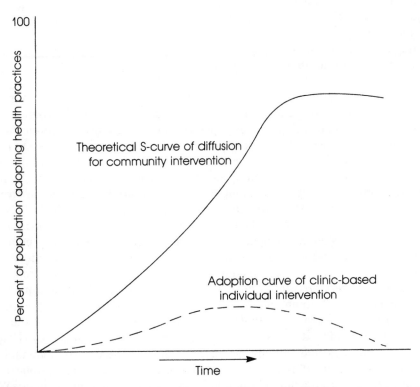

**FIGURE 14-1.** Comparison of the theoretical S-curve of diffusion through community-directed intervention with the usual adoption curve of clinic-based individual intervention. *(From Farquhar, J.W. The community-based model of life style intervention trials. American Journal of Epidemiology, August 1978, 108, 103–111.)*

the effectiveness of some mass immunization programs. Expectations of others regarding appropriate maternal behavior in seeing that children are immunized against major infectious diseases may be more responsible for a high level of participation than actual fear of illness or disability from lack of immunization. Ubel[4] has stressed the ultimate impact of even a 3- to 5-percent population change per year in any specific health practice. This rate of change is sufficient to create a social milieu supportive of the "target practice" within only a few years, since there is accelerating social pressure for the desired behavior to become modal. Positive group influences can be effectively used in community programs.

Community-based programs currently exist in a variety of areas within prevention and health promotion. These include:[5]

- Accident prevention
- Early detection of disabilities among children
- Immunization
- Case finding and contact investigation (communicable diseases)
- Substance abuse control
- Suicide prevention
- Family planning
- Industrial hygiene and occupational health
- Environmental sanitation and pollution control

While many of the above programs have been in existence for some time, increasing attention is being given to the cost effectiveness of such programs, and their impact on the health status of populations is being closely scrutinized.

Community programs for risk reduction and lifestyle change represent recent community initiatives. By and large these programs are experimental in nature and are available in a very limited number of geographic areas. The Stanford Three-Community Study is an example of a community-based program directed at risk modification.[6] This program, which was targeted on reducing risk for cardiovascular disease, is described in detail in Chapter 7. Use of the mass media (e.g., radio, television, newspapers, and direct mail) in providing health education about risk factors and ways of reducing risk was the major mode of intervention applied in the study. Two communities served as the experimental groups and one community served as the control. Groups of high-risk individuals within each of the experimental communities were also given face-to-face intervention or personalized health teaching. Follow-up studies indicated that use of the mass media had resulted in decreased risk in the experimental communities (15 to 20 percent), while risk had actually increased slightly in the control community (7 percent). Estimation of risk was based on plasma cholesterol, systolic blood pressure, weight, frequency of smoking, and electrocardiogram findings. While some changes were apparent in the level of dietary fat intake, the change in level of risk appeared to be a result primarily of the rate of smoking cessation. Men receiving face-to-face instruction in addition to mass media were slightly more successful in reducing risk than were individuals who received mass media intervention only.

The results of the Stanford Three-Community Study support the potential effectiveness of community-based programs in altering collective and individual behavior. The social group dynamics that played a part in the success of the program need to be analyzed carefully in order to provide greater insight into the support and diffusion effects of community-based efforts in prevention and health promotion.

In a related study, Miller and Cantor[7] examined the effectiveness of differing forms of mass media in disseminating health information on cancer, substance abuse, and sickle cell anemia to a target community. The study was conducted in 1978 in a county in South Carolina. A preliminary survey of exposure to mass media within the geographic area indicated that 95 to 97 percent of the residents owned a radio; 97 to 100 percent owned a television; and 78 to 97 percent read the newspaper. In the community survey, which followed repeated presentation of educational material via all three forms of mass media, residents were queried concerning receipt of the health education information. Findings indicated that overall the newspaper was the most effective means of disseminating information about all three major health problems. In exploring patterns of dissemination of information regarding each of the major diseases, differences were noted. In small towns as opposed to urban areas, television was more effective than either radio or newspaper in disseminating information about cancer prevention. In providing information about substance abuse, newspaper and television were superior to radio throughout the county. However, information about sickle cell anemia was more frequently acquired from the newspaper or radio than from television. Interesting differences also emerged based on race. Black participants received information on all three health problems more frequently on radio than did white participants, indicating differential patterns of exposure to mass media.

The results of this study emphasize the importance of population characteristics in determining the most effective program of information dissemination within a community. The most effective approach, of course, is to use all three mass media if monies permit. However, if this is not possible, careful attention to lifestyle patterns and use of mass media by the target population is critical in order to maximize potential for altering collective and individual behavior through health education efforts. Pilot surveys preceding major community campaigns are essential for accurate assessment of potential program impact.

## EXPANDING CHOICES AND BEHAVIORAL OPTIONS

Knowledge of the need for lifestyle change and actual changes made often do not coincide. Thus, knowing is not directly related to doing. Limits in choice of health-promoting options may be perceived or real. For example, an individual does not control personal reactions to environmental stress because he or she believes that control of neuroendocrine changes and levels of muscle tension is not possible. In reality, such control is possible, but beliefs in lack of control create perceptual barriers. On the other hand, a worker near retirement with years of seniority and repeated exposure to asbestos may be unable to transfer to another job without loss of pension and social security benefits. Options for working in an occupational environment with decreased health hazards are limited by economic and social constraints representing a real barrier.

Limited health-promoting choices are encountered frequently in circumstances of everyday living. The cafeteria or vending machine areas in work settings frequently offer few options for adequate nutrition intake. Cigarettes are readily available in vending machines, but finding a vending machine with fresh fruits may be impossible. Bars and saloons abound on every corner in most towns and cities, yet finding an intimate environment in which fruit juices or low-calorie, caffeine-free, nourishing drinks are served is difficult. Many of the habitual behaviors that threaten health are an institutionalized part of the American way of living; consider the morning sweet roll, the candy bar, and soft drinks. To exaggerate the problem, frequently health-damaging options are not only more readily accessible but also more attractively packaged and less costly than health-promoting options.

Milio[8] contends that health-damaging options are even more accessible in relation to health-promoting options among low-income groups than among groups with higher levels of income:

> *Low-income Americans are not only more vulnerable to acute disease relative to their affluent counterparts, but also sustain more of the chronic degenerative illnesses and accidents which are integral to the affluence of the wider society. The cigarettes, sucrose, cars, pollutants and tensions are readily available to the poor, while at the same time they are deprived of the level of protection afforded by the quality of food, shelter and environment which sustain the more affluent.*

Both individuals and organizations make choices based on cost versus actual or perceived gain. Perceptions of gain are often present-oriented; little attention is given to future consequences. For example, the cessation of smoking may be perceived as more painful than the benefit of having healthy lungs 15 to 25 years hence. For industry, the profit available from the manufacture of tobacco products appears to offset their potential lethal affects. The essence of a capitalistic society is to maximize gain and minimize loss. Thus, the accumulation of valued resources—often but not necessarily monetary rewards—provides powerful profit motivation irrespective of the personal or societal health risks involved in the long run.

In discussing the impact of industry on personal health options, Navarro[9] has pointed out the limited control available to many workers over their occupational environment and thus over their own personal health. Eighty percent of Americans have little control over the setting in which they work, since actual control of work environments is in the hands of 5 percent of the population that own 75 percent of organized industry and business. This 5 percent exerts an overwhelming amount of influence over economic and political institutions because of the capital they control. Problems that are collectively and politically caused cannot be solved solely by personal health services or self-reliance. Since disease is partly a collective and political phenomenon, it requires a collective and political response.[10]

Milio[11] has presented six propositions that place personal choice making in the context of societal option setting. These propositions emphasize the importance of the social context in achieving major changes in health status for a significant proportion of any target population. The propositions are as follows:

1. The health status of populations is the result of deprivation and/or excess of critical health-sustaining resources.
2. Behavioral patterns of populations are a result of habitual selection from limited choices, and these habits of choice are related to (a) actual and perceived options available and (b) beliefs and expectations developed and refined over time by socialization, formal learning, and immediate experience.
3. Organizational behavior (decisions or policy choices made by governmental/ nongovernmental, national/nonnational; nonprofit/for profit, formal/nonformal organizations) sets the range of options available to individuals for personal choice making.
4. The choice making of individuals at a given point in time concerning potentially health-promoting or health-damaging selections is affected by their efforts to maximize valued resources.
5. Social change may be thought of as changes in patterns of behavior resulting from shifts in the choice making of significant numbers of people within a population.
6. Health education, as the process of teaching and learning health-supporting information, can have little significantly extensive impact on behavior patterns, that is, on personal choice-making groups of people, without the easy availability of new, or newly perceived, alternative health-promoting options for investing personal resources.

The American population experiences many chronic illnesses that are partially caused by excesses or deprivation. Many of these illnesses are unrelated to socioeconomic status, while others are clearly more prevalent in low-income groups. Malnutrition is a good example. It is prevalent at all socioeconomic levels but for different reasons. Malnutrition among the affluent results from consumption of calorie-rich, nutrient-poor foods that have popular appeal or are convenient to eat or prepare. Individuals and families that can afford to eat frequently in restaurants where food costs are high often consume nutrient-poor meals that are cost effective for restaurants to offer. Food eaten outside the home is likely to be high in fat and simple carbohydrates but low in protein, complex carbohydrates, vitamins, and minerals. Lower socioeconomic groups are often malnourished because of deprivation due to inability to purchase nutritious foods with limited resources. In addition, low-income individuals may not fully understand how to invest their food dollar for maximum nutritional quality.

Patterns of eating behavior within the family of orientation also enter into choices among health-related options. Because of the creation of preferences for convenient, high-carbohydrate, high-fat foods, as opposed to more nourishing ones, health may be threatened. It becomes a vicious cycle, with even the limited monies available spent for "junk foods," which individuals have learned to prefer and which provide a sense of immediate gratification.

If individuals act out of habit or feel "powerless" in controlling their environment, they will continue to limit personal options even when a broader range of options actually becomes available. The person who purchases a sweet roll every morning during coffee break is often unlikely to purchase a granola bar or a package of raisins even if those options are available, unless he or she is convinced of the personal advantages of the change. The factory worker who can purchase coffee at minimal cost is unlikely, because of limited resources, to purchase milk or fruit juice as snacks during the day. American society offers many illustrations of how, through socialization, individuals and groups have come to prefer health-damaging rather than health-promoting habits and patterns. Social groups can serve as strong reinforcers of many undesirable health habits.

The importance of organizational behavior in setting the range of options available to individuals cannot be overly stressed. Resistance of industry to the control of toxic substances to minimize hazards to the health of workers is readily apparent in organizational responses to government regulatory action. Many law suits have been filed by industries against the Environmental Protection Agency (EPA) to show technical defects in the laws and thus negate the need for compliance with federal regulations. As a result, despite the passage of numerous laws, the EPA has set permanent standards for only four hazardous air pollutants (vinyl chloride, asbestos, beryllium, and mercury) and six toxic water pollutants in its 9 years of existence.[12]

Organizational control of advertising, production, and pricing policies sets the parameters of choice for many Americans. Advertising appeals to the emotions, priorities, preferences, and even self-concept of many Americans. Influential, attractive, and successful people are used to promote products that are actually health damaging or that divert resources away from more desirable purchases that are health promoting. Control of production dictates the products and related services that will be available for purchase and the extent of safety of those products. The current campaign to promote the safety of toys manufactured for children is evidence of the need for continuing efforts to insure that the products offered to the public are safe and not detrimental to health. Another vivid example of the impact of production on individual behavior is in auto safety. Even with reduced speed limits of 55 miles per hour, cars made to go 120 miles per hour will be driven at that speed by irresponsible individuals. With lowered speed limits and interest in fuel conservation, cars of lower horsepower are beginning to appear on the market.

Milio[13] has proposed that choice-making behavior at any point in time reflects individual efforts to maximize valued resources. The "value atmosphere or hierarchy" characteristic of the society or a particular segment of society within which the individual resides will determine those resources that are valued and consequently maximized. Some values are characteristic of all societies, e.g., the values of survival, safety, security, and self-esteem. Other values may assume differing importance. For instance, within the United States, "success" is highly valued and is inculcated in children as a value early in life. Health has been less frequently taught to children as an important value since health often is viewed as an enabling factor rather than an important end in itself. That is, good health enables the individuals to pursue values that represent more important life goals. Any society that is to markedly change the health status of its people must see health as a primary value rather than as a secondary goal. If health is seen as an important resource to be maximized, significant changes will occur in values, self-care practices, and choice-making behavior among large segments of the population.

In the interest of energy conservation or out of habit, most individuals select the most convenient and accessible options to meet their needs at any point in time. Milio[14] proposes that health-promoting choices be made easier and health-damaging options more difficult. For instance, in restaurants and in grocery stores, nourishing foods should be the norm rather than the exception. Most restaurants have only one low-calorie option and fast-food restaurants generally none. Grocery stores offer shelf after shelf of nutritiously "empty" foods and a smaller number of high-protein, high-fiber, high-vitamin, and mineral options. When nutritious food products are offered, they are generally priced higher than the food products low in nutrients. Making nutritious foods more readily accessible and lower in cost increases the probability of health-promoting choices.

Once health-promoting options become more available, they must be accepted and approved by referent groups within society (the relevant collectives) in order to make individual health-promoting choices easier. Not only convenience and availability of health-promoting options but also their social acceptance will create expectations for healthier lifestyles.

Interested lay individuals, concerned health professionals, and informed health policy makers are essential for constructive social change supportive of health and well-being. Social or structural change within any society consists of a number of phases. Each phase requires different strategies in order to bring that phase to successful completion. The phases are not always mutually exclusive and sequential in their occurrence, but all must occur before social change is clearly evident. The phases are as follows:

1. Social awareness or increased sensitization to an existing problem on the part of a significant portion of the population
2. Acknowledgment of the threat posed by the problem to individual health and general welfare
3. Preliminary (pilot) attempts to decrease the societal impact of the problem (takes into account relevant knowledge and economic and political factors)

4. Evaluation of the success of problem-solving protocols
5. Organization or reorganization within society to deal with the problem
6. Dissemination (voluntary or mandatory) of rules, regulations, and procedures throughout society for solving the problem
7. Resolution of the societal problem through organizational change
8. Continued monitoring of problem status to maintain or augment resolution

Individual behavior change occurs gradually, but organizational behavior change proceeds at an even slower pace. The bureaucracy inherent in organizational structures, resistance from vested interest groups and monetary expenditures required for change all retard progress. Continual prodding and sustained efforts are required of groups attempting to make social changes relevant to health in order to accomplish specific health-promoting goals.

## ENVIRONMENTAL CONTROL

The chemical environment in which Americans live is primarily controlled by organizations rather than by individuals. While individuals can control their own use of food additives, pest-control substances, and aerosol sprays, the majority of chemicals are encountered within the larger environment. For example, one in four Americans is exposed to health hazards on the job while at least one million workers are exposed to carcinogenic substances.[15] Four million workers contract occupational diseases every year, and 100,000 annually die from them.[16]

Higginson[17] has addressed the importance of environmental factors in the etiology of human cancer. Currently, exogenous and environmental stimuli are considered to play a role in at least 30 to 40 percent of human cancers within the United States. In industrialized societies it is unknown to what extent material gain has been associated with unforeseen environmental hazards.

Current cancer patterns represent reactions to substances present in the environment 20 to 50 years ago, often making the exact substance(s) responsible for the development of cancer hard to identify. Reactions of human populations to newly manufactured chemicals will only be evident after years of continuing exposure. While animal studies provide some useful information about toxicity, reactions of human populations may differ from laboratory findings. Examples of cancers thought to be partially caused by the cultural, occupational, or physical environment include the following:

> *Lung cancer* — smoking (cultural environment), asbestos (occupational contaminant), side stream smoke, and air pollution (physical environment)
>
> *Esophageal and liver cancer* — excessive drinking (cultural environment) exaggerated by occupational environment, e.g., exposure to specific chemicals associated with liver pathology
>
> *Skin cancer* — excessive exposure to sun without adequate protection

(cultural environment, e.g., looking tan, and occupational environment, e.g., farming)

*Colon cancer* — exposure to high fat content in diet, low fiber, and charcoal-broiled meats (cultural environment)[18]

While the above associations have not been based on experimental studies with human populations, strong epidemiologic evidence exists for such links.

Cancers clearly of occupational origin appear to represent at least 5 to 7 percent of all tumors in industrialized states. Not only do workers suffer exposure in the immediate environment, but industrial chemicals have become widespread in the general environment, resulting in higher than anticipated exposures on the part of large populations. It is unknown to what extent the presence of a wide variety of chemicals of industrial origin in the general environment is responsible for nonoccupationally related cancers. Information on human health effects of long-term exposure to low levels of air pollution is crucial for the establishment of rational standards for air pollutants. The effects of interaction of pollutants must also be considered.[19] For instance, exposure to asbestos appears to potentiate the carcinogenic effects of cigarettes. See Table 14-1 for data on this interaction.

In looking at environmental control from an even broader perspective, the EPA estimates that fully one-third of the 1500 active ingredients in pesticides are toxic, although only five are restricted. In the matter of toxic substances alone, every week new threats or side effects of toxic substances are discovered that were not previously suspected. Adequate testing procedures are not currently available for determining the full extent of toxic effects of many substances, nor are adequate laws available that require the testing of products and technologies that go on the market to make sure that they are safe before there is wide distribution and use.[20]

It has been estimated by the EPA that 20 percent of the 70,000 chemicals in commercial use are carcinogens. For example, cadmium, which is not yet regulated, has been linked to birth defects, cancer, and damage to kidneys and liver. Cadmium is discharged into sewage systems from electroplating and rubber tire industries (from deteriorating tires) and poses a threat to water supplies. Of the recommended limits for 100 chemicals proposed by the National Institute for Occupational Safety and Health (NIOSH), only 23 have been promulgated. Bureaucracy and industrial pressures retard the process, making it difficult to take statutory mandates into implementation.[21]

With an incidence of cancer at 300 per 100,000 per year, or one in four Americans during their lifetime, control of environmental carcinogens is critical. It is interesting to note that in migrants, the cancer pattern of the adopted country becomes apparent during that individual's lifetime or at the latest in the second generation. While individual susceptibility of racial or genetic origin to specific cancers cannot be ruled out, it appears highly likely that environmental factors play a strong role in causation. With deaths from malignant neoplasms much lower in other countries than in the United States, attention must be given to the potential health-damaging effects that accompany industrialization.

**TABLE 14-1   CALCULATIONS ON RELATIVE IMPORTANCE OF RISK FACTORS FOR
CANCER OCCURRING IN A POPULATION OF 100 MILLION MALES IN A YEAR\***

|  | Incidence per $10^5$ | Number of Cases Observed | Relative Risk Ratio Assumed |
|---|---|---|---|
| **Lung Cancer** | | | |
| Nonsmokers (say 30% of population) | 8 | 2,500 | 1 |
| General population (including smokers and nonsmokers) | 60 | 60,000 | 7 |
| All smokers (say 70% of population) | 85 | 57,000 | 10 |
| Heavy smokers (say 25% of population) | 130 | 32,500 | 15 |
| Nonsmoking asbestos† workers (assuming 10,000 persons at risk) | 16 | 2.4 | 2 |
| Smoking asbestos workers (assuming 30,000 persons at risk) | 560 | 210 | 70 |
| **Angiosarcoma** | | | |
| General population | 0.014 | 30 | 1 |
| Vinyl chloride workers (assuming 20,000 persons at risk) | 6‡ | 1.2 | 400 |

\*Calculations are based on relative ratio studies and should only be regarded as an approximation
of the situation in a modern industrial society. Calculations that include comparative risks would
not, however, modify the overall conclusions, although they might affect the individual figures.
†At present insufficient data are available to compare cancer ratios in nonsmoking asbestos
workers with nonsmoking controls, but for illustrative purposes a relative risk of 2 has been assumed.
‡Based on very small figures.
From Higginson, J. A hazardous society? Individual versus community responsibility in cancer prevention. *American Journal of Public Health*, April 1976, *66*, 359–366. With permission.

Control of environmental hazards demands not only the actions of legislative
bodies and organized industry and business but also the efforts and collaboration
of an informed public. Therefore, accurate information about risks should be made
available to the public as soon as possible and expressed in a clear and concise
way. This will enable individuals to decide to what extent a particular hazard or
activity accelerates or retards the occurrence of cancer and other chronic diseases.
It is only as the public becomes an organized collective (or a number of collectives), that major changes will be made in regard to cultural, occupational, and
physical environments to improve the quality of life and health for all.

## VOLUNTARY CHANGE VERSUS LEGISLATIVE POLICY

It has been stated that matters that benefit survival and security are predominantly subject to regulatory decisions while matters where risks are not clearly vital to general health and welfare are issues for personal decision and action. In our society, even vital risks may be left to individual decision, providing that they do not infringe on the rights of others. The question can be posed as to what government's role is in legislating environmental and behavioral changes that promote good health and increased longevity. If the government uses the means at its disposal for regulating changes in behavior it may be faced with problems of an ethical nature. On the other hand, education and individualized approaches may fall short in widely inducing changes in self-damaging behaviors.

Government involvement in lifestyle reform is to some extent supported by the long-standing role of the federal government as a health care provider. Faced with the costs of almost insatiable demands for health care, it could be cost effective for the government to consider legislation that required individuals to assume more self-care responsibility. While such federal regulations might be cost effective if health-promotion interventions are shown to substantially reduce health care costs, many individuals would resist legislation of preventive and health-promotion measures as unethical or undue intrusion upon individual freedom. Ethical issues, including individual autonomy, must be thoughtfully considered in matters of health.

It is clear that emphasis on individual responsibility for health without social support for the necessary changes may present even greater ethical dilemmas. Crawford[22] has stressed the importance of avoiding approaches to prevention and health promotion that cultivate a "blame the victim" attitude in health care services or policy decisions. Such a dilemma could occur if focus was primarily shifted to the need for changes in individual lifestyles without careful examination of societal and environmental factors that affect individual and family health behavior. Concern has been expressed that the focusing of attention on the health-damaging effects of individual lifestyles will distract the government from examining other health threats such as unsafe work conditions, environmental health hazards, and social and commercial determinants of injurious behavior.

Legislation of healthful patterns of living is not new. Various public health and labor laws with that intent have been in existence for hundreds of years. Without constructive health policy that requires prohibitions and negative sanctions as well as mandates for desired behaviors, the health of the public would be markedly endangered. Where should the line be drawn between voluntary efforts/incentives and regulation? Green[23] has suggested the following guidelines for such a decision:

1. To the extent that behavior is only a risk to the individual, incentives should be used to change behavior.
2. To the extent that behavior threatens the health of others, regulations rather than incentives should be used to change behavior.

Public participation in the decision about what to regulate is critical in order to prevent decisions for coercion without adequate representation of the public. The public bears the ultimate responsibility as a collective to facilitate environmental and societal changes conducive to health. It is for this reason that health and health-related legislation should be promulgated and written so that it can be understood by average citizens and their elected representatives. Legislation should be based on the public's understanding of facts, not on emotion.

While government regulation is sometimes deemed necessary for the public good, self-direction is valued by Americans because most individuals believe that they themselves are the best judge of what is good for them, and the process of choosing is considered a good in itself even when the outcomes are health-damaging. Some persons may voluntarily opt for a brief life span full of unhealthy practices. It can be argued that if the practices are nondetrimental to others and carried out in full awareness of the consequences, these people should be allowed to pursue the course they want. However, the role of society is to make sure that individuals have as much information as possible on which to base informed decisions concerning life style and health related behavior. Approaches to maintaining social conditions that support informed and voluntary choice include the following:[24]

- Make sure that individuals and groups are well aware of the consequences of their acts and the extent to which given behaviors are health promoting or health damaging.
- Create conditions in which health-related decisions can be made free from social or commercial manipulation.
- Structure situations for choice making in which individuals are not under severe mental stress or compulsion.
- Prevent undue external constraints on individual choice making.

Before resorting to government regulation, voluntary approaches to behavior change should be considered. If individuals are informed about specific health-promoting or health-damaging behaviors through mass media or other approaches to health education, they may engage in self-regulating behavior in sufficient numbers to decrease the incidence of a particular health problem. Voluntary control programs can also be offered that provide incentives for health-promoting behaviors as opposed to health-damaging behaviors. One type of incentive program that is becoming increasingly widespread is the company-sponsored fitness program as a fringe benefit for employees and families. Rolm Corporation in Santa Clara, California, offers a recreational facility for its 2000 workers; it consists of two racquetball-handball courts, an exercise room, a game room, a sauna, a steam bath, two pools, a volleyball court, two lighted tennis courts, a basketball half-court, an 800-yard track, and an exercise course. Prudential Insurance Company in Houston has a quarter-mile jogging track on the roof to complement an indoor exercise room.

Noel Fenton, the president of Acurex Corporation in Mountain View, California, states that potential employees are more impressed by a gym, tennis courts, and swimming pool than by other fringe benefits. A 43-year-old machinist at Goodyear Tire and Rubber Company in Akron, Ohio, believes that the gym and sports program are the best fringe benefits that he has. He states that if one can keep fit and keep oneself from having health problems, it is a lot better benefit than having hospital care paid for after one becomes ill.[25]

Other types of incentives include paying employees by the mile to walk or jog. Hospital Corporation of American in Nashville pays exercisers by the mile: 16 cents for runners and walkers, 4 cents for bicyclists and 64 cents for swimmers. Employees at Schwartz Meat Company in Norman, Oklahoma, can earn up to a month's extra pay per year if both husband and wife participate in a fitness plan. Cropnell[26] has provided information on a safety initiative program within the Harvester's Farmall Tractor Plant in Rock Island, Illinois. Each time that the company reaches a million manhours without an accident, gifts are given to every employee. Along with tangible rewards has gone a comprehensive educational program in occupational safety.

Such incentive programs within industry offer a means of changing collective health behavior. Not only is there an incentive to perform safely on the job and stay physically fit, but there is also motivation to see that fellow workers or family engage in similar behaviors. Peer pressure and the support of the work collective appear to be successful approaches to sustaining individual health behaviors.

If voluntary efforts at behavior change fail and the health and welfare of large groups of individuals are at stake, legislation or government regulation may be necessary. Behavior changes to be legislated should be ethically evaluated before the formulation and enactment of relevant legislation. The primary goals of legislated health behavior reform include the following:[27]

> *Maintenance and improvement of the general welfare*
> *Fair distribution of the financial burden caused by illness*
> *Improvement of the environment in which people work and live in order to enhance the quality of life*

At present, conclusions concerning the impact of preventive/promotive interventions on health have been based on association data. Better epidemiologic evidence and prospective studies are needed before far-reaching government or voluntary efforts are made to change potentially health-damaging aspects of lifestyle. The error of equating associations with causality can lead to misdirected legislative efforts and needless coercion, intrusiveness, and deprivation.[28]

In deciding whether lifestyle changes to enhance health should be voluntary or mandatory our society has a complex dilemma with no easy answer. The extent of coercion used must also be considered. Is it coercive (and if so, to what extent) to increase cigarette tax in order to help defray the cost of smoking-induced disease? Would such a move also imply that highly refined sugar products and high-cholesterol foodstuffs should also be taxed more heavily to pay for the cost of obesity and atherosclerosis-induced health problems? Should tax on large, high-speed automobiles be proportionately higher than taxes on smaller cars with limited speed and greater fuel economy? Should overweight individuals pay higher taxes than individuals of normal weight, with the excess taxes and interest to be paid back at the time the target individual loses weight and arrives at the norm for his or her height–weight category? Which health behaviors or lifestyle changes should be voluntary and which should be mandatory through enactment of legislation has not yet been determined. It remains to be seen what the voluntary/mandatory blend will be in terms of illness prevention and health promotion.

## SUMMARY

The focus of this chapter has been on society as a collective, and the impact of the cultural, occupational, and physical environments on the health status of individuals and families. Prevention and health promotion are both individual and social problems and consequently must be dealt with at both levels. Individual changes in behavior without a supportive environment to make continuing enactment of change possible will result in frustration and failure of health-promotion efforts.

A balanced approach to prevention and health promotion within the United States requires avoidance of a "blame the victim" ideology to the exclusion of concerns for the quality of the environment. On the other hand, environmental and occupational control measures should not be funded to the exclusion of funds for personal health services and community-based programs that facilitate health-promoting changes in individual lifestyles. It is the responsibility of professional nurses to become well informed on prevention/promotion issues so that they can play a significant role in supporting appropriate voluntary and legislative initiatives.

## REFERENCES

1.  Vuori, H. The medical model and the objectives of health education. *International Journal of Health Education*, 1980, *23*, 12–19.
2.  Weigel, G. Paper presented at the Center for the Study of Democratic Institutions, Chicago, Ill., 1958.
3.  Farquhar, J.W. The community-based model of life style intervention trials. *American Journal of Epidemiology*, August 1978, *108*, 103–111.
4.  Ubel, E. Health behavior change: A political model. *Preventive Medicine*, 1972, *1*, 209–221.
5.  Jonas, S. Hospitals adopt new role. *Hospitals*, October 1979, *53*, 84–86.
6.  Farquhar, *op. cit.* p. 107.
7.  Miller, M.C., & Cantor, A.B. A comparison of mass media effectiveness in health education. *International Journal of Health Education*, 1980, *23*, 49–54.
8.  Milio, N. A framework for prevention: Changing health-damaging to health-generating patterns. *American Journal of Public Health*, May 1976, *66*, 435–439.

9. Navarro, V. Justice, social policy and the public's health. *Medical Care*, May 1977, *15*, 363–370.
10. *Ibid.*, p. 364.
11. Milio, *op. cit.*, p. 436.
12. Smith, R.J. Toxic substances: EPA and OSHA are reluctant regulators. *Science*, January 5, 1979, *203*, 28–32.
13. Milio, *op. cit.*, p. 437.
14. *Ibid.*, p. 438.
15. Culliton, B.J. Toxic substances legislation: How well are laws being implemented? *Science*, September 1978, *201*, 1198–1199.
16. Navarro, *op. cit.*, p. 366.
17. Higginson, J. A hazardous society? Individual versus community responsibility in cancer prevention. *American Journal of Public Health*, April 1976, *66*, 359–366.
18. Brammer, S.H., & DeFelice, R.L. Dietary advice in regard to risk for colon and breast cancer. *Preventive Medicine*, 1980, *9*, 544–549.
19. Aubry, F., Gibbs, G.W., & Becklake, M.R. Air pollution and health in three urban communities. *Archives of Environmental Health*, September–October 1979, *34*, 360–368.
20. Cahn, R. The case for an environmental ethic. *The Center Magazine*, March 1980, *13*, 5–13.
21. Smith, *op. cit.*, p. 29.
22. Crawford, R. You are dangerous to your own health: The ideology and politics of victim blaming. *International Journal of Health Services*, 1977, *7*, 663–680.
23. Green, L.W. National policy in the promotion of health. *International Journal of Health Education*, 1979, *22*, 161–168.
24. Wikler, D.I. Persuasion and coercion for health: Ethical issues in government efforts to change lifestyle. *Milbank Memorial Fund Quarterly*, Summer 1978, *56*, 303–338.
25. As companies jump on fitness bandwagons. *U.S. News and World Report*, January 28, 1980, pp. 36–39.
26. Cropnell, S.G. Awards and incentives add zest to safety performance. *Occupational Hazards*, August 1980, pp. 33–36.
27. Wikler, *op. cit.*, p. 306.
28. Meenan, R.F. Improving the public's health: Some future reflections. *The New England Journal of Medicine*, 1976, *294*, 45–46.

# CHAPTER 15
# Economic Issues in Prevention and Health Promotion

## ALBERT R. PENDER

The current trend toward increased emphasis on prevention and health promotion within the United States is one of the most promising changes in health care delivery in recent years. While this movement is viewed by some health professionals and consumers as the "second epidemiologic revolution,"[1] others are more conservative in their appraisal. Whether changes in the environment and individual lifestyles will significantly decrease the incidence of chronic illness, improve health status, and increase longevity can only be determined through careful analysis of the impact of such changes on large segments of the population.

The potential for changing the health status of Americans through expanded prevention and health-promotion services was recognized in the recommendations of the 1977 Health Report to the White House Summit on Inflation.[2] Those recommendations were:

1. Encourage use of ambulatory care and place increased emphasis on preventive medicine through the restructuring of insurance benefit packages and through the development of prepaid group practice.
2. Increase the supply of primary care physicians, nurse practitioners, and physician assistants to extend primary care capabilities.
3. Explore alternative patterns of health care delivery.
4. Increase consumer education activities.

While the major thrust of the above recommendations is toward changing the health care delivery system (institutional change), the need for modification of individual behavior is also addressed. Some health economists believe that changing individual behavior will be more successful than attempts at major institutional change because of the political and economic impediments to large-scale changes in established social institutions.[3] Still others see efforts directed toward modifying individual behavior as a fragmented, inconsistent, and unpredictable way of dealing with major health problems. It appears that both individual and institutional changes will be required if health-promotion and prevention strategies are markedly to alter the health status of the American people and decrease costs within the health care delivery system.

Questions relevant to the cost of health care that must be addressed by individuals and groups responsible for establishing health policy include the following:

- Can Americans develop and effectively make use of a future-oriented, less technologically intense health care system?
- Are prevention and health promotion efficient uses of national economic resources?
- Can health-promotion and prevention services significantly increase the health status of the American population?
- What will be the degree of difference between potential (theoretical) effectivenss and observed (actual) effectiveness of prevention and health-promotion strategies?
- What financial incentives currently exist or can be offered to promote use of prevention and health-promotion services as opposed to only curative services?

The discussion that follows will present information relevant to these concerns in an attempt to assist nurses and other health care providers in thinking critically about the economic issues that impact on health care delivery and consumer acceptance of prevention and health-promotion services.

## THE COST OF ILLNESS

Total health care expenditures within the United States increased from $60.6 billion in 1969 to $162.6 billion in 1977. These expenditures represented 8.8 percent of the 1977 Gross National Product (GNP), or $737 per person within the United States. Of this amount, $721 per capita was spent for treatment of illness, while only $16 per capita was spent for prevention or health promotion.[4] These figures represent the direct costs of health care and do not include other associated indirect costs. Calculation of indirect costs are generally based on the economic value of the individual in terms of losses in productivity or wages due to morbidity and mortality. Adding both direct and indirect costs of illness together, total monetary expenditures amounted to 18 percent of the GNP in 1977. This figure is projected to rise to 22 to 25 percent by 1985. Continued rise at the current inflation rate will result in direct costs alone of $416.4 billion by the year 2000.[5]

The cost of hospital care, which accounts for 40 percent of health care expenditures, has been rising even more rapidly than the total national health care bill. The average cost of $144.46 for a hospital room in 1975 rose to $208.70 in 1977. This represents a 12-percent annual increase, which has been the prevailing inflation rate for hospital care since 1965.[6] Figure 15-1 presents an interesting picture of national expenditures for illness care and preventive care and associated

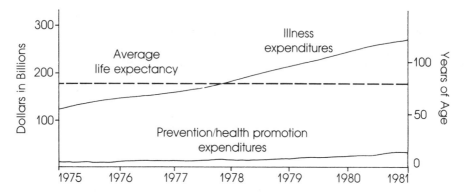

**FIGURE 15-1.** Life expectancy trend versus national expenditures for illness care, 1940–75.

changes in life expectancy. While expenditures for prevention are barely percep-tible at the bottom of the graph, illness expenditures have been rising consistently. The increased cost of care without proportional health benefits leads one to ponder the wisdom of continuing current patterns for health care expenditures.

Another approach to looking at the cost of health care is to examine ex-penditures related to specific causative factors or disease etiology. For example, Luce and Schweitzer[7] have provided interesting information about the cost of smoking and alcohol abuse. Given the current epidemiologic evidence concerning the link between smoking and cancer, cardiovascular diseases, and respiratory diseases, the smoking factors for each of three major health problems within the United States have been calculated. Estimates are based on national morbidity and mortality data. The smoking factor or extent to which smoking contributes to the morbidity and mortality associated with each health problem is presented below.

| Disease | Smoking Factor (%) |
|---|---|
| Neoplasms | 20.0 |
| Circulatory disorders | 25.0 |
| Respiratory disorders | 40.0 |
| Accidents (e.g., fires) | 1.1 |

Using these percentage figures, the direct cost for smoking-related disorders was calculated to be $8.2 billion, which represents 7.8 percent of national direct health care costs (adjusted to 1976 prices). Luce and Schweitzer concluded that when indirect costs (lost earnings due to illness or disability) were added to direct costs, the total cost of smoking-related illness was $27.5 billion, or 11.3 percent of the total costs of illness in 1976. That same year, Americans spent $15.7 billion for all tobacco products, with $5.8 billion of that amount collected as taxes by all levels of government. In total (excluding taxes) during 1976, Americans spent $37.4 billion in purchasing tobacco products or in treating the health-damaging consequences of their use. Costs related to smoking might well be substantially reduced by appropriate interventions to change smoking behavior. The cost effectiveness ratio for smoking cessation programs has been estimated to be 1:1.8.

Alcohol abuse is another expensive health problem of increasing frequency among adults and adolescents within the United States. The direct costs of treating alcoholism plus related disorders was $11.9 billion in 1976, with indirect costs of $20.6 billion resulting from lost earnings. Additional costs of $11.5 billion were also incurred because of alcohol-related motor vehicle accidents, crimes, and fire losses. This resulted in a total estimated cost of alcohol abuse in 1976 of $44.2 billion. The amount spent on the purchase of alcoholic beverages was $30 billion, for a total outlay of $74.2 billion. Fortunately, alcoholism is receiving increasing attention as a risk factor for a number of major illnesses and as a significant health problem in its own right. Data currently available on the cost effective ratio of alcohol treatment programs is impressive at 1:2.3

The cost of surgical treatment for a variety of pathologic disorders should also be examined. The United States has one of the highest rates of elective surgery in the world, with twice as many surgeons and twice as many operations in proportion to population as Great Britian. In England, the hysterectomy rate is 40 percent that of the United States. A 1976 Congressional report extrapolating from data collected in a number of small studies, concluded that 2.4 million unnecessary surgical procedures were performed in 1974, at a cost of $4 billion ($1 billion paid by Medicare). It was estimated that these procedures resulted in 11,900 unnecessary deaths. Because of methodologic problems in the above study, follow-up studies correcting for area differences, biases of selection, and errors of projection will undoubtedly yield lower yet significant figures indicating that there is a substantial amount of unnecessary surgery and needless expenditure of health care dollars within the United States.[8]

The high cost of illness, including potentially preventable health problems, is apparent from the preceding discussion. Treatment of illness is in almost all cases technologically intensive or service (personnel) intensive, thus increasing total costs. This discussion of the costs of illness will provide the context for examining the potential cost effectiveness of prevention and health-promotion services in the present chapter.

## EVALUATING THE ECONOMIC IMPACT OF PREVENTION AND HEALTH PROMOTION

Because of inflation in health care costs, new programs are being critically scrutinized as never before, with competition for health care dollars exceptionally keen. The question must be raised whether prevention and health-promotion efforts can change the current picture of health care expenditures.

The approach most commonly used in exploring the economic impact of new types of health services is that of cost-effectiveness analysis, a derivative of cost/benefit analysis. While this approach has its limitations in that it does not take into consideration the pain, suffering, and human unhappiness caused by illness, it does offer a standardized approach for looking at the potential impact of various prevention and health-promotion interventions on life expectancy and health care costs. In cost-effectiveness analysis, the value of an individual is based on his or her contribution to the GNP by wages earned. Such an approach provides a common monetary unit that allows the impact of many different types of health care programs to be compared.

Before programs or services can be evaluated, they must be clearly defined. This is particularly important with prevention and health-promotion interventions since they are not technologically intensive and thus are less likely to be identified by health consumers as discrete episodes of health care. For example, physical examination and screening procedures are the primary strategies that consumers associate with prevention and health promotion. Health education, dietary counseling, risk appraisal, or stress management are less well recognized as circumscribed health services since technical instrumentation is not clearly a part of these interventions. In other words, nothing is done "to the individual." For this reason, a clear understanding of the goals and parameters of specific prevention and health-promotion interventions is critical in order to evaluate their impact on health successfully.

Shepard and Thompson[9] have identified six important steps in evaluating health services for cost effectiveness:

1. Identify the epidemiologic or causal link between illness/health and the target intervention.
2. Define precisely the program to be analyzed, its focus, processes, and limits.
3. Compute the net monetary cost for prevention/promotion and/or treatment of illness under the proposed program.
4. Identify possible negative effects of the program (iatrogenesis) and compute cost of morbidity/mortality or disability.
5. Compute the health effects or benefits.
6. Establish policy or make program decisions based on net costs and net health effects.

A given health goal may be achieved by using a number of different intervention strategies, all with different cost/effectiveness ratios. Cost/effectiveness analysis allows comparison of community-based programs with each other or with personal health services or mass media efforts. Monetarization of costs and benefits facilitates comparison.

Specific health effects that have been used as measures of the impact of health programs include the following:[10]

*Additional years of healthy survival*
*Postponement of death (morbidity may still be present)*
*Improvement in health without affecting longevity*
*Negative effects, such as disability*

The measure(s) used to determine the effectiveness of a given prevention or health-promotion program depend(s) on the major potential impact of the intervention as determined from whatever epidemiologic data are available at that point in time.

Both short-term and long-term effects of prevention and health-promotion interventions must be assessed. For many programs, costs are incurred now and benefits derived later. Reconciling the two in dollars and cents is generally handled by a procedure called *discounting*. While monetary costs can be reconciled as part of cost/effectiveness analysis, the question must also be asked whether consumers are willing to spend as much to protect themselves from a health problem with 20 years' latency as to protect themselves from a health problem with 3 to 5 years' latency. Consumer values and attitudes will affect the acceptance and marketability of any given prevention or health-promotion service and consequently its actual rather than potential impact on health.

The impact of health promotion programs is more difficult to evaluate than that of prevention or treatment programs since specific disease threats are not the focus and effects on clients are general in nature rather than targeted. Health-promotion programs aim for *positive* changes in a variety of behavioral, sociologic, and physiologic parameters. Use of only morbidity and mortality statistics for evaluation provides an inappropriate, disease-oriented estimate of impact.

Factors that affect the cost/effectiveness ratio of various prevention and health-promotion interventions are the magnitude of the problem, the number and effectiveness of intervention methods currently available, the number of cases preventable with current intervention methods, the cost of prevention versus the cost of cure or care in illness, the potential savings from promotive/preventive interventions (the rate of adoption must be considered) compared with treatment (low medical compliance must be considered) and the appropriate target populations for intervention.[11]

The importance of selecting appropriate populations for intervention cannot be stressed too strongly. A good illustration of the importance of this decision is in the use of mammography for detection of breast cancer. In women under 50 years of age, mammography appears to add very little to the probability of detecting new cases and may actually be a causative factor in cancer of the breast. Because of the increased incidence of breast cancer in women after 50 years of age, the usefulness of mammography for detection may outweigh the human and economic costs of treatment/induced cancer. In addition, the decreased number of years for potential exposure after 50 years of age lowers the frequency of iatrogenic carcinoma.[12]

Another example of the need for appropriately targeted intervention is in the area of hypertension. Review of research data available favors treatment of high diastolic pressures, particularly in young men and older women. The potential value of initiating treatment early for men appears especially impressive. However, before such decisions are made it is imperative that more data be obtained concerning the risks posed by life-long courses of pharmacologic therapy, their effect on health, and health care expenditures. Better demonstration of the relationship between decreased blood pressure and decreased risk of cardiovascular disorders is also crucial, especially in mild hypertension where uncertainty over type of treatment and treatment efficacy currently exists.

Still another important consideration related to the economic impact of promotive/preventive care is the dose–response relationship. Not only must differing approaches to intervention such as mass screening, screening at risk populations, mass education, personal health services, and environmental measures be considered as possible modes of intervention, but the extent of each intervention necessary to produce desired effects must be determined.[13] Questions to be asked include the following:

- Should intervention be short-term, long-term, continuous, or intermittent to maximize effectiveness and control cost?
- At what point does the dose result in diminishing returns or negative effects?
- What factors alter the dose–response relationship (decrease or increase extent of dose necessary)?
- After reviewing dose–response relationship of various interventions, which offers the higher human and/or cost advantage?

Cost studies can provide valuable information helpful to consumers, providers, and third-party payers in choosing between personal health services, mass education, or environmental control as approaches to health promotion/protection. While all the above interventions will undoubtedly have their place in promotive/preventive care, third-party payers are increasingly concerned about the impact of new types of services and the responsible use of new insurance benefits. As causal links between various factors and health are identified and appropriate programs are developed, health care providers, third-party payers, large purchasers of insurance, and the public will have to be educated concerning the efficacy of various intervention strategies. Willingness of third-party payers to offer new benefits for prevention and health promotion to enrollees will undoubtedly increase as cost effectiveness data become available concerning specific interventions.

The bottom line in considering cost/effectiveness of any prevention and health-promotion effort is what the public is willing to pay directly or indirectly for access to such services. While alternative modes of care and new preventive/promotive services can be made available, they must enter the quasi-free market place and compete for dollars now spent by government, third-party payers, and consumers on treatment services.[14] Can money spent on curative or supportive care be diverted to health-promoting and prevention options? It is only as the public learns to value promotive/preventive services and is willing to pay directly or demand insurance coverage for them that such services will have an impact on personal and family health.

## POTENTIAL VERSUS ACTUAL EFFECTIVENESS

Differentiating between the potential (optimal) and actual effectiveness of a prevention or health-promotion intervention is critical to realistic estimation of the cost/effectiveness ratio. Potential effectiveness can be defined as the impact of an intervention if all eligible individuals take full advantage of the service/program and derive maximum benefits. Such a response to any health program is highly unlikely. The actual effectiveness of an intervention is a product of its efficacy in altering health status, morbidity, or mortality and the probability of people gaining access to the service or engaging in the recommended behavior(s). The difference between the two types of effectiveness is clearly indicated in the following equations:

- *Potential Effectiveness* = Identification and intervention with all eligible individuals × maximal participation and health benefits from intervention
- *Actual Effectiveness* = Identification and intervention with a finite number of eligible individuals × limited rate of participation and partial health benefits from intervention

As an example, in 1976 the National Cancer Institute estimated that there were 60 million smokers in the United States. Evaluation of past antismoking efforts indicates a 25-percent success rate. If 50 percent of the 60 million smokers were reached with antismoking interventions, 7.5 million rather than 60 or 30 million would be the realistic effectiveness figure in estimating the actual effectiveness of a new antismoking intervention. If alcohol abuse was the target of intervention, the estimated success rate from previous experience is approximately 30 percent. If half of the 9 million alcoholics took advantage of the intervention, 1.5 million would be the estimated effectiveness figure on which prediction of success should be based (incidentally, the success rate of current interventions for alcohol abuse is less well established than that for antismoking efforts).[15]

Screening programs for hypertension constitute another example of the contrast between potential and actual effectiveness of preventive care. Screening for hypertension is relatively inexpensive, yet many individuals do not successfully control their hypertension after detection. Failure to adhere to medical regimens is common among 55 to 85 percent of the hypertensive population and is frequently due to the cost of life-long therapy or the side effects experienced. Noncompliance greatly compromises the cost effectiveness of screening programs.[16] Interventions to improve compliance with medical regimens or the development of alternative means of hypertension control (e.g., relaxation, stress management) may be a more productive and economically feasible approach to the problem of hypertension than increased funding for extensive nation-wide screening programs.[17]

Consumer resistance to the introduction of seat belts to decrease highway accidents is still another vivid illustration of the difference between potential effectiveness and actual effectiveness of a preventive measure. Based on the fact that studies have shown a decrease of 35 to 50 percent in fatal traffic accidents and severe injuries when seat belts were worn,[18] major consumer education efforts were mounted to increase their use. Despite this campaign, consumers reacted to the inconvenience and discomfort of seat belts and reversed legislative requirements for interlock systems in all cars (a system where seat belts had to be locked before car would start). The cost effectiveness of seat belt installation and public education efforts was greatly reduced by lack of acceptance of the accident-prevention measure by consumers.

The probability of acceptance and use of new prevention and health-promotion measures must be determined before accurate estimates of cost/effectiveness can be calculated. The actual rather than the potential effectiveness of a new intervention determines the extent to which public and private resources should be invested in facilities and personnel for implementation.

## EFFECTIVENESS OF SECONDARY PREVENTION

The early detection of diseases (periodic screening) for which primary prevention is not yet available has been the major approach to decreasing morbidity and mortality. The ratio of costs to benefits determines the economic impact of any specific screening program. Screening for chronic illness involves the following cost factors in order to mount a comprehensive program:[19]

- Cost of persuading people to be screened
- Cost of transportation and time devoted to screening visits
- Cost of the professionals, facilities, and equipment used in screening
- Cost of follow-up and treatment of people who are found abnormal on the screen
- Cost of any deleterious (iatrogenic) effects of the screen, their follow-up, and treatment

Additional aspects of screening that must be considered in cost/effectiveness analysis include optimal spacing to minimize cost while maximizing benefits, appropriate selection of target population groups to be screened, pay policies for screening services, and ratio of number screened to number engaging in follow-up. Numerous screening efforts for major chronic illnesses and metabolic defects have been initiated in recent years. Several of these programs will be reviewed in terms of their cost and effects on health status.

Shapiro[20] reported the results of a randomized clinical trial in the Health Insurance Plan of Greater New York to determine whether periodic screening with mammography in addition to palpation would result in reduced mortality from cancer. The picture emerging from the long-term New York study is a 10-percent reduction in mortality from breast cancer when mammography is used in addition to palpation. Interestingly, all the gains from use of mammography in screening were at age 50 or above. Mortality rates in the study and control groups were the same for women under 50 years of age. The decrease in mortality reported in this study represents a considerable savings in terms of earnings that would have been cut short by death or disability. In addition, the cost of more complex medical services necessary to treat advanced disease is also decreased.

Dickinson et al.[21] provided data relevant to the effectiveness of screening programs for cervical cancer. Since the introduction of the Papanicoleau smear and an increase in annual screening rate to 30 percent of women at risk above 30 years of age, 3 years have been added to the life expectancy of women. The mortality rate from cervical cancer went from 9.3 per 100,000 in 1954 to 6.2 per 100,000 in 1969. An increased life expectancy of 3 years, associated earnings, and lower costs of medical therapy support the cost effectiveness of periodic Pap smears for women at risk below 35 years of age and all women over 35 years of age.

Cancer of the colon (large bowel) accounts for approximately 15 percent of the incidence of cancer and 13 percent of the mortality rate from malignant diseases. It is fairly evenly distributed among males and females and results in a total annual cost of $3.5 billion. Direct costs of medical care and treatment total $800 million, and decreased earnings and productivity account for $27 billion indirect costs. Colon cancer screening can be quite simply conducted through a stool guaiac screening test for occult blood. The cost of the test is estimated at $2 by the National Cancer Institute. The estimated cost/effectiveness ratio for screening individuals over 55 years of age is 1:8.38. This means saving $8.38 in treatment costs or lost earnings for every $1 spent for early detection. A stool guaiac test could be conducted on all persons over 55 years of age for a cost of approximately $80 million. Early detection is estimated to improve survival by 20 percent and reduce direct medical care costs by 50 percent. In this instance, a relatively inexpensive screening test offers highly cost-effective benefits as well as decreasing the extent of human suffering associated with malignant disease.[22]

Cretin[23] reports the results of a comparative study in which the cost effectiveness of screening for elevated cholesterol followed by education about a low-cholesterol diet was compared with the cost effectiveness of coronary care units and mobile coronary care units following cardiovascular accidents. The per person benefits of increased life expectancy (decreased mortality) was used as the basis for comparing the cost effectiveness of screening with treatment strategies. While all interventions significantly increased life expectancy by a little less than a year, neither screening nor treatment methods were clearly superior. Screening, as opposed to treatment interventions, decreased the number of hospitalizations by decreasing the incidence of myocardial infarction. The report pointed out the need for better methods of comparing the cost/effectiveness of prevention and treatment approaches to chronic health problems.

Screening has been proposed for school-age children in order to identify those in the upper tail of the cholesterol curve. The estimated cost of screening per child (10 years of age) is $1. Intervention costs were assumed to include an initial physician visit the first year ($15), six visits with a counselor for dietary instruction and management ($10 a visit), and subsequent annual physician visits until age 20 ($15 a visit). The preventive cost factor was based on the assumption that those children in the upper 5 percent of the cholesterol distribution would be recommended for treatment and that 50 percent of those identified as having high cholesterol would comply with dietary recommendations.

Another interesting example of cost-effective prevention is the use of metabolic screening in newborns. Screening for 31 inborn metabolic errors is now possible. The cost of screening for all amino acid disorders detectable at birth for which dietary alterations provide protection from retardation or mental deterioration is $2 per child. The cost of screening for hypothyroidism is $1 per infant. The total cost of screening is far less than the cost of institutionalization or care for retarded individuals as a result of the metabolic errors.[24]

Alderman and Kristein[25] reported on the cost effectiveness of a work-based hypertension program. Total cost of the hypertension screening and follow-up program was $94,187 for 1 year. This represented a cost of $250 per capita for all individuals treated and a cost of $363 per capita for all individuals who were controlled (BP decrease to 148/90 on follow-up) or improved (10 percent decrease in diastolic). At the 1 year follow-up, 60 percent were controlled and 74 percent were improved or controlled. It is estimated that hypertensive individuals spend approximately $250 on medical care annually and may experience an average loss in wages of $794 a year because of illness or premature death. This total amount of $1044 a year is obviously greater than the cost of intervention, even when calculated conservatively on the basis of controlled or improved ($362 per capita) rather than total patients.

The total direct and indirect costs of illness and disability associated with hypertension were estimated to be $16 billion in 1977. It appears that $6 to $8 billion of this could be saved by a national screening program (cost: $5 million) and a relatively high rate of successful treatment. This would result in a cost/effectiveness ratio of 1:2.[26]

A study by Haynes et al.[27] indicated the critical importance of appropriate follow-up after detection of hypertension. He found that individuals newly diagnosed as hypertensive who did not bring blood pressure under control had an 80-percent increase in work absenteeism because of illness. This was attributed to heightened awareness of the existing problem and resultant anxiety rather than to disease pathology. When individuals were informed that they had hypertension but no means were offered for helping them cope constructively with the problem, they undoubtedly felt threatened and helpless and adopted the sick role more easily and frequently. Thus, cost-effectiveness analysis of hypertension screening must include the costs of appropriate follow-up and the cost of detection without intervention.

Other types of secondary prevention programs in addition to screening also show cost effectiveness. Five-year findings of the Hypertension Detection and Follow-up Program sponsored by the National Heart, Lung, and Blood Institute of the National Institutes of Health serves as an example of successful prevention.[28] A sample of more than 10,000 individuals with elevated blood pressures was assigned either to a systematic progressive medical regimen to lower their blood pressure, referred to as Stepped Care, or to Referred Care, which consisted of follow-up by local physicians. In Stepped Care, a medical regimen was followed that commenced with diuretic therapy and progressed to other antihypertension medications as needed to maintain blood pressure within recommended limits.

For the group entering the study with diastolic blood pressures between 90 and 104 mm Hg (mild hypertension), mortality was 20 percent lower in the Stepped Care group than in the Referred Care group. The 5-year mortality rates indicated that deaths from all causes was 17 percent less for participants in Stepped Care than for those in Referred Care. These results support the importance of early detection, counseling, and management of hypertension, particularly for individuals with mild elevations in blood pressure and the economic impact of such efforts.

Another prevention effort currently underway in which preliminary results look promising is the Multiple Risk Factor Intervention Trial.[29] The aim in the program is to change health behaviors of men at high risk for cardiovascular disorders through intensive counseling. Although final results of the study will not be available until 1983, preliminary findings indicated that the program has been successful in decreasing the incidence of smoking, bringing high blood pressure under control, and, to a lesser extent, decreasing serum cholesterol levels. These changes represent potential savings in treatment costs and fewer economic losses as a result of nonproductivity (morbidity or mortality).

The economic impact of education for self-care is evident from the work of Zapka and Averill.[30] They report on an innovative approach to the prevention of need for medical management of upper respiratory infections. The clinic that served as the site of the study offered an educational program on the self-care of colds that included information on rest, fluids, salt gargle, use of over-the-counter medications, and general information on self-care. The cost of managing upper respiratory infections following introduction of the self-care educational sessions was $1.37 per capita, as compared with $9.03 per capita before initiation of the program. During the second year of the program, costs of management were $0.75 per capita, rather than a potential $11.02 for medical management. This resulted in a cost/effectiveness ratio of 1:14.7. Savings during the first year of the program totaled $20,260, and they were $25,860 during the second year of the program. It appears that cold self-care may decrease the incidence of prolonged upper respiratory infections as well as decrease the use of medical services for a health problem that could be managed by individuals themselves.

Another cost-effective approach to prevention is the use of child-resistant containers for medications. The cost of producing the child-proof caps is only slightly greater than the cost of traditional caps. However, on clinical trials of the caps, the incidence of accidental poisoning among children was decreased by 75 to 90 percent.[31] This represents considerable savings in the need for emergency care of poisoning victims and resultant disabilities incurred from the deleterious effects of harmful substances.

In summary, early detection of disease and other preventive measures can be effective in lowering health care costs. Continuing evaluation of new screens and other preventive measures as they become available will provide data helpful in the development of prevention programs and in the formulation of related health policy.

## EFFECTIVENESS OF HEALTH PROMOTION

The cost effectiveness of health promotion has received much less attention in the literature than has the cost effectiveness of prevention. A major investigation of the impact of health promotion on life expectancy was the epidemiologic study conducted by Belloc and Breslow[32] at the Human Population Laboratory of Alameda County, California, in 1965, with subsequent follow-ups in 1970 and 1974. The relationships between seven health-promoting practices and personal health status were assessed. The seven health habits included never smoking cigarettes, regular physical activity, moderate or no use of alcohol, 7 to 8 hours sleep regularly, maintaining proper weight, eating breakfast, and not eating between meals. The significant positive association between these seven health habits and health status was independent of age, sex, and income level.

A $5\frac{1}{2}$ year follow-up study revealed a strong relationship between health habits and life expectancy. The average number of years remaining at age 45 for men in the zero to three health-practices group was 21.6 years, compared to 33.1 years for men in the six to seven health-practices group. This represented a difference of more than 11 years. Among women, the difference between the two health-practice groups was 7 years.[33] Table 15-1 provides an overview of the data on life expectancy for various age groups.

In 1974 a $9\frac{1}{2}$ year follow-up study was conducted to determine the stability of the seven health habits over time and to determine whether the health practices/health status relationship was still evident. Of the original sample of 6928 persons,

**TABLE 15-1   AVERAGE REMAINING LIFETIME, USING DEATH RATES OF THREE HEALTH PRACTICE GROUPS**

|  |  | Number of Health Practices | | |
| --- | --- | --- | --- | --- |
|  | AGE | 0–3 | 4–5 | 6–7 |
| Men | 45 | 21.63 | 28.15 | 33.08 |
|  | 55 | 13.77 | 20.21 | 24.95 |
|  | 65 | 10.61 | 13.71 | 17.41 |
|  | 75 | 7.43 | 10.23 | 11.22 |
|  | 85 | 6.47 | 5.82 | 5.04 |
| Women | 45 | 28.58 | 34.08 | 35.84 |
|  | 55 | 20.02 | 25.11 | 27.83 |
|  | 65 | 12.35 | 17.30 | 19.87 |
|  | 75 | 8.63 | 11.70 | 12.50 |
|  | 85 | 4.63 | 7.50 | 7.61 |

Data abstracted from Table X, p. 79, in Belloc, N.B., Relationship of health practices and mortality. *Preventive Medicine*, 1973, 2, 67–81. Based on $5\frac{1}{2}$ years of follow-up of persons covered in a household survey, Alameda County, California, 1965.

5722 were contacted by means of questionnaire for the second follow-up. Seventy-eight percent of the survivors of the 1965 study responded.[34]

The study results indicated considerable stability of the seven health practices over time. Of the men, 72 percent still practiced 0 to 3 health practices, with only 7 percent moving from poor (zero to three) to good (six to seven) health practices. Of those practicing six to seven health habits in 1965, 77 percent remained the same or had made only a slight change. Only 3 percent had changed from good to poor health practices over the 9-year period. Similar results were apparent for women.

Analysis of the data also revealed that the relationship between health practices and life expectancy persisted over time. After a 9-year interval, men following six to seven health practices had a standardized mortality ratio (SMR) of 37 percent of that of men engaging in zero to three health practices. Women following six to seven health practices had an SMR of 50 percent that of women following zero to three health practices.

While conclusions concerning direct cause-and-effect relationships cannot be drawn from this descriptive study, the results offer encouragement for selecting and testing the impact of various changes in lifestyle on health care costs and life expectancy. If the increased life expectancy identified in this study was converted to added years of productivity in wages and earnings, the economic advantage of the identified health practices would be formidable.

Because of the few studies that address the impact of lifestyle change on health care costs, this is a fertile area for further research efforts. Both programs to promote lifestyle change, and the resultant positive health practices should be evaluated to determine their impact on health status.

## IMPACT OF DECREASING THE LEADING CAUSES OF DEATH

In order to acquire a more holistic view of the impact of prevention and health promotion on the economy of the United States, the prevention potential for major chronic diseases and the effect of lowered mortality from these major causes of death (e.g., cardiovascular diseases, cancer, accidents, etc.) must be considered. Gori and Richter[35] present interesting data on prevention potential for major chronic illnesses. Their calculations are based on comparison of mortality rates in the United States with those of countries with the lowest or next-to-lowest mortality rates from major chronic disease among industrialized countries. Table 15-2 presents data concerning the prevention potential for five major causes of death. As an example, deaths from cardiovascular and renal diseases account for 51 percent of total mortality within the United States. If mortality rates were to be lowered to the minimum mortality rate among industrialized countries, the U.S. mortality rate would be decreased by 77 percent. If the U.S. mortality rate were to be lowered to the next-to-lowest rate, a 39-percent decrease in mortality would occur. Deaths from malignant neoplasms have a prevention potential of 25 to 77 percent. Actual prevention as opposed to prevention potential would of

**TABLE 15-2   MORTALITY FROM THE FIVE MAJOR CAUSES OF DEATH IN 1973 WTHIN THE UNITED STATES AND PREVENTION POTENTIAL CALCULATED BY COMPARING U.S. MORTALITY RATE WITH NEXT-TO-THE-LOWEST (MIN) AND LOWEST (MAX) RATE AMONG INDUSTRIALIZED COUNTRIES**

| Cause | Number of Deaths | Percent of Total Mortality | Pevention Potential (%) | |
| --- | --- | --- | --- | --- |
| | | | MIN | MAX |
| Major cardiovascular renal diseases | 1,012,341 | 51 | 39 | 77 |
| Malignant neoplasms | 351,055 | 18 | 25 | 77 |
| Accidents—motor vehicle and other | 115,821 | 6 | 38 | 39 |
| Diseases of the respiratory system | 92,267 | 5 | 17 | 38 |
| Diabetes mellitus | 38,208 | 2 | 63 | 74 |

From Gori, R., & Richter, B. Macroeconomics of disease prevention in the United States. *Science,* 1978, *200,* 1124–1130. Copyright 1978 by the American Association for the Advancement of Science.

**TABLE 15-3   LIFE EXPECTANCY BEFORE AND AFTER ELIMINATION OF MINIMUM PREVENTABLE PORTION OF FIVE MAJOR CAUSES OF DEATH**

| Age | Remaining Years of Life Expected | | Difference (%) |
| --- | --- | --- | --- |
| | BEFORE* | AFTER | |
| 0 | 70.75 | 74.22 | 4.90 |
| 10 | 62.57 | 66.00 | 5.48 |
| 20 | 53.00 | 56.41 | 6.43 |
| 30 | 43.71 | 46.95 | 7.41 |
| 40 | 34.52 | 37.65 | 9.07 |
| 50 | 25.93 | 28.84 | 11.22 |
| 60 | 18.34 | 20.52 | 11.89 |
| 70 | 12.00 | 13.23 | 10.25 |
| 80 | 7.10 | 7.94 | 11.83 |

*Based on 1969–71 U.S. mortality data.
From Gori, G. & Richter, B. Macroeconomics of disease prevention in the United States. *Science,* 1978, *200,* 1124–1130. Copyright 1978 by the American Association for the Advancement of Science.

course depend on the efficacy of preventive measures and their rate of acceptance and adoption by the public.

With such dramatic changes in mortality rates, the size and mean age of the population would increase. The projected changes in life expectancy after elimination of the minimum preventable portion of five major causes of death within the United States is presented in Table 15-3. The health status of a population with an increased average age is unknown. It is expected that health-promotion efforts would result in a healthier even though older population. The possibility must also be considered that older individuals would suffer from new causes of morbidity and mortality that would impose costs for treatment, palliation, and supportive care. Thus, while prevention might offer considerable potential for improved health status and longevity gains, it is unclear at this point as to whether health-care costs would be decreased in the long run. Prevention and health-promotion efforts could have three possible outcomes: (1) decrease the cost of health care within the United States, (2) result in no significant change in health care costs, or (3) increase the cost of health care for the American population.

The question must also be raised concerning whether healthy individuals would be allowed to work later in life, rather than only until the present mandatory retirement age of 65 years. If older individuals were allowed to work, what would be their rate of disability, absenteeism, and productivity? If the social security program remained the same and older individuals were not allowed to work, pensions and social security payments would be made to a larger segment of the total population, necessitating increased taxes to meet future retirement expenditures. The increase in social security beneficiaries with no change in the benefit program before and after elimination of the minimal preventable portion of major causes of death is depicted in Table 15-4.

**TABLE 15-4   SOCIAL SECURITY BENEFICIARIES (THOUSANDS) BEFORE AND AFTER GRADUAL ELIMINATION OF MINIMUM PREVENTABLE PORTION OF MAJOR CAUSES OF DEATH**

| Year | Before | After | Difference (%) |
|------|--------|-------|----------------|
| 1980 | 26,527 | 26,530 | 0.01 |
| 1985 | 28,914 | 29,007 | 0.32 |
| 1990 | 30,995 | 31,599 | 1.95 |
| 1995 | 32,096 | 33,908 | 5.65 |
| 2000 | 32,446 | 35,442 | 9.23 |
| Tax rate needed (%) | | | |
| | 11.81 | 13.41 | 13.55 |

From Gori, G. & Richter, B. Macroeconomics of disease prevention in the United States. *Science*, 1978, *200*, 1124–1130. Copyright 1978 by the American Association for the Advancement of Science.

**TABLE 15-5 LIFE EXPECTANCY (ê₁) AT VARIOUS AGES FOR THE TOTAL POPULATION AFTER CARDIOVASCULAR DISEASE, MALIGNANT NEOPLASMS, AND MOTOR VEHICLE ACCIDENTS ARE COMPLETELY ELIMINATED: UNITED STATES, 1967–71**

| Exact Age (in years) | Life Expectancy Without Elimination | Cardiovascular Disease | | Malignant Neoplasms | | Motor Vehicle Accidents | |
|---|---|---|---|---|---|---|---|
| | | $\hat{e}_1$ | GAIN | $\hat{e}_1$ | GAIN | $\hat{e}_1$ | GAIN |
| 0 | 70.81 | 83.17 | 12.36 | 73.33 | 2.52 | 71.51 | 0.70 |
| 1 | 71.29 | 83.89 | 12.60 | 73.85 | 2.56 | 72.00 | 0.71 |
| 5 | 67.53 | 80.16 | 12.63 | 70.08 | 2.55 | 68.21 | 0.68 |
| 10 | 62.67 | 75.32 | 12.65 | 65.20 | 2.53 | 63.31 | 0.64 |
| 15 | 57.79 | 70.46 | 12.67 | 60.31 | 2.52 | 58.41 | 0.62 |
| 20 | 53.10 | 65.83 | 12.73 | 55.61 | 2.51 | 53.59 | 0.49 |
| 25 | 48.47 | 61.28 | 12.81 | 50.98 | 2.51 | 48.84 | 0.37 |
| 30 | 43.81 | 56.67 | 12.86 | 46.30 | 2.49 | 44.10 | 0.29 |
| 35 | 39.17 | 52.08 | 12.91 | 41.64 | 2.47 | 39.40 | 0.23 |
| 40 | 34.62 | 47.55 | 12.93 | 37.04 | 2.42 | 34.81 | 0.19 |
| 45 | 30.23 | 43.14 | 12.91 | 32.56 | 2.33 | 30.38 | 0.15 |
| 50 | 26.04 | 38.88 | 12.84 | 28.23 | 2.19 | 26.16 | 0.12 |
| 55 | 22.10 | 34.82 | 12.72 | 24.08 | 1.98 | 22.19 | 0.09 |
| 60 | 18.47 | 31.02 | 12.55 | 20.18 | 1.71 | 18.54 | 0.07 |
| 65 | 15.14 | 27.46 | 12.32 | 16.55 | 1.41 | 15.19 | 0.05 |
| 70 | 12.14 | 24.19 | 12.05 | 13.25 | 1.11 | 12.18 | 0.04 |
| 75 | 9.50 | 21.19 | 11.69 | 10.31 | 0.81 | 9.53 | 0.03 |
| 80 | 7.32 | 18.61 | 11.29 | 7.88 | 0.56 | 7.34 | 0.02 |
| 85 | 5.61 | 16.40 | 10.79 | 5.97 | 0.36 | 5.62 | 0.01 |
| 90 | 4.54 | 14.75 | 10.21 | 4.76 | 0.22 | 4.55 | 0.01 |
| 95 | 4.16 | 13.47 | 9.31 | 4.29 | 0.13 | 4.16 | 0.00 |
| 100 | 2.84 | 11.38 | 8.54 | 2.93 | 0.09 | 2.84 | 0.00 |

From Tsai, S., Lee, E., & Hardey, R. The effect of a reduction in leading cause of death: Potential gain in life expectancies. *American Journal of Public Health*, October 1978, *68*, 966–971.

Tsai, Lee, and Hardey[36] have also presented data on the added years of life expectancy following total elimination of the leading causes of death. The calculated gains in life expectancy are presented in Table 15-5. The largest gains in life expectancy appear to be due to decreased mortality from cardiovascular disorders, with lower gains in relation to decreased mortality from malignant neoplasms and motor vehicle accidents. Since complete elimination of mortality due to the major chronic diseases may not be possible, added life expectancy for varying degrees (percentages) of elimination of mortality among individuals of working age is depicted in Table 15-6. This table should be interpreted with caution since all individuals 15 to 65 years of age have been grouped together, obscuring age specific differences.

TABLE 15-6   ADDED YEARS OF LIFE FOR WORKING AGED BY REDUCING
CARDIOVASCULAR DISEASE, MALIGNANT NEOPLASMS, AND MOTOR VEHICLE
ACCIDENTS: UNITED STATES, 1969–71

| Cause of Death and Race/Sex Group | Percent Elimination (working ages, 15–65 yr) | | | | | |
|---|---|---|---|---|---|---|
| | 10 | 20 | 30 | 50 | 70 | 100 |
| Major cardiovascular diseases | | | | | | |
| Total population | 0.09 | 0.18 | 0.27 | 0.45 | 0.63 | 0.91 |
| White males | 0.11 | 0.23 | 0.35 | 0.58 | 0.83 | 1.20 |
| White females | 0.04 | 0.08 | 0.13 | 0.22 | 0.31 | 0.45 |
| Nonwhite males | 0.16 | 0.32 | 0.49 | 0.83 | 1.17 | 1.71 |
| Nonwhite females | 0.12 | 0.25 | 0.37 | 0.63 | 0.89 | 1.29 |
| Malignant neoplasms | | | | | | |
| Total population | 0.06 | 0.12 | 0.17 | 0.29 | 0.41 | 0.59 |
| White males | 0.06 | 0.11 | 0.17 | 0.28 | 0.39 | 0.56 |
| White females | 0.06 | 0.12 | 0.17 | 0.29 | 0.41 | 0.59 |
| Nonwhite males | 0.07 | 0.13 | 0.20 | 0.33 | 0.47 | 0.68 |
| Nonwhite females | 0.07 | 0.13 | 0.20 | 0.34 | 0.47 | 0.68 |
| Motor vehicle accidents | | | | | | |
| Total population | 0.04 | 0.08 | 0.12 | 0.20 | 0.28 | 0.40 |
| White males | 0.06 | 0.12 | 0.18 | 0.30 | 0.42 | 0.60 |
| White females | 0.02 | 0.04 | 0.06 | 0.10 | 0.14 | 0.19 |
| Nonwhite males | 0.06 | 0.12 | 0.18 | 0.31 | 0.43 | 0.62 |
| Nonwhite females | 0.02 | 0.03 | 0.05 | 0.09 | 0.12 | 0.18 |

From Tsai, S., Lee, E., & Hardey, R. The effect of a reduction in leading cause of death: Potential gain in life expectancies. *American Journal of Public Health, October 1978, 68,* 966–971.

Increases in health status or level of wellness may also result from partial elimination of major chronic illnesses that are not reflected in the life-expectancy tables based on mortality and morbidity. New methods for assessing the impact of elimination of chronic diseases on quality as well as quantity of life are essential. In addition, the long-term effects of prevention and health-promotion interventions on the total population must be determined, as well as their impact on health and health-related (e.g., social security) costs.

## FINANCIAL INCENTIVES FOR PREVENTION

Current insurance coverage offers little in the way of incentives to increase motivation for self-care or ambulatory care as opposed to illness care in the hospital setting. As Figure 15-1 illustrates, rapidly increasing health (illness) expenditures have not markedly altered the life expectancy of Americans for a number of years. Additional expenditures for care in illness are not likely to result in significant changes in the quality of life for the American population or in major changes in morbidity and mortality. How can increasing amounts of money be spent annually to pay for a health care system that does not commensurately improve health? It appears that unless economic incentives can be developed to encourage decreased use of medical services and increased attention to health-promotion and preventive measures, there is little hope of containing costs or of improving the well-being of the American people.[37]

Ninety percent of the population has insurance coverage for hospital care, yet few have coverage for health promotion or ambulatory care not related to a specific diagnosis or medical complaint. While the federal government itself extols health promotion and disease prevention, it prohibits reimbursement by Medicare for many preventive services. Medicare–Medicaid now pays 42 percent of the total national medical care bill; this includes 53 percent of hospitalization costs and 33 percent of personal health care expenditures. Federal expenditures on prevention represented only 1 percent of total health expenditures in 1974 and between 2 to 3 percent of the health budget in 1977.

Insurance benefits, both public and private, in 1976 covered only 60 percent of physician visits and other ambulatory care services outside of the hospital setting.[38] In general, present reimbursement patterns tend to limit consumer choice among alternative systems of health care delivery and among various health care providers, thus restricting access to prevention and health-promotion services.

The current organizational structure for health care within the United States has also presented barriers to the delivery of prevention and health-promotion services to rural and urban populations. Feldman et al.,[39] in exploring factors related to the financial viability of 101 rural primary care centers, found that providing a high proportion of services covered by third party pay were positively correlated with self-sufficiency of the centers. Financial solvency was negatively related to the number of outreach programs that the center provided. The centers that did not offer community or home-based care were 37-percent more self-sufficient than were those that offered such care. Since prevention and health-promotion services are often more successfully carried out in community and family settings, the financial disadvantage to primary care centers for offering such services should be of critical concern to consumers, health professionals, and individuals responsible for formulating health policy.

In the same study, per capita income was negatively associated with financial viability. The higher the family income within the geographic area of the center, the lower the self-sufficiency. Individuals with higher incomes, rather than using the local center, traveled to nearby cities and towns for medical services. It appears that the centers were viewed as second-rate care. The question can also be raised as to whether prevention and health-promotion services will be viewed as second-rate care because of their low technologic intensity and strong emphasis on augmenting client's own self-care competencies.

Efforts to develop Health Maintenance Organizations (HMOs) and other arrangements for prepaid care have not attracted significant numbers of health care providers or consumers. HMOs were conceived as health care plans or services that would place heavy emphasis on prevention and health promotion and as a result decrease the cost of care for illness. In addition, such an approach to care was directed toward increasing both the quality of life for clients and the years of life expectancy. It is interesting to note that in a study of 8000 Medicaid families, the rate of surgical admissions and general hospital use was approximately twice as high as for a comparable group of individuals under practice plans of an HMO.[40] In still another study of the incidence of tonsillectomies, the probability of the surgery varied from 41 percent for Blue Cross–Blue Shield subscribers to 10 percent for subscribers to prepaid groups plans. In 1971 the U.S. Civil Service Commission reported that employees in group practice plans had hospitalization rates that were only 40 percent of the rates of subscribers to Aetna Health Insurance and only 46 percent of the rates of those enrolled under Blue Cross–Blue Shield.[41] It appears that HMOs and other prepaid plans can significantly lower the use of hospital and medical services. Whether this is a direct result of initially screening subscribers, health-promotion and prevention services provided by the group practice plan and subsequent changes in the health status of the insured population or a predisposition among HMOs toward more conservative treatment can only be determined from further empirical studies.

Economic incentives for use of health-promotion and preventive services may meet with success if the economic advantage is individualized and brought directly to consumers. The following suggestions for financial incentives are offered:

- Expand insurance coverage to ambulatory care services directed toward prevention and health promotion.
- Offer partial premium refunds at end of each insurance period for maintaining good health or improving health status.
- Offer decreased insurance rates for active participation in community or individual health-promotion programs.
- Offer health-promotion and prevention services or facilities as part of employee fringe benefits.
- Develop a sliding scale for insurance premiums based on the extent of involvement in health-promotion and prevention activities or practices.
- Provide prevention and health promotion guidelines and literature free of charge to insurance subscribers.

Considerable attention should be given to financial incentives that will encourage the public to use potentially less expensive forms of health care, such as prevention and promotion services, and thus decrease the costs of care in illness. Concrete ways of increasing the incidence of positive, health-promoting practices within the population need to be identified and implemented.[42,43]

## MANPOWER FOR PREVENTION AND HEALTH PROMOTION

Provision of appropriate prevention and health-promotion services to the public on a nationwide basis will require the use of a variety of health care personnel. While physicians have been concerned traditionally with care in illness, the emphasis of professional nursing has been on assisting clients in maintaining and regaining health even in the presence of a physical disease or disability. Professional nurses are in a key position to synthesize the knowledge from the physical and behavioral sciences in developing competencies and skills necessary to provide prevention and health-promotion services. Nurses should assume the leadership in developing, planning, and implementing such services for individuals, families, and community groups.

The skills of nurses, physicians, nutritionists, physical-fitness specialists, psychologists, health educators, physical therapists, and other health professionals will be required to provide the range of services necessary for health promotion and prevention. The important consideration for cost effectiveness is that the expertise of each type of health care provider be well utilized in order to facilitate quality care at reasonable cost.

## SUMMARY

This chapter has provided information relevant to the potential economic impact of prevention and health-promotion services on the American public. With inflation in health care costs, it is imperative that better use of professional and client resources be achieved. Health professionals and consumers must be clear on the appropriate health personnel to deliver a variety of prevention and health-promotion services in the most effective and efficient way. Attention must also be given to the continuity of care provided and costs and benefits for various interventions.

Increased federal expenditures on prevention and health-promotion programs are needed in order to allow for adequate evaluation of their impact. Improved measures of health status must also be developed in order to determine the extent to which various prevention and health-promotion strategies impact on the quality of life as well as on life expectancy. The results of studies conducted to date look promising in regard to the potential of prevention and health-promotion services for improving the health status of the American people.

## REFERENCES

1. McGinnis, J.M. Trends in disease prevention: Assessing the benefits of prevention. *Bulletin of the New York Academy of Medicine,* January–February 1980, *56,* 38–44.
2. Zubkoff, M. *Health: A victim or cause of inflation.* New York, Prodist, 1977.
3. Battistella, R.M. Disease prevention and health education. In Battistella, R.M., & Rundall, T.G. (Eds.), *Health care policy in a changing environment.* Berkeley, Calif.: McCutchan, 1978, pp. 274–293.
4. Gibson, R., & Fisher, C. National health expenditures: Fiscal year 1977. *Social Security Bulletin,* July 1978, *41,* 3–20.
5. Scheffler, R.M. The economic evidence on prevention. In *Healthy people: The Surgeon General's report on health promotion and disease prevention.* (U.S. Public Health Service Publ. No. 79-55071). Washington, D.C.: Government Printing Office, 1979.

6. Kristein, M.M., Arnold, C.B., & Wynder, E.L. Health economics and preventive care. *Science,* February 1977, *195,* 457–462.

7. Luce, B.R., & Schweitzer, S.O. Smoking and alcohol abuse: A comparison of their economic consequences. *New England Journal of Medicine,* 1978, *298,* 569–571.

8. *Cost and quality of health care: Unnecessary surgery.* Report by a Subcommittee of the House of Representatives Committee on Interstate and Foreign Commerce. Washington, D.C.: Government Printing Office, 1976.

9. Shepard, D.S., & Thompson, M.S. First principles of cost-effectiveness analysis in health. *Public Health Reports,* November–December 1979, *94,* 535–543.

10. *Ibid.,* p. 538.

11. Peddecord, K.M. Competing for acute care dollars: The economics of risk reduction. *Family and Community Health,* May 1980, *3,* 25–40.

12. Lave, J.R., & Lave, L.B. Measuring the effectiveness of prevention, Part I. *Milbank Memorial Fund Quarterly,* Spring 1977, *55,* 273–289.

13. Breslow, L. Risk factor intervention for health maintenance. *Science,* May 1978, *200,* 908–912.

14. Peddecord, *op. cit.*

15. Luce & Schweitzer, *op. cit.*

16. Stason, W.B., & Weinstein, M.C. Public health rounds at the Harvard School of Public Health: Allocation of resources to manage hypertension. *New England Journal of Medicine,* 1977, *296,* 732–739.

17. *Ibid.*

18. Robertson, L.S. Factors associated with seat belt use in 1974 starter-interlock equipped cars. *Journal of Health and Social Behavior,* 1975, *16,* 173–177.

19. Lave, J.R., & Lave, L.B. Cost-benefit concepts in health: Examination of some prevention efforts. *Preventive Medicine,* 1978, *7,* 414–423.

20. Shapiro, S. Measuring the effectiveness of prevention, Part II. *Milbank Memorial Fund Quarterly,* Spring 1977, *55,* 291–305.

21. Dickinson, L., Mussey, M.E., & Kurland, L.T. Evaluation of the effectiveness of cytologic screening for cervical cancer. II: Survival parameters before and after inception of screening. *Mayo Clinic Proceedings,* 1972, *47,* 545–549.

22. Fielding, *op. cit.*

23. Cretin, S. Cost/benefit analysis of treatment and prevention of myocardial infarction. *Health Services Research,* Summer 1977, 174–189.

24. Fielding, J.E. Successes of prevention. *Milbank Memorial Fund Quarterly,* 1978, *56,* 274–302.

25. Alderman, M.H., & Kristein, M.M. *Costs of a work-site hypertension program.* Unpublished paper, 1978.

26. Kristein, Arnold, & Wynder, *op. cit.*

27. Haynes, R.B., Sackett, D.L., Taylor, D.W., *et al.* Increased absenteeism from work after detection and labeling of hypertensive patients. *New England Journal of Medicine,* 1978, *299,* 741–744.

28. Five-year findings of the hypertension detection and follow-up program. I. Reduction in mortality of persons with high blood pressure, including mild hypertension. *JAMA,* 1979, *242,* 2562–2571.

29. Multiple Risk Factor Intervention Trial (MRFIT). National study of primary prevention of coronary heart disease. *JAMA,* 1976, *235,* 825–827.

30. Zapka, J., & Averill, B.W. Self care for colds: A cost-effective alternative to upper respiratory infection management. *AJPH,* August 1979, *69,* 814–816.

31. Breault, H.J. Five years with 5 million child-resistant containers. *Clinical Toxicology,* 1974, *7,* 91–95.

32. Belloc, N.B., & Breslow, L. Relationships of physical health status and health practices. *Preventive Medicine,* August 1972, *1,* 409–421.

33. Belloc, N.B. Relationship of health practices and mortality. *Preventive Medicine,* 1973, *2,* 67–81.

34. Breslow, L., & Enstrom, J.E. Persistence of health habits and their relationship to mortality. *Preventive Medicine,* 1980, *9,* 469–483.

35. Gori, G., & Richter, B. Macroeconomics of disease prevention in the United States. *Science,* 1978, *200,* 1123–1130.

36. Tsai, S., Lee, E., & Hardey, R. The effect of a reduction in leading causes of death: Potential gain in life expectancies. *AJPH,* October 1978, *68,* 966–971.

37. Kristein, Arnold, & Wynder, *op. cit.*

38. Lee, P.R. Paying for primary care—time for a change? *American Journal of Medicine,* March 1980, *68,* 319–321.

39. Feldman, R., Deitz, D.M., & Brooks, E.F. The financial viability of rural primary health care centers. *AJPH,* October 1978, *68,* 981–988.

40. Caus, C., Cooper, B., & Hirschman, C. *Contrasts in HMO and fee-for-service performance.* Washington, D.C.: Office of Research and Statistics, Social Security Administration, December 1975.

41. Federal Employees Health Benefits Program. *Report for fiscal year ended June 30, 1971.* Washington, D.C.: Bureau of Retirement, Insurance, and Occupational Health, U.S. Civil Service Commission, 1971.

42. Kristein, M.M. Economic issues in prevention. *Preventive Medicine,* 1977, *6,* 252–264.

43. Schweitzer, S. Cost effectiveness of early disease detection. *Health Services Research,* Spring 1974, *9,* 22–32.

# CHAPTER 16
# Establishing Nurse–Client Relationships for Illness Prevention and Health Promotion

Throughout this book, a comprehensive approach to illness prevention and health promotion has been presented that should be an integral part of professional nursing practice in all care environments. In order to provide quality care, professional nurses must take into consideration the level of health of a client as well as potential health threats. In addition, clients must be viewed within the holistic context of family, society, and the environment. The concepts of health promotion, prevention, continuity of care, family support, self-determination, and self-management are no longer exclusive or unique to community health nursing. Such concepts represent critical dimensions of all sound professional nursing practice.[1]

An understanding of the factors that influence health-protecting and health-promoting behaviors of clients is critical to the development of effective nurse–client relationships directed toward prevention and health promotion. The Health Belief Model and Modified Health Belief Model described in Chapter 3 and the proposed Health Promotion Model presented in Chapter 4 provide conceptual frameworks for the provision of nursing care directed toward these ends. A number of studies support the usefulness of the Health Belief Model in predicting health-protecting (preventive) behavior. However, the proposed modifications of the model need further empirical testing. Both the Health Belief Model and the Modified Health Belief Model address the determinants of health behavior when the threat of a specific disease is the focus. Actions taken within this conceptual framework are directed toward avoiding potential harm resulting from acute or chronic illness. In contrast, the Health Promotion Model is proposed as an explanation of the factors that affect behavior directed toward enhancing personal health and well-being, strengthening interpersonal relationships, and developing a healthier and more fulfilling lifestyle. A specific disease is not the focus. Attaining higher levels of health is the primary challenge.

While the variables within the Health Promotion Model represent a synthesis of research findings to date concerning factors affecting health-promoting behavior, the proposed model must be systematically studied in order to determine its predictive potential. The extent to which altering factors within the model increase the incidence of health-promoting behavior and decrease the incidence of health-damaging behavior must also be determined. At present, the Health Promotion Model can serve the heuristic purposes of concept integration as a basis for practice and hypothesis generation as a basis for research. Identifying and explaining relationships between nursing strategies and changes in client behavior is critical to expand the scientific basis for professional nursing practice.

## INTEGRATING ILLNESS PREVENTION AND HEALTH-PROMOTION STRATEGIES INTO NURSING PRACTICE

At this point, the reader should be familiar with a number of nursing strategies useful in providing illness-prevention and health-promotion services to clients. Questions may still remain concerning the settings in which such care can be provided and how preventive/promotive care can be incorporated into professional nursing practice. In the following discussion, answers to these questions will be proposed and alternative practice settings considered.

Many settings in which nurses currently practice provide opportunities for the provision of care directed toward illness prevention and health promotion. Time spent in direct client contact in hospital-based patient-education programs, community clinics, health departments, schools, business/industry, and home settings can be productively used for health assessment, anticipatory counseling, and instruction in self-care. Illness-prevention and health-promotion activities can be carried out with individual clients, families, or communitiy groups. To provide such services in any setting, nurses must be motivated, assertive, realistic in planning, and creative in approaches to care of clients.

Hospitals, the setting in which most nurses practice, are becoming increasingly interested in the role that their staffs can play in the promotion of health within the community. Patient-education programs and outpatient or ambulatory care clinics can fulfill a vital role in preparing individuals to care for themselves better. Many hospitals are actively involved in offering wellness workshops, well adult clinics, and well child clinics to facilitate efforts of individuals and families to adopt more healthful lifestyles. Discharge planning or teaching interactions with individual patients during hospitalization provide additional opportunities for health promotion. The individual who is ill may exhibit a high level of readiness to learn about preventing the recurrence of illness or maintaining and promoting health.

Nurses working in community clinics or carrying client caseloads within health departments have numerous opportunities to assist clients in gaining greater competence in self-care. Child health clinics, community health programs, senior citizen centers, and residential or day care centers offer appropriate populations and settings for the provision of prevention and health-promotion services. Schools also provide a prime setting for nurse-initiated programming directed toward prevention and health promotion. Not only are children highly receptive to health information if interestingly presented (pictures, films, games, and action projects), they represent the group most likely to benefit from such care. Many health-damaging behaviors that are apparent among adults developed early in childhood or during adolescence. Teaching positive health practices to children during their early years, in contrast to changing health-damaging behaviors during adult years, offers potential cost savings in terms of decreased illness and increased productivity. The quality of life during later years can also be greatly enhanced by decreasing the episodes of illness that thwart growth and by increasing self-care skills to promote self-actualization (realization of personal potential). Nurses have only begun to tap the possibilities that schools offer as a setting for primary care, health education, and health counseling directed toward illness prevention and health promotion.

Business and industry as settings for preventive/promotive care offer an advantage similar to that of the schools in that nursing service can be provided where people are and where they spend many of their waking hours. Access to services is convenient for clients at work settings since appointments may be made immediately before or after work or during the lunch hour. The cost of transportation for health care is minimized and the services provided are generally covered by company health insurance programs. Since the health of workers directly affects their productivity, employers are becoming increasingly interested in the development of employee benefit programs that include prevention and health-promotion services. In addition, unions may negotiate for such services as part of labor–management contracts.

Another setting for nurse-provided prevention and health-promotion services is the medical group practice. Increasingly, consumers are demanding more comprehensive health care services from physicians. As a result, physicians in group practices are developing collegial relationships with professional nurses to expand the range of services provided to clients. Nurses within these settings may be baccalaureate, masters, or doctorally prepared, and they are responsible for assessing, teaching, counseling, and providing direct care to clients. They often provide services such as risk appraisal, health education, nutrition counseling, stress management, counseling in human sexuality, and lifestyle modification. The medical group practice setting has the advantages of providing ready access to a large population of clients and ease of referral between physician and nurse. Negotiations for such a practice relationship may be initiated either by nurses or by physicians.

Health Maintenance Organizations (HMO) represent a unique form of group practice (prepaid) that places particular emphasis on prevention and health promotion. An HMO cannot fully accomplish its purpose unless the talents and expertise of a variety of health professionals are used. Professional nursing care that incorporates the strategies presented in this book should be an integral part of the health services offered in all HMOs. While prepaid plans have been slow in catching on within the United States, such arrangements offer the potential for providing quality care to populations and at the same time decreasing health care costs.

Two other settings for the provision of health-promotion and prevention services to clients must also be discussed: the nurse group practice and independent practice. In increasing numbers, nurses are incorporating in professional groups and contracting to provide services to hospitals, large physician groups, schools, businesses, and industries. The parameters of services to be provided and the cost of the service contract to the purchaser are clearly delineated, usually in the form of a legal contract. This arrangement provides the opportunity for nurses to offer those services to clients that they deem appropriate for prevention and health promotion while maintaining considerable autonomy in professional practice. To date, nurse group practice has had limited visibility within the health care system. However, the potential of this approach for providing direct care to clients should be further developed.

A final practice arrangement to be described is that of independent or private practice. In this arrangement, each nurse–client contract for services (verbal or written) is negotiated between the specific client (individual, family, or community group) and the professional nurse. Independent practice may be of a continuing nature, providing nursing services to clients throughout the life span, or short-term, providing specific services to clients (e.g., stress management, weight control) over a period of weeks or months. The parameters of practice and the duration and nature of client contact will depend on the characteristics of the population served and the areas of expertise of the professional nurse. Generally, in private practice, sources of referral are needed to achieve an adequate client load. Referrals may come through physicians, county health departments, hospitals, or other health agencies within the community. Advertising the services available can also increase lay awareness of nurses in private practice, while ''word of mouth'' communication from clients can be highly effective in building a caseload.

Nurses in private practice must be clear on how services provided will be reimbursed. At this point, the federal government and private insurers have not formulated general policies for direct reimbursement of nurses for prevention and health-promotion services. Pilot studies of differing approaches to reimbursement are currently being conducted in a variety of health care settings. Nurses interested in independent practice as a setting for providing prevention and health-promotion services to clients are referred to several helpful resources in the nursing literature.[2–4]

Health-promotion and prevention services can be offered in a variety of care settings, ranging from the traditional to the more innovative or progressive. In all settings, professional nurses should be actively involved in assessing the needs of clients for such care and in developing appropriate programs to meet their needs. In offering a comprehensive program for prevention and health promotion, nurses should optimally make use of their own professional skills as well as the skills of other health personnel to provide quality services to clients.

## THE NURSE–CLIENT RELATIONSHIP

Regardless of the arrangements for practice (e.g., setting, reimbursement policies), the nurse–client relationship that must be established to provide preventive/promotive care consists of a number of phases. The patterns of nurse–client interaction should represent a "helping relationship" rather than a social relationship with which the client may be more familiar. The phases of a helping relationship can be identified as initial phase, transition phase, working phase, termination, and follow-up. Successful implementation of all phases is necessary to provide individualized care and continuity of care for clients. The helping relationship can be initiated by the nurse or by the client and results from a recognized need for professional services to achieve a particular health goal. The contract for services may be formal or informal, but it indicates a mutual commitment on the part of nurse and client to work toward common health priorities. The ultimate aim of the helping process is to increase clients' competencies for care of themselves and to enhance their capacities for healthy, productive, and meaningful living.

### Initial Phase

This phase of the nurse–client relationship begins with the first contact. Early interactions provide an opportunity for the nurse to explore with the client the nature of the services needed and the ways in which such services can be appropriately provided. Mutual understanding of the client's health goals and expectations from the relationship provide the basis for quality care. It is important to stress that when clients seek services from the health care system, they are asking for assistance, not abdicating their rights as individuals.[5] The orientation of the professional nurse must be one of sustaining and enhancing the independence of clients while facilitating further development of self-care competencies.

The nurse should be aware of his or her own "helping style" and evaluate its impact on clients with differing personalities, backgrounds, and lifestyles. Self-awareness on the part of the nurse concerning how he or she works with clients is critical for meaningful self evaluation and improvement of helping skills.

During the initial phase of the relationship, the interest of the client in improving health should be aroused. (It is at this time, too, that the client assesses the nurse as a professional in terms of expertise, trustworthiness, reliability, and helpfulness.[6]) It is during this early phase of the relationship that the nurse comes to understand the many frames of reference of the client: personal, social, cultural, and environmental. Familiarity with the client's life experience is essential in order to provide meaningful assistance to the client in integrating new health practices into his or her lifestyle.

In the initial phase of the relationship, the nurse assists the client in making informed choices concerning actions to take for health protection and promotion. Such decisions are made through health assessment, values clarification, health education for self-care, and development of a Health Protection/Promotion Plan. As a result of these activities, the client and nurse have a clearer understanding of the competencies of each, the goals to be achieved, and the mutal obligations that each brings to the nurse–client relationship.

It is generally during this phase of the relationship that attitudes developed by the client as a result of previous contacts with the health care system are most apparent. Traumatic experiences or negative reactions from health care professionals in prior encounters can result in hesitancy on the part of the client to establish an open and honest relationship with the nurse. The extent to which the nurse can convey concern, respect, and unconditional positive regard for the client will determine the potential productivity of the helping relationship and the length of the initial phase.

**Transition Phase**

This phase represents a critical period for the client in terms of continuation of the nurse–client relationship. Commitment to the helping relationship as a means of attaining personal health goals may fluctuate. During this period, the client may vacillate between enthusiasm and apathy, between acceptance and rejection, and between open and guarded communication with the nurse.[7] This is particularly true of clients with low self-esteem or of those who have difficulty in establishing close relationships with others. Some suggestions for stabilizing the client's commitment to the helping relationship at this time include establishing client-centered objectives and goals, working with issues important to the client, continuing contact with the client by phone or mail when face-to-face contact is not possible, including the family more extensively in the plan of care, and establishing very specific nurse–client contracts to facilitate commitment to prevention and health-promotion activities.[8]

Getting further into the client's frame of reference can be particularly critical at this point. Questions to be asked include these: How does the client view him- or herself, his or her social roles, his or her significance to others, and his or her goals or ambitions? Additional insight into the client's feelings and thoughts permits the nurse to help the client in dealing with ambivalency and in moving into the working phase of the relationship.

**Working Phase**

The initial and transition phases of the helping relationship take place during the decision-making period of health behavior; the working phase, termination, and follow-up coincide with the action component. In reality, the working phase of the relationship is the most intensive period of action. Considerable energies are expended by both client and nurse in marshalling personal, social, and environmental resources to achieve identified health goals.

Self-exploration begun during the initial phase of the relationshp may continue into this phase, with the client developing increased sensitivity to personal feelings, concerns, and body states. In addition, new insights into personal assets, attitude/behavior incongruencies, and level of self-esteem may occur. Personal involvement in initiating health-protecting and health-promoting actions often gives the client new feelings of control, enhanced perceptions of self-worth, and new opportunities for growth and self-actualization. Self-discovery is a continuing experience during the working phase of the helping relationship. Such discovery leads to new appreciation of the many dimensions of healthy, happy, and productive living. It may take considerable time for some adults to achieve a better understanding of themselves, their needs, their goals, and their priorities. Yet unless they experience themselves, their capacity for understanding others and the world around them will be limited.[9] The nurse's role during periods of self-discovery is critical. She should be ready to listen, reflect the client's thinking, and accept unconditionally what the client is learning about him- or herself.

Sustained contact through regularly scheduled visits is important during the working phase to allow the client to implement various action alternatives and evalute their success. The support of significant others as well as that of the nurse is particularly important to the client at this time when attempts may be made to develop congruency between values, attitudes, and behaviors, to make major changes in lifestyle, and to maintain consistency in positive health practices. It is critical that there be systematic use and evaluation of the Health Protection/Promotion Plan and modification of the plan as needed to facilitate client progress toward health goals during the working phase of the helping relationship. Knowledgeable use of specific action strategies identified earlier in this book can facilitate client movement toward higher levels of health and well-being. Strategies suggested for the action phase include the implementation of an individualized exercise and physical-fitness program, good nutrition and weight control, stress management, modification of lifestyle, and building meaningful social support systems.

During the working phase of the nurse–client relationship, the time commitment of the client goes far beyond periodic appointments with the nurse. Concerted efforts at self-monitoring, self-management, and evaluation of progress toward valued health goals must take place on a continuing basis within the home setting. Family and significant others should be actively involved whenever possible in providing support and reinforcement during the action phase as well as providing cues for appropriate client behaviors. Progress should be well rewarded through tangible or social reinforcements. Lack of progress may signal changes that need to be made in the plan of care, such as the time frame for implementation or the specific nursing strategies used.

Since the working phase is a time of intense commitment on the part of both nurse and client, the relationship developed should be rewarding: satisfying yet challenging. While the nurse functions in an educative, supportive, or counseling role, the client is primarily responsible for the direction and extent of changes made to achieve a healthier lifestyle. In reality, the client bears the major responsibility for appropriate self-care to prevent disease and promote health.

**Termination Phase**

The support and assistance offered in the helping relationship can create a sense of dependency, even when every effort is made to maintain the independence of the client. The satisfactions derived from the relationship may make the experience of terminating the intensive working phase a difficult one. The client and nurse may make attempts to prolong the relationship or express ambivalence, anger, and grief during this phase.

The termination phase can be handled more easily if, in initial contacts with clients, the length of the working phase can be clearly identified. As an example, the author informs her clients during the first visit that relaxation training and biofeedback sessions will occur over a 13- to 16-week period, with appointments tapering off in frequency during the following 6 months. This not only sets parameters for the working phase but allows gradual rather than abrupt termination of the relationship. If the family has been included in implementation of the Health Protection/Promotion Plan, gradual fading of the nurse from the working relationship and increasing support and participation of the family in prevention and health-promotion activities can ease the impact of termination.

During the termination phase, the client should be assisted in assessing the progress made and in developing future plans for self-care. The client should have a sense of pride in his or her progress and the goals accomplished. No new material should be introduced during this phase of the relationship.[10] Synthesis of information and stabilization of new behaviors that have been learned are the focus of nurse and client actions during this time. It may be helpful to provide the client with materials to be used in reviewing what has been learned. An example of such materials are the cassette tapes on relaxation that the author provides to clients following completion of the relaxation and biofeedback program. Such materials can be used in the home for "refresher sessions." The possibility for future contact with the nurse should always be left open.

If the client feels the need to see the nurse at a later date, he or she should be made to feel free to do so. Clients should never feel abandoned when the working phase of the helping relationship is completed. The advantages of the intensive relationship with the nurse should outweigh the disadvantages of termination. The ultimate goal of the nurse–client relationship is to help clients manage their own lives and health more successfully.

**Follow-up Phase**

Periodic contacts with the nurse over time can facilitate continued practice of health behaviors. Such contacts can reinforce the progress of the client or provide refresher sessions for review and refinement of positive health practices. The very nature of most health-protecting and health-promoting behaviors require their continued performance throughout the life span. While the intensive phase of client–nurse contact may terminate, the responsibility of the client for self-care remains. Continuity of care can be achieved by the nurse through periodic follow-up visits with clients every 6 months or at other appropriate time intervals.

Follow-up can be handled by repeat appointments with the nurse in the clinic setting, by home visits by the nurse, or by letter or telephone. Whenever possible, face-to-face contact between client and nurse is preferred to allow direct communication of further progress toward health goals or new problems or difficulties encountered. If time allows, the home of the client offers an ideal place for follow-up, enabling the nurse to evaluate the progress of the client within his or her own environment. The extent to which family members or significant others actively support and/or participate in positive health behaviors developed by the client can be more readily determined from a home visit than in the clinic setting.

Follow-up should be handled systematically, with clients contacted by card or telephone for appointments on a periodic basis. The follow-up phase, while freeing the nurse to work intensively with new clients, also maintains supportive relationships with past clients. Thus, the possibility remains that former clients will reactivate the working phase of the relationship as needed.

Through the helping relationship, the nurse teaches the client self-care, supports and reinforces the client as he or she learns, facilitates continuation of positive health practices, and promotes the client's efforts to achieve a meaningful and productive lifestyle. Planning, implementation, and continuation of health-protecting and health-promoting behaviors throughout the client's life span has the potential for extending longevity for the client and greatly increasing the quality of life experienced.

## CONCLUSION

This book has offered the reader a conceptual view of health-protecting and health-promoting behaviors and recommended specific nursing strategies for use with clients. In addition, the nature of the nurse–client relationship for illness prevention and health promotion has been discussed. Emphasis on prevention and the promotion of health are not passing fads, they represent new directions in health care delivery. The extent to which nursing will find a place in the development and delivery of such services depends on the creative investigative and practice efforts of talented individuals within the nursing profession. Nurses can maintain an illness orientation in the care that they provide or accept the challenge to explicate effective nursing strategies for promoting positive health practices. The impact of society and the environment on personal health status also mandates that nurses accept the responsibility for developing and supporting health policies that increase the range of health-promoting options and decreases the range of health-damaging options available to individuals within society.

Throughout this book, an attempt has been made to integrate theory and practice as a framework for providing health-protecting and health-promoting care to clients. Theory that lacks utility in practice is useless, and practice without theory is pointless. It is only when both are logically and systematically integrated that the goals of any professional discipline can be realized.

## REFERENCES

1. Robischon, P. Prevention and chronic illness. In Spradley, B.W. (Ed.), *Contemporary community nursing*. Boston: Little, Brown, 1975, p. 37.
2. Bullough, B. *The law and the expanding nursing role* (2nd ed.). New York: Appleton, 1980.
3. Jacox, A., & Norris, C. (Eds.). *Organizing for independent nursing practice*. New York: Appelton, 1977.
4. Koltz, C.J. *Private practice in nursing: Development and management*. Germantown, Md.: Aspen Systems Corporation, 1979.
5. Archer, S.E., & Fleshman, R. *Community health nursing: Patterns and practice*. North Scituate, Mass.: Duxbury Press, 1975, p. 331.
6. Smitherman, C. *Nursing actions for health promotion*. Philadelphia: Davis, 1981, p. 66.
7. *Ibid.*, p. 67.
8. Archer & Fleshman, *op. cit.*, pp. 329–330.
9. Dunn, H.L. High-level wellness for man and society. In Spradley, B.W. (Ed.), *Contemporary community nursing*. Boston: Little, Brown, 1975, p. 27.
10. Smitherman, *op. cit.*, p. 70.

# Appendix
# SUMMARY CHART OF SELECTED NUTRIENTS

| Nutrients | Importance | Sources | Deficiency Symptoms | Toxicity Level |
|-----------|-----------|---------|---------------------|----------------|
| Choline | Important in normal nerve transmission<br><br>Aids metabolism and transport of fats<br><br>Helps regulate liver and gallbladder | Egg yolks<br>Organ meats<br>Brewer's yeast<br>Wheat germ<br>Soybeans<br>Fish<br>Legumes<br>Lecithin | Fatty liver<br>Hemorrhaging kidneys<br>High blood pressure | No known oral toxicity, even with intake as high as 50,000 mg daily for 1 week |
| Folic acid (folacin) | Important in red blood cell formation<br><br>Aids metabolism of proteins<br><br>Necessary for growth and division of body cells | Dark-green leafy vegetables<br>Organ meats<br>Brewer's yeast<br>Root vegetables<br>Whole grains<br>Oysters<br>Salmon<br>Milk | Poor growth<br>Gastrointestinal disorders<br>Anemia<br>$B_{12}$ deficiency | No toxic effects. Single doses up to 400 $\mu$g are available without prescription |
| Inositol | Necessary for formation of lecithin<br><br>May be indirectly connected with metabolism of fats, including cholesterol<br><br>Vital for hair growth | Whole grains<br>Citrus fruits<br>Brewer's yeast<br>Molasses<br>Meat<br>Milk<br>Nuts<br>Vegetables<br>Lecithin | Constipation<br>Eczema<br>Hair loss<br>High blood cholesterol | No known toxicity. Single doses up to 500 mg are available without prescription |

| | Function | Sources | Deficiency/Symptoms | Notes |
|---|---|---|---|---|
| Niacin (nicotinic acid, niacinamide) | Necessary for carbohydrate, fat, and protein metabolism<br>Helps maintain health of skin, tongue, and digestive system | Lean meats<br>Poultry and fish<br>Brewer's yeast<br>Peanuts<br>Milk and milk products<br>Rice bran<br>Desiccated liver | Dermatitis<br>Nervous disorders | 100–200 mg nicotinic acid orally or 30 mg intravenously may produce side effects for some individuals. No effects with niacinamide |
| PABA | Aids bacteria in producing folic acid<br>Acts as a coenzyme in the breakdown and use of proteins<br>Aids in formation of red blood cells<br>Acts as a sunscreen | Organ meats<br>Wheat germ<br>Yogurt<br>Molasses<br>Green leafy vegetables | Fatigue<br>Irritability<br>Depression<br>Nervousness<br>Constipation<br>Headache<br>Digestive disorders<br>Graying hair | Single doses of 100 mg are available without prescription. Continued high ingestion may be toxic. |
| Pangamic acid | Helps eliminate hypoxia<br>Helps promote protein metabolism<br>Stimulates nervous and glandular system | Brewer's yeast<br>Rare steaks<br>Brown rice<br>Sunflower, pumpkin, and sesame seeds | Diminished oxygenation of cells | 500 mg tolerated daily with no toxic effect |
| Carbohydrate | Provides energy for body functions and muscular exertions<br>Assists in digestion and assimilation of foods | Whole grains<br>Sugar, syrup, and honey<br>Fruits<br>Vegetables | Loss of energy<br>Fatigue<br>Excessive protein breakdown<br>Disturbed balance of water, sodium, potassium, and chloride | Intake should not exceed what is needed to maintain desirable weight. |

| Nutrients | Importance | Sources | Deficiency Symptoms | Toxicity Level |
|---|---|---|---|---|
| Fat | Provides energy<br>Acts as a carrier for fat-soluble vitamins A, D, E and K<br>Supplies essential fatty acids needed for growth, health, and smooth skin | Butter and margarine<br>Vegetable oils<br>Fats in meats<br>Whole milk and milk products<br>Nuts and seeds | Eczema or skin disorders<br>Retarded growth | Intake should not exceed what is needed to maintain desirable weight. |
| Protein | Necessary for growth and development<br>Acts in formation of hormones, enzymes, and antibodies<br>Maintains acid–alkali balance<br>Source of heat and energy | Meats, fish, and poultry<br>Soybean products<br>Eggs<br>Milk and milk products<br>Whole grains | Fatigue<br>Loss of appetite<br>Diarrhea and vomiting<br>Stunted growth<br>Edema | Intake should not exceed what is needed to maintain desirable weight |
| **Vitamins**<br>Vitamin A (carotene) | Necessary for growth and repair of body tissues<br>Important to health of the eyes<br>Fights bacteria and infection<br>Maintains healthy epithelial tissue<br>Aids in bone and teeth formation | Liver<br>Eggs<br>Yellow fruits and vegetables<br>Dark-green fruits and vegetables<br>Whole milk and milk products<br>Fish–liver oil | Night blindness<br>Rough, dry, scaly skin<br>Increased susceptibility to infections<br>Frequent fatigue<br>Loss of smell and appetite | 50,000 or more IU may be toxic if there is no deficiency. 10,000 IU is the maximum single dose that can be bought without a prescription. |

| Vitamin | Functions | Sources | Deficiency Symptoms | Toxicity |
|---|---|---|---|---|
| Vitamin B complex | Necessary for carbohydrate, fat, and protein metabolism<br>Helps functioning of the nervous system<br>Helps maintain muscle tone in the gastrointestinal tract<br>Maintains health of skin, hair, eyes, mouth, and liver | See individual B vitamins | Dry, rough, cracked skin<br>Acne<br>Dull, dry, or gray hair<br>Fatigue<br>Poor appetite<br>Gastrointestinal tract disorders | See individual B vitamins; relatively nontoxic |
| Vitamin B₁ (thiamine) | Necessary for carbohydrate metabolism<br>Helps maintain healthy nervous system<br>Stabilizes the appetite<br>Stimulates growth and good muscle tone | Brewer's yeast<br>Whole grains<br>Blackstrap molasses<br>Brown rice<br>Organ meats<br>Meats, fish, and poultry<br>Egg yolks<br>Legumes<br>Nuts | Gastrointestinal problems<br>Fatigue<br>Loss of appetite<br>Nerve disorders<br>Heart disorders | No known oral toxicity. Single doses of up to 500 mg are available without prescription. |
| Vitamin B₂ (riboflavin) | Necessary for carbohydrate, fat, and protein metabolism<br>Aids in formation of antibodies and red blood cells<br>Maintains cell respiration | Brewer's yeast<br>Whole grains<br>Blackstrap molasses<br>Organ meats<br>Egg yolks<br>Legumes<br>Nuts | Eye problems<br>Cracks and sores in mouth<br>Dermatitis<br>Retarded growth<br>Digestive disturbances | No known oral toxicity. Single doses of 100 mg are available without prescription. |

| Nutrients | Importance | Sources | Deficiency Symptoms | Toxicity Level |
|---|---|---|---|---|
| Vitamin B$_6$ (pyridoxine) | Necessary for carbohydrate, fat, and protein metabolism<br>Aids in formation of antibodies<br>Helps maintain balance of sodium and phosphorus | Meats<br>Whole grains<br>Brewer's yeast<br>Blackstrap molasses<br>Wheat germ<br>Legumes<br>Green leafy vegetables<br>Desiccated liver | Anemia<br>Mouth disorders<br>Nervousness<br>Muscular weakness<br>Dermatitis<br>Sensitivity to insulin | No known oral toxicity. Single doses up to 100 mg are available without prescription. |
| Vitamin B$_{12}$ (cyanocobalamin) | Essential for normal formation of blood cells<br>Necessary for carbohydrate, fat, and protein metabolism<br>Maintains healthy nervous system | Organ meats<br>Fish and pork<br>Eggs<br>Cheese<br>Milk and milk products | Pernicious anemia<br>Brain damage<br>Nervousness<br>Neuritis | No known oral toxicity even with intake as high as 600–1200 $\mu$g |
| Vitamin B$_{13}$ (orotic acid) | Needed for metabolism of some B vitamins | Root vegetables<br>Liquid whey | Degenerative disorders | No known toxicity |
| Biotin | Necessary for carbohydrate, fat, and protein metabolism<br>Aids in use of other B vitamins | Egg yolks<br>Liver<br>Unpolished rice<br>Brewer's yeast<br>Whole grains<br>Sardines<br>Legumes | Dermatitis<br>Grayish skin color<br>Depression<br>Muscle pain<br>Impairment of fat metabolism<br>Poor appetite | No known oral toxicity. Single doses up to 50 $\mu$g are available without prescription. |

| Nutrient | Functions | Sources | Deficiency Symptoms | Notes |
|---|---|---|---|---|
| Pantothenic acid | Aids in formation of some fats<br>Participates in the release of energy from carbohydrates, fats, and protein<br>Aids in the use of some vitamins<br>Improves body's resistance to stress | Organ meats<br>Brewer's yeast<br>Egg yolks<br>Legumes<br>Whole grains<br>Wheat germ<br>Salmon | Vomiting<br>Restlessness<br>Stomach stress<br>Increased susceptibility to infection<br>Sensitivity to insulin | 10,000–20,000 mg as a calcium salt may have side effects in some people |
| Vitamin C | Maintains collagen<br>Helps heal wounds, scar tissue, and fractures<br>Gives strength to blood vessels<br>May provide resistance to infections<br>Aids in absorption of iron | Citrus fruits<br>Rose hips<br>Acerola<br>Cherries<br>Alfalfa seeds, sprouted<br>Cantaloupe<br>Strawberries<br>Broccoli<br>Tomatoes<br>Green peppers | Bleeding gums<br>Swollen or painful joints<br>Slow-healing wounds and fractures<br>Bruising<br>Nosebleeds<br>Impaired digestion | Essentially nontoxic. 5000–15,000 mg daily over a prolonged period may have side effects in some people. |
| Vitamin D | Improves absorption and use of calcium and phosphorus required for bone formation<br>Maintains stable nervous system and normal heart action | Salmon<br>Sardines<br>Herring<br>Vitamin-D fortified milk and milk products<br>Egg yolks<br>Organ meats<br>Fish liver oils<br>Bone meal | Poor bone and tooth formation<br>Softening of bones and teeth<br>Inadequate absorption of calcium<br>Retention of phosphorus in kidney | 25,000 IU may be toxic in some individuals over extended period of time. 400 IU is the maximum single dose that can be purchased without a prescription. |

| Nutrients | Importance | Sources | Deficiency Symptoms | Toxicity Level |
|---|---|---|---|---|
| Vitamin E | Protects fat-soluble vitamins<br>Protects red blood cells<br>Essential in cellular respiration<br>Inhibits coagulation of blood by preventing blood clots | Cold-pressed oils<br>Eggs<br>Wheat germ<br>Organ meats<br>Molasses<br>Sweet potatoes<br>Leafy vegetables<br>Desiccated liver | Rupture of red blood cells<br>Muscular wasting<br>Abnormal fat deposits in muscles | Essentially nontoxic. 4–12 g (4000–30,000 IU) of tocopherol for prolonged periods produces side effects in some persons. |
| Vitamin K | Necessary for formation of prothrombin<br>Needed for blood coagulation | Green leafy vegetables<br>Egg yolks<br>Safflower oil<br>Blackstrap molasses<br>Cauliflower<br>Soybeans | Lack of prothrombin, increasing the tendency to hemorrage | Synthetic vitamin K may have side effects in newborn infants. Available in alfalfa tablet form. |
| Bioflavonoids | Help increase strength of capillaries | Citrus fruits<br>Fruits<br>Black currants<br>Buckwheat | Tendency to bleed and bruise easily | No known toxicity |
| **Minerals**<br>Calcium | Sustains development and maintenance of strong bones and teeth | Milk and milk products<br>Green leafy vegetables | Tetany<br>Softening bones<br>Back and leg pains<br>Brittle bones | Excessive intakes of calcium may have side effects in certain persons. |

| Mineral | Functions | Food Sources | Deficiency | Toxicity |
|---|---|---|---|---|
| | Assists normal blood clotting, muscle action, nerve function, and heart function | Shellfish<br>Molasses<br>Bone meal | | No known oral toxicity |
| Chlorine | Regulates acid–base balance<br>Maintains osmotic pressure<br>Stimulates production of hydrochloric acid<br>Helps maintain joints and tendons | Table salt<br>Seafood<br>Meats<br>Ripe olives<br>Rye flour | Loss of hair and teeth<br>Poor muscular contractibility<br>Impaired digestion | Daily intake of 14–28 g of salt (sodium chloride) is considered excessive. Excess intake of chlorine may have adverse effects. |
| Chromium | Stimulates enzymes in metabolism of energy and synthesis of fatty acids, cholesterol, and protein<br>Increases effectiveness of insulin | Corn oil<br>Clams<br>Whole-grain cereals<br>Brewer's yeast | Depressed growth rate<br>Glucose intolerance in diabetics<br>Atherosclerosis | No known toxicity |
| Cobalt | Functions as part of vitamin $B_{12}$<br>Maintains red blood cells<br>Activates a number of enzymes in the body | Organ meats<br>Oysters<br>Clams<br>Poultry<br>Milk<br>Green leafy vegetables<br>Fruits | Pernicious anemia<br>Slow rate of growth | Excessive intake of cobalt may have side effects in certain people. Available by prescription only. |

425

| Nutrients | Importance | Sources | Deficiency Symptoms | Toxicity Level |
|---|---|---|---|---|
| Copper | Aids in formation of red blood cells<br>Part of many enzymes<br>Works with vitamin C to form elastin | Organ meats<br>Seafood<br>Nuts<br>Legumes<br>Molasses<br>Raisins<br>Bone meal | General weakness<br>Impaired respiration<br>Skin sores | 20 times RDA over prolonged period may cause toxicity. |
| Fluorine | May reduce tooth decay by discouraging the growth of acid-forming bacteria | Tea<br>Seafood<br>Fluoridated water<br>Bone meal | Tooth decay | Excessive intake of fluorine may have side effects in some persons |
| Iodine | Essential part of the hormone thyroxine<br>Necessary for the prevention of goiter<br>Regulates production of energy and rate of metabolism<br>Promotes growth | Iodized salt | Enlarged thyroid gland<br>Dry skin and hair<br>Loss of physical and mental vigor<br>Cretinism in children born to iodine-deficient mothers | Up to 1000 $\mu$g daily produced no toxic effects in persons with a normal thyroid. |
| Iron | Necessary for hemoglobin and myoglobin formation<br>Helps in protein metabolism<br>Promotes growth | Organ meats and meats<br>Eggs<br>Fish and poultry<br>Blackstrap molasses<br>Cherry juice<br>Green leafy vegetables | Weakness<br>Paleness of skin<br>Constipation<br>Anemia | 100 mg daily over prolonged period of time may be toxic in some individuals |

| Mineral | Function | Sources | Deficiency Symptoms | Toxicity |
|---|---|---|---|---|
| Magnesium | Acts as a catalyst in the use of carbohydrates, fats, protein, calcium, phosphorus, and possibly potassium | Dried fruits<br>Desiccated liver<br>Seafood<br>Whole grains<br>Dark-green vegetables<br>Molasses<br>Nuts<br>Bone meal | Nervousness<br>Muscular excitability<br>Tremors | 30,000 mg daily may be toxic in certain individuals with kidney malfunctions. |
| Manganese | Enzyme activator<br>Plays a part in carbohydrate and fat production<br>Necessary for normal skeletal development<br>Maintains sex-hormone production | Whole grains<br>Green leafy vegetables<br>Legumes<br>Nuts<br>Pineapples<br>Egg yolks | Paralysis<br>Convulsions<br>Dizziness<br>Ataxia<br>Blindness and deafness in infants | Excessive intake may have side effects in certain people. Single doses of up to 60 mg are available without prescription. |
| Molybdenum | Acts in oxidation of fats and aldehydes<br>Aids in mobilization of iron from liver reserves | Legumes<br>Whole-grain cereals<br>Milk<br>Liver<br>Dark-green vegetables | Premature aging | 5–10 ppm is considered toxic. |
| Phosphorus | Works with calcium to build bones and teeth<br>Uses carbohydrates, fats, and proteins | Fish, meats, and poultry<br>Eggs<br>Legumes<br>Milk | Loss of weight and appetite<br>Irregular breathing<br>Pyorrhea | No known toxicity |

427

| Nutrients | Importance | Sources | Deficiency Symptoms | Toxicity Level |
|---|---|---|---|---|
| | Stimulates muscular contractions | Milk products<br>Nuts<br>Whole-grain cereals<br>Bone meal | | |
| Potassium | Works to control activity of heart muscles, nervous system, and kidneys | Lean meats<br>Whole grains<br>Vegetables<br>Dried fruits<br>Legumes<br>Sunflower seeds | Poor reflexes<br>Respiratory failure<br>Cardiac arrest | No known toxicity |
| Selenium | Works with vitamin E<br>Preserves tissue elasticity | Tuna<br>Herring<br>Brewer's yeast<br>Wheat germ and bran<br>Broccoli<br>Whole grains | Premature aging | 5–10 ppm is considered toxic. |
| Sodium | Maintains normal fluid levels in cells<br>Maintains health of the nervous, muscular, blood, and lymph systems | Seafood<br>Table salt<br>Baking powder and baking soda<br>Celery<br>Processed foods<br>Milk products<br>Kelp | Muscle weakness<br>Muscle shrinkage<br>Nausea<br>Loss of appetite<br>Intestinal gas | Excessive sodium intake may have adverse effects<br>Intake of 14–28 g of sodium chloride (salt) is considered excessive. |

| Mineral | Functions | Sources | Deficiency Symptoms | Notes |
|---|---|---|---|---|
| Sulfur | Part of amino acids<br>Essential for formation of body tissues<br>Part of the B vitamins<br>Plays a part in tissue respiration<br>Necessary for collagen synthesis | Fish<br>Eggs<br>Meats<br>Cabbage<br>Brussel sprouts | | Not available for over-the-counter sales |
| Vanadium | Inhibits cholesterol formation | Fish | | No known toxicity |
| Zinc | Component of insulin and male reproductive fluid<br>Aids in digestion and metabolism of phosphorus<br>Aids in healing process | Sunflower seeds<br>Seafood<br>Organ meats<br>Mushrooms<br>Brewer's yeast<br>Soybeans | Retarded growth<br>Delayed sexual maturity<br>Prolonged healing of wounds | Relatively nontoxic. 50 mg available without prescription |
| Water | Part of blood, lymph, and body secretions<br>Aids in digestion<br>Regulates body temperature<br>Transports nutrients and body wastes | Fruit juices<br>Fruits<br>Vegetables | Dehydration | |

# Index